Kidney Diseases: Management and Emerging Therapies

Kidney Diseases: Management and Emerging Therapies

Editor: Kevin Lewis

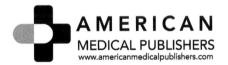
AMERICAN
MEDICAL PUBLISHERS
www.americanmedicalpublishers.com

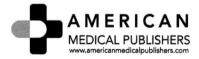
AMERICAN
MEDICAL PUBLISHERS
www.americanmedicalpublishers.com

Cataloging-in-Publication Data

Kidney diseases : management and emerging therapies / edited by Kevin Lewis.
   p. cm.
Includes bibliographical references and index.
ISBN 978-1-63927-710-0
1. Kidneys--Disease. 2. Kidneys--Diseases--Treatment. 3. Kidneys--Disease--Diagnosis.
4. Kidneys--Diseases--Prevention. 5. Nephrology. I. Lewis, Kevin.
RC902 .K533 2023
616.61--dc23

American Medical Publishers,
41 Flatbush Avenue,
1st Floor, New York,
NY 11217, USA

ISBN 978-1-63927-710-0 (Hardback)

Contents

Preface

The main aim of this book is to educate learners and enhance their research focus by presenting diverse topics covering this vast field. This is an advanced book which compiles significant studies by distinguished experts in the area of analysis. This book addresses successive solutions to the challenges arising in the area of application, along with it; the book provides scope for future developments.

Kidney diseases are the diseases that can affect or damage the kidneys. Diabetes and hypertension are the major risk factors for kidney disease and can cause kidney failure. Diabetes causes higher levels of sugar in blood that damages the kidneys and decreases their ability to filter waste and fluid from the blood, causing kidney disease over time. High blood pressure is the second most common cause of kidney failure, after diabetes. It narrows the blood vessels which reduces the blood flow and obstructs the normal functioning of kidneys. Eating healthy, being physically active and taking medicine on time can help slow the progression and prevent damage to kidneys. Renin-angiotensin system blockade, glycemic and blood pressure control are generally used therapeutic approaches for managing kidney diseases, but there are emerging therapies which focus on delaying fibrosis development and reducing inflammation. Furthermore, certain lifestyle changes, like managing stress, weight, and diet are also helpful in the management and prevention of kidney diseases. The aim of this book is to present researches that have transformed the study of kidney diseases. It attempts to understand the various interventions used for the management of kidney diseases as well as the emerging therapies.

It was a great honour to edit this book, though there were challenges, as it involved a lot of communication and networking between me and the editorial team. However, the end result was this all-inclusive book covering diverse themes in the field.

Finally, it is important to acknowledge the efforts of the contributors for their excellent chapters, through which a wide variety of issues have been addressed. I would also like to thank my colleagues for their valuable feedback during the making of this book.

Editor

Hemodynamic Predictors for Sepsis-Induced Acute Kidney Injury

Oana Antal [1,2,*], Elena Ștefănescu [1,2], Monica Mleșnițe [1,2], Andrei Mihai Bălan [1], Alexandra Caziuc [1] and Natalia Hagău [1]

[1] Department of Anaesthesia and Intensive Care, "Iuliu Hațieganu" University of Medicine and Pharmacy, No 3-5 Clinicilor Street, Cluj-Napoca, 400005 Cluj, Romania; stefanescuelena2004@yahoo.com (E.S.); monicamle@icloud.com (M.M.); balanandreimihai@yahoo.com (A.M.B.); alex.8610@gmail.com (A.C.); hagaunatalia@gmail.com (N.H.)
[2] Department of Anaesthesia and Intensive Care, Cluj Emergency Clinical County Hospital, No 3-5 Clinicilor Street, Cluj-Napoca, 400005 Cluj, Romania
* Correspondence: antal.oanna@gmail.com

Abstract: The aim of our study was to assess the association between the macrohemodynamic profile and sepsis induced acute kidney injury (AKI). We also investigated which minimally invasive hemodynamic parameters may help identify patients at risk for sepsis-AKI. We included 71 patients with sepsis and septic shock. We performed the initial fluid resuscitation using local protocols and continued to give fluids guided by the minimally invasive hemodynamic parameters. We assessed the hemodynamic status by transpulmonary thermodilution technique. Sequential organ failure assessment (SOFA score) (AUC 0.74, 95% CI 0.61–0.83, $p < 0.01$) and cardiovascular SOFA (AUC 0.73, 95% CI 0.61–0.83, $p < 0.01$) were found to be predictors for sepsis-induced AKI, with cut-off values of 9 and 3 points respectively. Persistent low stroke volume index (SVI) ≤ 32 mL/m^2/beat (AUC 0.67, 95% CI 0.54–0.78, $p < 0.05$) and global end-diastolic index (GEDI) < 583 mL/m^2 (AUC 0.67, 95% CI 0.54–0.78, $p < 0.05$) after the initial fluid resuscitation are predictive for oliguria/anuria at 24 h after study inclusion. The combination of higher vasopressor dependency index (VDI, calculated as the (dobutamine dose $\times$ 1 + dopamine dose $\times$ 1 + norepinephrine dose $\times$ 100 + vasopressin $\times$ 100 + epinephrine $\times$ 100)/MAP) and norepinephrine, lower systemic vascular resistance index (SVRI), and mean arterial blood pressure (MAP) levels, in the setting of normal preload parameters, showed a more severe vasoplegia. Severe vasoplegia in the first 24 h of sepsis is associated with a higher risk of sepsis induced AKI. The SOFA and cardiovascular SOFA scores may identify patients at risk for sepsis AKI. Persistent low SVI and GEDI values after the initial fluid resuscitation may predict renal outcome.

Keywords: sepsis-induced AKI; advanced hemodynamic monitoring

1. Introduction

Sepsis is still an important cause of morbidity and mortality in the intensive care unit (ICU) [1]. The combination of acute kidney injury (AKI) and sepsis carries an even higher mortality; sepsis-induced AKI was found to be a significant independent factor for mortality [2]. Sepsis is the leading cause of AKI in critically ill patients with a reported incidence of around 42.1% [3].

The pathophysiology of sepsis AKI is multifactorial, involving hemodynamic, microcirculatory, and inflammatory mechanisms [4]. Fluid management is a fundamental step in the management of this condition; it was already demonstrated that a successful goal-directed therapy decreases the risk of developing sepsis AKI [5].

Early identification and optimal management of patients at risk for sepsis AKI may lower the associated morbidity and mortality. The altered macrohemodynamic profile is one of the multiple triggers for sepsis induced AKI. The central role of the hemodynamic management in the prevention and treatment of patients with or at risk of sepsis AKI was already stated [6], but there is only limited research regarding the ability of the hemodynamic parameters in identifying the risk of AKI in the septic setting [7–9].

Advanced hemodynamic monitoring may be an essential tool in diagnosing the hemodynamic alterations and in achieving hemodynamic coherence [10,11]. Transpulmonary thermodilution technique was proven to be a reliable tool in assessing the hemodynamic status and in guiding fluid resuscitation in the critically ill [12,13]. By measuring cardiac output (CO) and its components (preload, afterload, and contractility) and by tailoring our interventions accordingly, we may improve diagnosis, treatment, and outcome.

The aim of our study was to find advanced hemodynamic parameters that may help in the early identification of patients at risk of developing sepsis AKI.

2. Patients and Methods

This prospective observational study was carried out between 2016 and 2017, in a mixed surgical and medical ICU of a university hospital. The protocol was approved by the Ethics Committee of the University of Medicine and Pharmacy of Cluj-Napoca (no 119/6.03.2015). We obtained individual informed consent from each patient or from next of kin before data acquisition.

2.1. Study Patients

Seventy-one consecutive septic patients [14,15], recruited in the emergency department (ED) or hospital ward, were included in this study. Sepsis was defined as a life-threatening organ dysfunction caused by a dysregulated host response to infection, clinically defined as a qSOFA (quick sequential organ failure assessment) > 2, in the presence of suspected infection [15]. Organ dysfunction was defined as an acute change in total sequential organ failure assessment (SOFA) score of 2 points or greater secondary to infection [15]. Septic shock was defined by persisting hypotension requiring vasopressors to maintain a MAP of 65 mm Hg or higher and a serum lactate level greater than 2 mmol/L (18 mg/dL) despite adequate volume resuscitation [15].

All patients included in this study had no previous history of acute kidney disease or end-stage renal disease with oliguria or anuria, and had a normal urinary output prior to this hospital admission.

Patients were excluded if aged ≥80, previously known with cardiac failure NYHA III or IV, significant aortic valvular disease, severe pulmonary hypertension or cor pulmonale, hepatic failure, renal failure, known vascular disease, severe anaemia with no consent for red blood cells (RBCs) transfusion, or prone position. We used these complex exclusion criteria in order to avoid all factors that could bias the hemodynamics of the patients [16–19]. Both spontaneous breathing and mechanically ventilated patients were included in the study.

2.2. Data Collection

Time zero (T_0) was defined as the time of study inclusion in the intensive care unit (ICU). H_3, H_6, and H_{24} were defined as the 3rd, 6th, and 24th hour after study inclusion. Sepsis onset was defined as the moment when the patient with suspected infection met at least two points from the qSOFA or SOFA scores [15]; the time interval between sepsis onset and study inclusion time (T_0) was less than two hours.

Fluid resuscitation in this time interval was carried out following local protocols (Supplemental Material 1A). Protocol compliance was achieved in all patients.

From T_0 to H_3 fluid resuscitation was carried out according to the same local protocols (Supplemental Material 1A). Starting with the 3rd h (H_3) to the 24th h (H_{24}) after study inclusion, all patients continued to be resuscitated using minimally invasive hemodynamic monitoring parameters obtained through transpulmonary thermodilution techniques (EV1000, Edwards Lifesciences©, Irvine, CA, USA) and the local protocol (Supplemental Material 1B). Calibrations in the first 24 h were performed at H_3, H_6, and H_{24}, and at any time the vasoactive infusion was adjusted. Static hemodynamic parameters and clinical features were also used in the monitoring process. Compliance to the fluid resuscitation protocol was achieved in all patients.

We used the vasopressor dependency index (VDI), to express the relationship between the vasopressor infusion dose and MAP. VDI is calculated as following: ((dobutamine dose × 1) + (dopamine dose × 1) + (norepinephrine dose × 100) + (vasopressin × 100) + (epinephrine × 100))/MAP [20]. Epinephrine, norepinephrine, dobutamine, and dopamine are expressed as μg/kg/min and vasopressin as units/min.

We defined vasoplegia as the syndrome of pathological low systemic vascular resistance, manifested clinically through the need for vasopressors in order to maintain a blood pressure ≥65 mm Hg in the absence of hypovolemia [21].

Sequential organ failure assessment (SOFA), cardiovascular SOFA, and acute physiology and chronic health evaluation (APACHE II) scores were used to classify the illness severity [22,23], while the kidney disease improving global outcomes (KDIGO) and acute kidney injury network (AKIN) urinary output criteria were used to define sepsis related AKI [24,25]. The rationale for choosing this clinical parameter at the expense of creatinine levels was due to the early and high sensitivity in predicting AKI [26].

We defined AKI as oliguria or anuria which persisted 24 h after sepsis diagnosis, after adequate fluid resuscitation was performed and obstruction was ruled out [25].

According to the renal outcome at 24 h, we separated the patients in two groups: the oliguric/anuric group, 19 patients (oliguric/anuric patients at 24 h after enrollment) and the normal urinary output group, 49 patients (patients which were with normal diuresis both at the time of study inclusion and 24 h later and the patients which were initially oliguric/anuric but restored normal diuresis by the 24th h after enrollment). This stratification was performed after the exclusion of patients with mortality < 24 h and patients with continuous renal replacement therapies (CRRT).

2.3. Statistical Analysis

For the statistical analysis we used IBM SPSS Statistics (version 23.0, IBM Corp, Armonk, NY, USA) MedCalc statistical software (version 17.9, MedCalc Software, Ostend, Belgium) Microsoft Excel (2013, Microsoft Corporation, Redmond, WA, USA), and GraphPad Prism (6, GraphPad Software, La Jolla, CA, USA). Continuous variables were expressed as mean ± SD and categorical variables as numbers or percentages. For descriptive statistics we used tables and graphs. To compare means we used the Wilcoxon signed rank test and Mann–Whitney U test and independent samples t-test. Proportions were compared using the two-proportion Z-Test; Receiver operating characteristic (ROC) curve analysis was used to determine predicting factors and cutoff points; odds ratio (OR) and relative risk (RR) were used as measures of association; a $p < 0.05$ was considered to be statistically significant.

3. Results

All 71 patients were included in the statistical analysis. Their demographic and physiologic characteristics are shown in Table 1.

By the 3rd h after study inclusion (H_3) most of the macro hemodynamic parameters were in the targeted range (Supplemental Material 2). An improvement in microcirculation was also noted, as shown by the reduction in the number of patients with increased capillary refill time (CRT, $p < 0.05$ at 6 hours and $p < 0.01$ at 24 h), the reduction in the number of patients presenting oliguria/anuria ($p < 0.05$ at H_3 and $p < 0.01$ at H_6 and H_{24}), and the reduction in serum lactate level (for the septic shock patients, $p < 0.0001$ at H_{24}) (Supplemental Material 2). We considered the fluid resuscitation to be appropriate as we noticed an improvement in these macro- and micro-hemodynamic parameters.

Table 1. Clinical and demographic characteristics of the patients included in the study.

	All Patients Included in the Study	Oliguric/Anuric Group	Normal Urinary Output Group	p Value *
Number of patients N	71	19	52	
Age Mean ± SD	62.6 ± 14.7	61.4 ± 10.7	62.9 ± 15.1	0.57
Weight (actual) kg Mean ± SD	82.5 ± 20.0	88.5 ± 21.4	79.9 ± 19.6	0.14
Body Surface Area Mean ± SD	1.9 ± 0.2	2.0 ± 0.2	1.9 ± 0.2	0.09
Diagnosis N (%)				
Sepsis	37 (52.1)	13 (68.4)	21 (40.4)	0.03
Septic shock	34 (47.9)	6 (31.6)	31 (59.6)	0.03
Type of sepsis N (%)	N (%)			
Medical	26 (36.6)	8 (42.1)	19 (36.5)	0.66
Surgical	45 (63.4)	11 (57.9)	33 (63.5)	0.66
Ventilation N (%)	N (%)			
Mechanically ventilated	49 (69)	18 (94.7)	31 (59.6)	0.04
Spontaneous ventilation	22 (31)	1 (5.3)	21 (40.4)	0.04
PEEP for Mechanically ventilated at study inclusion (T_0) Mean ± SD	5.7 ± 1.1	6 ± 1.2	5.5 ± 0.9	0.16
SOFA Score at study inclusion (T_0) Mean ± SD points	9.5 ± 3.2	11.3 ± 2.9	8.8 ± 3.2	0.02
SOFA Score without renal SOFA at study inclusion (T_0) Mean ± SD points	7.1 ± 2.5	8.2 ± 2.2	6.8 ± 2.6	0.06
Cardiovascular SOFA at study inclusion (T_0) Mean ± SD points	2.8 ± 1.4	3.4 ± 1.2	2.5 ± 1.3	0.03
APACHE II Score at study inclusion (T_0) Mean ± SD points	21.9 ± 8.6	23.3 ± 8.5	20.8 ± 8.4	0.17
Heart Rate at study inclusion (T_0) Mean ± SD beats/min	105.0 ± 20.6	108.5 ± 19.2	101.6 ± 18.0	0.15
Mean arterial blood pressure (MAP) at study inclusion (T_0) Mean ± SD mm Hg	75.2 ± 13.6	74.3 ± 16.4	75.8 ± 12.8	0.68
Lactate at study inclusion (T_0) Mean ± SD mmol/l	2.52 ± 2.2	4.1 ± 2.0	3.5 ± 2.3	0.12
Norepinephrine at study inclusion (T_0) Mean ± SD mcg/kg/min	0.09 ± 0.1	0.18 ± 0.1	0.06 ± 0.07	0.001
VDI Mean ± SD at study inclusion (T_0)	0.14 ± 0.2	0.26 ± 0.27	0.08 ± 0.1	0.001
Creatinine Mean ± SD at study inclusion (T_0) μmol/l	218.3 ± 192.7	291.7 ± 226.3	192.76 ± 179.5	0.06
Urea Mean ± SD at study inclusion (T_0) mmol/l	16.4 ± 12.0	20.3 ± 13.7	14.6 ± 11.2	0.09

* p value between the oliguric/anuric group and the normal urinary output group.

The incidence of sepsis induced AKI in our study was 27.9%, as shown by the number of oliguric/anuric vs. normal urinary output patients (19 vs. 49).

When we compared the SOFA and cardiovascular SOFA scores at T_0 among the two groups we found statistically significant differences ($p < 0.05$).

The ROC curve analysis for the SOFA score identified a cutoff point of >9 points (AUC 0.74, SE 0.06, 95% CI 0.61–0.83, $p < 0.01$) and a cutoff point of >3 for the cardiovascular SOFA for identifying patients at risk of oliguria/anuria (AUC 0.73, SE 0.06, 95% CI 0.61–0.83, $p < 0.01$). The graphical representation is shown in Figure 1.

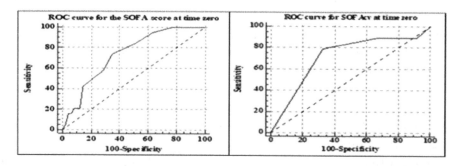

Figure 1. Receiver operating characteristic (ROC) curve analysis for Sequential organ failure assessment (SOFA) and cardiovascular SOFA at time zero.

If we compare the total fluid load (from T_0 to the H_{24}) among the two groups, we can observe that the anuric/oliguric patients received more fluids compared to the normal urinary output group (113.43 ± 72.73 versus 88.02 ± 50.06 (Figure 2A).

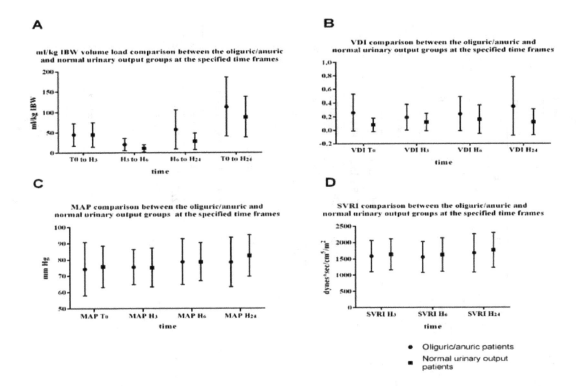

Figure 2. Comparison between the poor and normal urinary output groups at the specified time frames. (**A**) Fluid load, (**B**) vasopressor dependency index, (**C**) mean arterial blood pressure, (**D**) systemic vascular resistance index.

From T_0 to H_3 the fluid load was similar among the two groups (Figure 2A). Still the 3rd h minimally invasive hemodynamic evaluation showed a statistically significant lower stroke volume index (31.5 ± 9.3 compared to 37.0 ± 9.6, $p = 0.03$) and global end diastolic index (565.8 ± 133.6 versus 661.8 ± 158.4, $p = 0.03$) in the oliguric/anuric group compared to the normal urinary output group. The ROC curve analysis showed a cutoff point of 32 mL/m^2/beat for SVI (AUC 0.67, SE 0.07, 95% CI 0.54–0.78, $p < 0.05$) and a cutoff value of 583 mL/m^2 for GEDI (AUC 0.67, SE 0.07, 95% CI 0.54–0.78, $p < 0.05$) as predictive for oliguria/anuria at 24 h after study inclusion (Figure 3). There were no statistically significant differences in the MAP and SVRI among the two groups, even though the patients in the oliguric/anuric group had statistically significant more norepinephrine ($p < 0.001$, at T_0, and $p < 0.02$ at H_{24}, Table 2) and statistically significant higher VDI levels ($p < 0.001$, at T_0, and $p < 0.01$ at H_{24}, Table 2). Both the difference in norepinephrine infusion and the higher VDI were suggestive for a more severe vasoplegia in the oliguric/anuric.

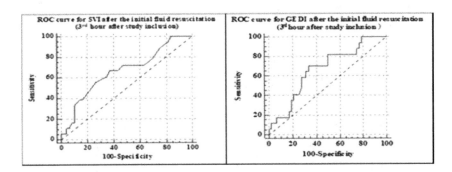

Figure 3. ROC curve analysis for the stroke volume index (SVI) and global end diastolic index (GEDI) after the initial fluid resuscitation.

Table 2. The hemodynamic parameters of the two groups of patients.

	T$_0$			H$_3$			H$_6$			H$_{24}$		
	Oliguric/ Anuric Group	Normal Urinary Output Group	p Value	Oliguric/ Anuric Group	Normal Urinary Output Group	p Value	Oliguric/ Anuric Group	Normal Urinary Output Group	p Value	Oliguric/ Anuric Group	Normal Urinary Output Group	p Value
SOFA Mean ± SD points	11.3 ± 2.9	8.8 ± 3.2	0.02	not calculated at the 3rd h			not calculated at 6th h			10.0 ± 2.5	7.2 ± 3.6	0.02
SOFAcv Mean ± SD points	3.4 ± 1.2	2.5 ± 1.3	0.03							3.0 ± 1.6	2.3 ± 1.5	0.03
SOFAr Mean ± SD points	3.1 ± 1.4	1.9 ± 1.6	0.03							2.7 ± 1.3	1.1 ± 1.3	0.00
SOFAp Mean ± SD points	2.4 ± 1.2	1.8 ± 1.2	0.02							2.1 ± 0.9	1.6 ± 1.0	0.12
APACHE II Mean ± SD points	23.3 ± 8.5	20.8 ± 8.4	0.17							not calculated at 24th h		
SBD Mean ± SD mm Hg	121.1 ± 23.9	117.5 ± 19.9	0.53	124.2 ± 18.5	123.0 ± 17.9	0.80	126.1 ± 17.3	127.9 ± 18.5	0.70	130.5 ± 17.9	130.1 ± 20.0	0.93
DBP Mean ± SD mm Hg	57.7 ± 14.5	55.6 ± 10.0	0.67	58.0 ± 11.9	55.0 ± 11.9	0.34	60.5 ± 12.0	56.5 ± 11.7	0.21	60.4 ± 12.3	59.5 ± 13.3	0.80
MAP Mean ± SD mm Hg	74.3 ± 16.4	75.8 ± 12.8	0.68	75.4 ± 10.9	75.2 ± 11.9	0.94	78.7 ± 14.1	78.6 ± 11.7	0.97	78.5 ± 15.2	82.4 ± 12.7	0.29
Heart rate Mean ± SD beats/min	108.5 ± 19.2	101.5 ± 17.9	0.15	101.7 ± 18.7	96.5 ± 18.3	0.26	100.1 ± 21.0	98.1 ± 19.5	0.90	101.1 ± 14.9	95.5 ± 17.4	0.25
CVP Mean ± SD mm Hg	8.5 ± 4.2	6.8 ± 4.7	0.08	10.7 ± 3.9	7.6 ± 4.9	0.006	11.2 ± 3.7	8.2 ± 4.9	0.01	7.7 ± 3.9	8.3 ± 4.6	0.96
CI Mean ± SD l/min	not monitored at time 0			3.2 ± 0.8	3.5 ± 0.9	0.20	3.1 ± 0.8	3.7 ± 0.9	0.03	3.2 ± 0.6	3.5 ± 0.7	0.23
SVI Mean ± SD mL/m²/beat				31.5 ± 9.4	37.0 ± 9.6	0.03	34.1 ± 12.2	38.0 ± 10.0	0.27	33.1 ± 8.6	38.0 ± 10.4	0.07
GEDI Mean ± SD mL/kg				565.8 ± 133.6	661.8 ± 158.4	0.037	530.9 ± 199.3	651.9 ± 203.0	0.07	605.1 ± 120.6	707.4 ± 153.6	0.009
ITBI Mean ± SD mL/m²				754.5 ± 215.6	764.6 ± 153.0	0.15	761.9 ± 247.0	858.3 ± 262.2	0.20	776.4 ± 247.8	931.4 ± 229.8	0.009
ELWI Mean ± SD mL/kg				7.9 ± 2.0	8.7 ± 3.3	0.88	8.88 ± 3.03	8.9 ± 4.0	0.49	8.8 ± 2.2	8.5 ± 3.0	0.45
GEF Mean ± SD				23.6 ± 8.7	22.3 ± 5.8	0.91	23.6 ± 9.8	22.7 ± 6.2	0.96	22.7 ± 7.0	21.1 ± 6.2	0.64
SVRI Mean ± SD dynes * sec/cm⁵/m²				1584.4 ± 477.4	1638.9 ± 476.4	0.97	1554.3 ± 472.3	1623.7 ± 512.1	0.85	1678.0 ± 588.0	1765.6 ± 536.0	0.69
Norepinephrine Mean ± SD mcg/kg/min	0.18 ± 0.19	0.06 ± 0.07	0.001	0.14 ± 0.14	0.08 ± 0.08	0.08	0.17 ± 0.16	0.10 ± 0.12	0.11	0.24 ± 0.30	0.12 ± 0.19	0.02
VDI Mean ± SD	0.26 ± 0.27	0.08 ± 0.1	0.001	0.19 ± 0.19	0.12 ± 0.13	0.14	0.24 ± 0.25	0.16 ± 0.21	0.19	0.35 ± 0.43	0.12 ± 0.19	0.01
Creatinine Mean ± SD) μmol/L	291.7 ± 226.3	192.76 ± 179.5	0.06	not monitored at these time frames						249.3 ± 191.8	184.8 ± 165.3	0.14
Urea Mean ± SD mmol/L	20.32 ± 13.7	14.6 ± 11.28	0.09							19.0 ± 10.7	15.3 ± 11.6	0.11
Mean urinary output Mean ± SD mL/kg/hour										0.12 ± 0.12	1.26 ± 0.75	<0.001
Lactate (septic shock patients) mean ± SD mmol/L	4.1 ± 2.0	3.5 ± 2.3	0.12	3.6 ± 2.0	3.6 ± 3.4	0.08	3.5 ± 1.5	3.7 ± 3.4	0.18	2.2 ± 1.2	2.5 ± 2.7	0.18

Table 2. *Cont.*

	T_0			H_3			H_6			H_{24}		
	Oliguric/ Anuric Group	Normal Urinary Output Group	p Value	Oliguric/ Anuric Group	Normal Urinary Output Group	p Value	Oliguric/ Anuric Group	Normal Urinary Output Group	p Value	Oliguric/ Anuric Group	Normal Urinary Output Group	p Value
Lactate clearance ≥ 10% (septic shock patients) %	not monitored between time of presentation and time zero			53.8	44.4	0.60	53.8	44.4	0.60	84.6	94.4	0.36
Capilary refill time > 3 sec %	31.60	16.30	0.16	26.30	10.10	0.09	21.10	6.2%	0.06	5.30	4.10	0.08

T_0: time zero, time of study inclusion; H_3, H_6, H_{24}: 3rd, 6th, and 24th h transpulmonary thermodilution calibrations performed in Ev1000. SOFAcv: cardiovascular SOFA; SOFAr: renal SOFA; SOFAp: pulmonary SOFA; SBD: systolic blood pressure; DBP: dyastolic blood pressure; MAP: mean arterial blood pressure; CVP: central venous pressure; CI: cardiac index; SVI: stroke volume index; GEDI: global end-dyastolic index; ITBI: intrathoracic blood index; ELWI: extravscular lung water index; GEF: global ejection fraction; SVRi: systemic vascular resistance index; VDI: vasopressor dependency index.

Patients who had an SVI lower than the cutoff value had a higher risk of remaining oliguric/anuric at 24 h than the patients with normal SVI (OR = 3.44, 95% CI 1.1–10.76, $p = 0.03$); the calculated relative risk (RR) was 2.46 (CI 1.05–5.79, $p = 0.03$).

The renal outcome upon discharge or at 28 days after admission showed a higher creatinine level in the anuric/oliguric group compared to the normal urinary output group (164.4 μmol/L ± 255.1 vs. 95.4 μmol/L ± 70.0, $p = 0.14$). The number of ICU days among the two groups showed no statistically significant difference (19.3 ± 14.4 in the oliguric/anuric group compared to 17.4 ± 13.9 in the normal urinary output group, $p = 0.70$).

The all-cause mortality for all patients included in the study was 30.9%. The all-cause mortality within the normal urinary output patients was 22.4%, while in the oliguric/anuric patients was 52.63%. The odds ratio was 3.84, 95% CI 1.24–11.80, $p = 0.01$; the RR was 2.43, 95% CI 1.19–4.59, $p = 0.01$.

4. Discussion

The main finding of our study is the fact that renal outcome in patients with sepsis and septic shock may be predicted by severe vasoplegia in the first 24 h of sepsis. A persistent low SVI (≤32 mL/m^2/beat) and low GEDI (<583 mL/kg) after the initial fluid resuscitation are also predictive for sepsis AKI. There are few studies which investigate the relationship between hemodynamics and progression of AKI during early phases of sepsis, and, from our knowledge, there are no studies which focus on the predicting value of vasoplegia, SVI or GEDI [7,8].

The cutoff values found on the ROC curves analysis for the stroke volume index and global end-diastolic volume are lower than the normal values specified by the manufacturer. The association between a low SVI and a low GEDI is suggestive for a low preload. Therefore, we may argue that the patients in the oliguric/anuric group did not receive enough fluids. But as shown in Figure 2A, not only they received similar amounts of fluids in the initial fluid resuscitation, but in the next few hours, they were given more fluids, in the attempt to restore normal GEDI, SVI, and urinary output. If we add the fact that patients in the oliguric/anuric group were having both statistically higher VDI and norepinephrine infusion rates to maintain the SVRI in clinically acceptable ranges (Table 2), and also a significantly higher pulmonary SOFA at time 0 ($p < 0.05$, Table 2), we may state that these patients were having a more severe vasoplegia with both enhanced vascular compliance and capillary leakage [27,28]. This group of patients has a high risk for fluid overload, a status associated with increased mortality in sepsis.

A high SOFA score (>9 points) and a high cardiovascular SOFA (>3 points) at time zero may be predictors for sepsis AKI. The cutoff values found for the SOFA and cardiovascular SOFA may represent tools for screening the septic patients at risk for AKI. The ease in obtaining these scores made them efficient screening methods for sepsis and septic complications [15,29].

We used only the urine output criterion to define AKI at 24 h after study inclusion. The rationale for choosing this clinical parameter at the expense of creatinine levels was due to the early and high sensitivity in predicting AKI [26]. Kellum et al. demonstrated that AKI defined by isolated oliguria (no SC criteria present) was surprisingly frequent and was associated with a long-term morbidity and mortality [30]. In their study they also emphasized that some of the critically ill patients may have fluid overload with impact on the measured serum creatinine levels [30]. The mean values of creatinine among the two groups at admission and 24 h later (as shown in Table 2) are higher in the oliguric/anuric group compared to the normal urinary output group, but don't show statistically significant differences.

The incidence of sepsis induced AKI found in our study was lower compared to other studies [2,5,31]. This could be since we stratified the patients according to the 24 h renal outcome, including only patients with stage 2 and 3 AKIN and KDIGO acute kidney injury scores. This could be a limitation of our study.

All-cause mortality for the patients included in the study was 30.9%, similar to the one found in other significant research on the subject [3,32]. AKI is known to be an independent risk factor for in-hospital mortality [2]. Our research showed that patients which developed AKI had twice the mortality rate of septic patients without AKI, in concordance with other important works [33,34]. A possible limitation in our study was the fact that we did not calculate mortality with adjustments for SOFA or APACHE II scores.

The renal outcome at 28 day or upon discharge among survivors was similar in the two studied groups, but a larger study is needed in order to confirm these findings. The number of ICU days among the two groups showed no statistically significant difference (19.3 ± 14.4 in the oliguric/anuric group compared to 17.4 ± 13.9 in the normal urinary output group, $p = 0.70$), but due to the small sample size, further research is needed to confirm this result.

Our study has several limitations. Due to the complex exclusion criteria, which had the purpose of reducing the bias generated by the hemodynamic monitoring (e.g., severe valvular diseases may impair the results of the transpulmonary thermodilution hemodynamic monitoring parameters), our results cannot be extrapolated to all septic patients. Moreover, the sample size was also limited, and the study is underpowered; more research is needed in order to confirm these results.

The lack of temporal relationship as AKI onset after sepsis onset is probably the biggest weakness in research method.

Another limitation of our study is related to the ROC AUC values which are modest, especially in the context of the multiple factors involved in the onset and persistence of oliguria and sepsis related AKI. Furthermore, the differences in baseline characteristics and number of patients in the two groups are possible factors for further errors. The results obtained through a case control experimental design, matched for selected baseline factors, could support the results obtained in this observational study; further research is needed.

5. Conclusions

Severe vasoplegia in the first 24 h of sepsis is associated with a higher risk of sepsis induced AKI. The SOFA and cardiovascular SOFA may help identify patients at risk for sepsis-induced AKI. Renal outcome in patients with sepsis and septic shock may be predicted by a persistent low SVI ($\leq$32 nmL/m^2/beat) and low GEDI (<583 mL/kg) after the initial fluid resuscitation. Further research is needed to confirm these results.

Author Contributions: Conceptualization, N.H. and O.A.; Methodology, N.H. and O.A.; Software, O.A. and A.C.; Validation, N.H.; Formal analysis, O.A.; Investigation, O.A., E.Ș., M.M., A.M.B.; Resources, O.A.; Data curation, O.A.; Writing—original draft preparation, O.A.; Writing—review and editing, N.H. and O.A.; Visualization, O.A.; Supervision, N.H. All authors have read and agreed to the published version of the manuscript.

Acknowledgments: The group of patients included in this study was used in another statistical analysis, published in J Crit Care Med (Târgu-Mureș) in 2019 (Antal O., Ștefănescu E., Mleșniţe M., Bălan A.M., Hagău N. Initial Fluid Resuscitation Following Adjusted Body Weight Dosing in Sepsis and Septic Shock. J Crit Care Med (Targu Mures) [ahead of print], but the purpose of the statistical analysis is entirely different.

References

1. Sakhuja, A.; Kumar, G.; Gupta, S.; Mittal, T.; Taneja, A.; Nanchal, R.S. Acute Kidney Injury Requiring Dialysis in Severe Sepsis. *Am. J. Respir. Crit. Care Med.* **2015**, *192*, 951–957. [CrossRef]
2. Oppert, M.; Engel, C.; Brunkhorst, F.M.; Bogatsch, H.; Reinhart, K.; Frei, U.; Eckardt, K.U.; Loeffler, M.; John, S.; German Competence Network Sepsis (Sepnet). Acute renal failure in patients with severe sepsis and septic shock-a significant independent risk factor for mortality: Results from the German Prevalence Study. *Nephrol. Dial. Transplant.* **2008**, *23*, 904–909. [CrossRef]
3. Bagshaw, S.M.; George, C.; Bellomo, R.; Committee, A.D.M. ANZICS Database Management Committee. Early acute kidney injury and sepsis: A multicentre evaluation. *Crit. Care* **2008**, *12*, R47. [CrossRef]
4. Montomoli, J.; Donati, A.; Ince, C. Acute Kidney Injury and Fluid Resuscitation in Septic Patients: Are We Protecting the Kidney? *Nephron Clin. Pract.* **2019**, *143*, 170–173. [CrossRef]
5. Plataki, M.; Kashani, K.; Cabello-Garza, J.; Maldonado, F.; Kashyap, R.; Kor, D.J.; Gajic, O.; Cartin-Ceba, R. Predictors of acute kidney injury in septic shock patients: An observational cohort study. *Clin. J. Am. Soc. Nephrol.* **2011**, *6*, 1744–1751. [CrossRef]
6. Prowle, J.R.; Bellomo, R. Sepsis-associated acute kidney injury: Macrohemodynamic and microhemodynamic alterations in the renal circulation. *Semin. Nephrol.* **2015**, *35*, 64–74. [CrossRef]
7. Poukkanen, M.; Wilkman, E.; Vaara, S.T.; Pettilä, V.; Kaukonen, K.M.; Korhonen, A.M.; Uusaro, A.; Hovilehto, S.; Inkinen, O.; Laru-Sompa, R.; et al. Hemodynamic variables and progression of acute kidney injury in critically ill patients with severe sepsis: Data from the prospective observational FINNAKI study. *Crit. Care* **2013**, *17*, R295. [CrossRef] [PubMed]
8. Badin, J.; Boulain, T.; Ehrmann, S.; Skarzynski, M.; Bretagnol, A.; Buret, J.; Benzekri-Lefevre, D.; Mercier, E.; Runge, I.; Garot, D.; et al. Relation between mean arterial pressure and renal function in the early phase of shock: A prospective, explorative cohort study. *Crit. Care.* **2011**, *15*, R135. [CrossRef] [PubMed]
9. Vallabhajosyula, S.; Sakhuja, A.; Geske, J.B.; Kumar, M.; Kashyap, R.; Kashani, K.; Jentzer, J.C. Clinical profile and outcomes of acute cardiorenal syndrome type-5 in sepsis: An eight-year cohort study. *PLoS ONE* **2018**, *13*, e0190965. [CrossRef] [PubMed]
10. Ince, C. Personalized physiological medicine. *Crit. Care.* **2017**, *21* (Suppl. 3), 308. [CrossRef]
11. Kidney Disease: Improving Global Outcomes (KDIGO). KDIGO Clinical Practice Guideline for acute kidney injury. Section 2: AKI definition. *Kidney Int. Suppl.* **2012**, *2*, 19–36.
12. Teboul, J.L.; Saugel, B.; Cecconi, M.; De Backer, D.; Hofer, C.K.; Monnet, X.; Perel, A.; Pinsky, M.R.; Reuter, D.A.; Rhodes, A.; et al. Less invasive hemodynamic monitoring in critically ill patients. *Intensive Care Med.* **2016**, *42*, 1350–1359. [CrossRef] [PubMed]
13. Taton, O.; Fagnoul, D.; De Backer, D.; Vincent, J.L. Evaluation of cardiac output in intensive care using a noninvasive arterial pulse contour technique (Nexfin1) compared with echocardiography. *Anaesthesia* **2013**, *68*, 917–923. [CrossRef] [PubMed]
14. Dellinger, R.P.; Levy, M.M.; Rhodes, A.; Annane, D.; Gerlach, H.; Opal, S.M.; Sevransky, J.E.; Sprung, C.L.; Douglas, I.S.; Jaeschke, R.; et al. Surviving Sepsis Campaign: International guidelines for management of severe sepsis and septic shock, 2012. *Intensive Care Med.* **2013**, *39*, 165–228. [CrossRef] [PubMed]
15. Singer, M.; Deutschman, C.S.; Seymour, C.W.; Shankar-Hari, M.; Annane, D.; Bauer, M.; Bellomo, R.; Bernard, G.R.; Chiche, J.D.; Coopersmith, C.M.; et al. The Third International Consensus Definitions for Sepsis and Septic Shock (Sepsis-3). *JAMA* **2016**, *315*, 801–810. [CrossRef]
16. Iwakiri, Y.; Shah, V.; Rockey, D.C. Vascular pathobiology in chronic liver disease and cirrhosis – Current status and future directions. *J. Hepatol.* **2014**, *61*, 912–924. [CrossRef]
17. Varin, R.; Mulder, P.; Tamion, F.; Richard, V.; Henry, J.P.; Lallemand, F.; Lerebours, G.; Thuillez, C. Improvement of endothelial function by chronic angiotensin-converting enzyme inhibition in heart failure: Role of nitric oxide, prostanoids, oxidant stress, and bradykinin. *Circulation* **2000**, *102*, 351–356. [CrossRef]
18. Laurent, S.; Cockcroft, J.; Van Bortel, L.; Boutouyrie, P.; Giannattasio, C.; Hayoz, D.; Pannier, B.; Vlachopoulos, C.; Wilkinson, I.; Struijker-Boudier, H.; et al. Expert consensus document on arterial stiffness: Methodological issues and clinical applications. *Eur. Heart J.* **2006**, *27*, 2588–2605. [CrossRef]
19. Mitchell, G.F.; Parise, H.; Benjamin, E.J.; Larson, M.G.; Keyes, M.J.; Vita, J.A.; Vasan, R.S.; Levy, D. Changes in arterial stiffness and wave reflection with advancing age in healthy men and women: The Framingham Heart Study. *Hypertension* **2004**, *43*, 1239–1245. [CrossRef]

20. Cruz, D.N.; Antonelli, M.; Fumagalli, R.; Foltran, F.; Brienza, N.; Donati, A.; Malcangi, V.; Petrini, F.; Volta, G.; Bobbio Pallavicini, F.M.; et al. Early use of polymyxin B hemoperfusion in abdominal septic shock: The EUPHAS randomized controlled trial. *JAMA* **2009**, *301*, 2445–2452. [CrossRef]

21. Lambden, S.; Creagh-Brown, B.C.; Hunt, J.; Summers, C.; Forni, L.G. Definitions and pathophysiology of vasoplegic shock. *Crit. Care* **2018**, *22*, 174. [CrossRef] [PubMed]

22. Vincent, J.L.; Moreno, R.; Takala, J.; Willatts, S. The SOFA (Sepsis-related Organ Failure Assessment) score to describe organ dysfunction/failure. On behalf of the Working Group on Sepsis-Related Problems of the European Society of Intensive Care Medicine. *Intensive Care Med.* **1996**, *22*, 707–710. [CrossRef] [PubMed]

23. Knaus, W.A.; Draper, E.A.; Wagner, D.P.; Zimmerman, J.E. APACHE II: A severity of disease classification system. *Crit. Care Med.* **1985**, *13*, 818–829. [CrossRef] [PubMed]

24. Kellum, J.A.; Lameire, N.; Aspelin, P.; Barsoum, R.S.; Burdmann, E.A.; Goldstein, S.L.; Herzog, C.A.; Joannidis, M.; Kribben, A.; Levey, A.S.; et al. Kidney Disease: Improving Global Outcomes KDIGO Acute Kidney Injury Work Group KDIGO clinical practice guideline for acute kidney injury. *Kidney Int. Suppl.* **2012**, *2*, 1–138.

25. Mehta, R.L.; Kellum, J.A.; Shah, S.V.; Molitoris, B.A.; Ronco, C.; Warnock, D.G.; Levin, A.; Acute Kidney Injury Network. Acute Kidney Injury Network: Report of an initiative to improve outcomes in acute kidney injury. *Crit. Care* **2007**, *11*, R31. [CrossRef]

26. Macedo, E.; Malhotra, R.; Bouchard, J.; Wynn, S.K.; Mehta, R.L. Oliguria is an early predictor of higher mortality in critically ill patients. *Kidney Int.* **2011**, *80*, 760–767. [CrossRef]

27. D'Orio, V.; Wahlen, C.; Naldi, M.; Fossion, A.; Juchmes, J.; Marcelle, R. Contribution of peripheral blood pooling to central hemodynamic disturbances during endotoxin insult in intact dogs. *Crit. Care Med.* **1989**, *17*, 1314–1319. [CrossRef]

28. Teule, G.J.; von Lingen, A.; Verwey von Vught, M.A.; Kester, A.D.; Mackaay, R.C.; Bezemer, P.D.; Heidenal, G.A.; Thijs, L.G. Role of peripheral pooling in porcine Escherichia coli sepsis. *Circ. Shock* **1984**, *12*, 115–123.

29. Trancă, S.; Petrișor, C.; Hagău, N.; Ciuce, C. Can APACHE II, SOFA, ISS, and RTS Severity Scores be used to Predict Septic Complications in Multiple Trauma Patients? *J. Crit. Care Med. (Targu Mures)* **2016**, *10*, 124–130. [CrossRef]

30. Kellum, J.A.; Sileanu, F.E.; Murugan, R.; Lucko, N.; Shaw, A.D.; Clermont, G. Classifying AKI by Urine Output versus Serum Creatinine Level. *J. Am. Soc. Nephrol.* **2015**, *26*, 2231–2238. [CrossRef]

31. Lopes, J.A.; Jorge, S.; Resina, C.; Santos, C.; Pereira, A.; Neves, J.; Antunes, F.; Prata, M.M. Acute renal failure in patients with sepsis. *Crit. Care* **2007**, *11*, 411. [CrossRef] [PubMed]

32. Fleischmann, C.; Thomas-Rueddel, D.O.; Hartmann, M.; Hartog, C.S.; Welte, T.; Heublein, S.; Dennler, U.; Reinhart, K. Hospital Incidence and Mortality Rates of Sepsis. An Analysis of Hospital Episode (DRG) Statistics in Germany from 2007 to 2013. *Dtsch. Arztebl. Int.* **2016**, *113*, 159–166. [CrossRef] [PubMed]

33. Bagshaw, S.M.; Uchino, S.; Bellomo, R.; Morimatsu, H.; Morgera, S.; Schetz, M.; Tan, I.; Bouman, C.; Macedo, E.; Gibney, N.; et al. Septic acute kidney injury in critically ill patients: Clinical characteristics and outcomes. *Clin. J. Am. Soc. Nephrol.* **2007**, *2*, 431–439. [CrossRef] [PubMed]

34. Bagshaw, S.M.; Mortis, G.; Doig, C.J.; Godinez-Luna, T.; Fick, G.H.; Laupland, K.B. One-year mortality in critically ill patients by severity of kidney dysfunction: A population-based assessment. *Am. J. Kidney Dis.* **2006**, *48*, 402–409. [CrossRef]

The Predictive Value of Hyperuricemia on Renal Outcome after Contrast-Enhanced Computerized Tomography

Ming-Ju Wu [1,2,3,4,*], **Shang-Feng Tsai** [1,5,6], **Cheng-Ting Lee** [1] and **Chun-Yi Wu** [1]

[1] Division of Nephrology, Department of Internal Medicine, Taichung Veterans General Hospital, Taichung 407, Taiwan
[2] School of Medicine, Chung Shan Medical University, Taichung 402, Taiwan
[3] Rong Hsing Research Center for Translational Medicine, Institute of Biomedical Science, College of Life Science, National Chung Hsing University, Taichung 402, Taiwan
[4] Graduate Institute of Clinical Medical Science, School of Medicine, China Medical University, Taichung 404, Taiwan
[5] Department of Life Science, Tunghai University, Taichung 407, Taiwan
[6] School of Medicine, National Yang-Ming University, Taipei 112, Taiwan
* Correspondence: wmj530@gmail.com

Abstract: The aim of this study was to determine whether elevated serum level of uric acid (sUA) could predict renal outcome after contrast-enhanced computerized tomography (CCT). We used a historical cohort of 58,106 non-dialysis adult patients who received non-ionic iso-osmolar CCT from 1 June 2008 to 31 March 2015 to evaluate the association of sUA and renal outcome. The exclusion criteria were patients with pre-existing acute kidney injury (AKI), multiple exposure, non-standard volume of contrast, and missing data for analysis. A total of 1440 patients were enrolled. Post-contrast-AKI (PC-AKI), defined by the increase in serum creatinine ≥ 0.3 mg/dL within 48 h or $\geq 50\%$ within seven days after CCT, occurred in 180 (12.5%) patients and the need of hemodialysis within 30 days developed in 90 (6.3%) patients, both incidences were increased in patients with higher sUA. sUA ≥ 8.0 mg/dL was associated with an increased risk of PC-AKI (odds ratio (OR) of 2.62; 95% confidence interval (CI), 1.27~5.38, $p = 0.009$) and the need of hemodialysis (OR, 5.40; 95% CI, 1.39~21.04, $p = 0.015$). Comparing with sUA < 8.0 mg/dL, patients with sUA ≥ 8.0 mg/dL had higher incidence of PC-AKI (16.7% vs. 11.1%, $p = 0.012$) and higher incidence of hemodialysis (12.1% vs. 4.3%, $p < 0.001$). We concluded that sUA ≥ 8.0 mg/dL is associated with worse renal outcome after CCT. We suggest that hyperuricemia may have potential as an independent risk factor for PC-AKI in patients receiving contrast-enhanced image study.

Keywords: uric acid; contrast media; acute kidney injury; hemodialysis; chronic kidney disease

1. Introduction

Post-contrast acute kidney injury (PC-AKI) is one of the most common causes of acute kidney injury (AKI), independently associated with both morbidity and mortality [1–6]. Early awareness of the risk factors to eliminate the potentially preventable AKI after contrast-enhanced image studies is a critical healthcare issue [7]. Although estimated glomerular filtration rate (eGFR) has been widely accepted to detect the high-risk patients of AKI after contrast-enhanced image studies, there are several episodes of PC-AKI that have developed in patients without advanced chronic kidney disease (CKD). Thus, further studies are needed to identify more risk factors for predicting PC-AKI.

Hyperuricemia has been linked to AKI and progression of CKD via both crystal-dependent and crystal-independent mechanisms [8]. Both urate and calcium phosphate crystals could induce oxidative stress and the expression of chemokine, and lead to the renal tubular epithelium and acute alterations in auto-regulation of renal blood flow which contribute to the decrease of renal perfusion and the subsequent injury of renal tubule [8–11]. Elevated serum level of uric acid has been reported as a novel marker for predicting AKI and mortality in several clinical settings, such as admission, percutaneous coronary intervention, and surgery, especially cardiovascular survey [12–19].

The traditional risk factors for predicting contrast-induced nephropathy include pre-existing renal disease, elderly people, diabetes mellitus, congestive heart failure, hypovolemic status, administration of nephrotoxic agents, or a large amount of contrast medium [20,21]. Metabolic syndrome and pre-diabetes have been proposed as new risk factors for contrast–induced nephropathy [22].

However, the predictive value of serum level of uric acid on the risk of PC-AKI after contrast-enhanced computerized tomography (CCT) has not been examined. The aim of this study was to determine whether serum uric acid could predict the risk of developing AKI and the need of dialysis after CCT, as well as the impact of PC-AKI on long-term change of renal function.

2. Patients and Methods

2.1. Study Design and Clinical Data Retrieval

We used a history cohort of 58,106 non-dialysis adult patients who received non-ionic iso-osmolar contrast, iodixanol (visipaque, Chicago, IL, USA), enhanced CT from 1 June 2008 to 31 March 2015 and had available a baseline serum level of creatinine and uric acid within two weeks before CCT to evaluate the association of serum uric acid and renal outcome. The exclusion criteria were patients with pre-existing AKI, recent exposure to contrast media within 30 days, volume of contrast medium ≠ 100cc (regular contrast volume for CCT), missing baseline serum creatinine, missing baseline serum uric acid (data within two weeks before CCT), and missing post-contrast serum creatinine within one week after CCT. The informed consent was waived because the study is on the basis of data collection from routine care. The institute review board of Taichung Veterans General Hospital approved this study (IRB TCVGH No: CE16164B).

There was no formal protocol for the prevention of contrast-induced nephropathy at this hospital at the time of this study. We calculated the eGFR using the four variables chronic kidney disease epidemiology collaboration (CKD-EPI) equation [23].

To find the cutoff values of baseline serum uric acid potentially associated with renal outcome, patients were classified into five groups stratified by baseline serum uric acid level: ≤3.9, 4–5.9, 6–7.9, 8–9.9, ≥10 mg/dL.

2.2. Outcome Variables

The renal outcome was determined by the primary and secondary endpoints. The primary renal endpoint was PC-AKI, which is defined by absolute increase of serum creatinine ≥0.3 mg/dL from baseline within 48 h or ≥50% within seven days after CCT, the Kidney Disease Improving Global Outcomes (KDIGO) criteria of AKI [1]. We did not include the criteria of urine volume of KDIGO criteria of AKI, because we could not collect enough data of urine volume in our study cohort. The secondary endpoint studied was the need of emergent hemodialysis after CCT. We identified the first procedure of hemodialysis within 30 days after CCT as PC-AKI requiring emergent hemodialysis. We also examined the differences in patient's characteristics, clinical factors, and incidence of AKI after CCT between serum uric acid ≥8.0 mg/dL and <8.0 mg/dL.

2.3. Statistical Analysis

All statistical analyses were performed using the SPSS software (Statistical Package for the Social Science, version 20.0, Armonk, NY, USA). Quantitative data are expressed as mean ± standard deviation. Nominal and categorical variables were compared using the chi-squared likelihood ratio or Fisher exact test with post-hoc analyses to detect difference between each pair with bonferroni. Continuous variables were compared using the nonparametric Wilcoxon test. Stepwise multivariate logistic regression analysis was used to examine the independent association of PC-AKI with patient-related characteristics and clinical factors. Association between serum uric acid ≥8.0 mg/dL and the risk of acute kidney injury and dialysis within 30 days after contrast-enhanced computerized tomography was calculated by odds ratio (OR) and 95% confidence interval (CI). A two-sided *p* value of <0.05 was set to represent the statistical significance.

3. Results

3.1. Study Population

A total of 1440 eligible patients who received CCT were enrolled in the final study cohort (Figure 1). The age of study subjects ranged from 20 to 98 years (mean age 66.2 ± 15.7 years) and 66.9% patients were male. Among them, 354 (24.6%) participants had serum uric acid ≥8 mg/dL and 865 (60.1%) participants had eGFR greater than 60 mL/min/1.73 m². Mean serum level of uric acid was 6.3 ± 2.7 mg/dL, mean serum creatinine level was 1.7 ± 2.1 mg/dL, and mean eGFR was 75.9 ± 48.0 mL/min/1.73 m². The average times of measurement of baseline serum uric acid and serum creatinine were 6.4 ± 3.2 days and 5.2 ± 3.7 days before CCT. The high incidence of comorbidities was observed and listed in Table 1. Four subgroups were created after stratification by baseline serum levels of uric acid. There were 270, 430, 386, 225, and 129 patients in the groups of serum uric acid ≤3.9, 4–5.9, 6–7.9, 8–9.9, and ≥10 mg/dL, respectively. Higher baseline serum uric acid was associated with higher prevalence of old age, stage 3~5 CKD, hypertension, coronary arterial disease, heart failure, atrial fibrillation, and chronic liver disease (Table 1).

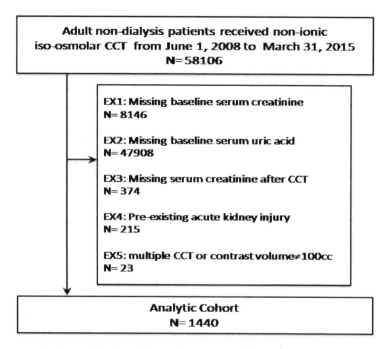

Figure 1. Study population selection flow diagram. CCT = Contrast-enhanced computerized tomography. EX = Exclusion.

Table 1. Baseline characteristics.

Serum Uric Acid (Number)	≤3.9 (N = 270)	4.0–5.9 (N = 430)	6.0–7.9 (N = 386)	8–9.9 (N = 225)	≥10 (N = 129)	Total (N = 1440)	p Value
Clinical characteristics							
Age (years)	63.2 ± 17.0	65.2 ± 15.5	67.5 ± 14.5	68.8 ± 14.5	67.5 ± 16.9	66.2 ± 15.7	<0.0001
Age ≥ 65 years *	131 (48.5%)	229 (53.3%)	244 (63.2%)	141 (62.7%)	76 (59%)	821 (57%)	<0.0001
Male sex *	176 (65.2%)	279 (64.9%)	254 (65.8%)	162 (72%)	93 (72.1%)	964 (66.9%)	0.233
Status of renal function							
Stage 1 CKD	175 (64.8%)	177 (41.2%)	71 (18.4%)	20 (8.9%)	8 (6.2%)	451 (31.3%)	
Stage 2 CKD	56 (20.7%)	135 (31.4%)	133 (34.5%)	60 (26.7%)	30 (23.3%)	414 (28.8%)	
Stage 3A CKD	14 (5.2%)	57 (13.3%)	72 (18.7%)	53 (23.6%)	19 (14.7%)	215 (14.9%)	<0.0001
Stage 3B CKD	10 (3.7%)	27 (6.3%)	43 (11.1%)	31 (13.8%)	33 (25.6%)	144 (10%)	
Stage 4 CKD	4 (1.5%)	14 (3.3%)	30 (7.8%)	29 (12.9%)	23 (17.8%)	100 (6.9%)	
Stage 5 CKD	11 (4.1%)	20 (4.7%)	37 (9.6%)	32 (14.2%)	16 (12.4%)	116 (8.1%)	
Comorbidity							
Cancer *	82 (30.4%)	141 (32.8%)	115 (29.8%)	77 (34.2%)	37 (28.7%)	452 (31.4%)	0.689
Diabetic mellitus *	93 (34.4%)	153 (35.6%)	132 (34.2%)	87 (38.7%)	49 (38%)	514 (35.7%)	0.786
Hypertension *	125 (46.3%)	233 (54.2%)	271 (70.2%)	154 (68.4%)	87 (67.4%)	870 (60.4%)	<0.0001
CAD *	48 (17.8%)	107 (24.9%)	127 (32.9%)	60 (26.7%)	47 (36.4%)	389 (27%)	<0.0001
Heart failure *	15 (5.6%)	30 (7%)	28 (7.3%)	14 (6.2%)	23 (17.8%)	110 (7.6%)	<0.0001
Atrial fibrillation *	27 (10%)	45 (10.5%)	59 (15.3%)	25 (11.1%)	35 (27.1%)	191 (13.3%)	<0.0001
CVA *	43 (15.9%)	100 (23.3%)	87 (22.5%)	47 (20.9%)	27 (20.9%)	304 (21.1%)	0.197
Chronic liver disease *	21 (7.8%)	34 (7.9%)	32 (8.3%)	24 (10.7%)	21 (16.3%)	132 (9.2%)	0.036
PAOD *	5 (1.9%)	19 (4.4%)	24 (6.2%)	14 (6.2%)	9 (7%)	71 (4.9%)	0.061
Shock *	30 (11.1%)	18 (4.2%)	14 (3.6%)	11 (4.9%)	14 (10.9%)	87 (6%)	<0.0001
GI bleeding *	12 (4.4%)	9 (2.1%)	15 (3.9%)	11 (4.9%)	9 (7%)	56 (3.9%)	0.098
Laboratory data							
Serum Albumin	3.0 ± 0.6	3.4 ± 0.8	3.4 ± 0.7	3.4 ± 0.7	3.3 ± 0.7	3.3 ± 0.7	<0.0001
Hemoglobin	10.3 ± 2.4	11.5 ± 2.6	11.3 ± 2.6	11.3 ± 2.6	10.8 ± 2.6	11.1 ± 2.6	<0.0001

CAD: Coronary arterial disease; CVA: Cerebral vascular attack; PAOD: Peripheral arterial occlusive disease; GI bleeding: Gastrointestinal bleeding. Data are expressed as mean ± standard deviation unless otherwise stated. * Data are n (%).

3.2. Renal Outcome Rates after CCT

In total, 180 (12.5%) patients developed PC-AKI, the primary endpoint, and 90 (6.3%) patients received emergent hemodialysis within 30 days. Not unexpectedly, the incidence of PC-AKI increased from 7.1% in stage 1 CKD to 29% in stage 4 CKD (Figure 2A, $p < 0.001$), but decreased to 17.2 in stage 5 CKD. The incidence of emergent hemodialysis within 30 days after CCT increased from 1.8% in stage 1 CKD to 38.8% in stage 5 CKD (Figure 2B, $p < 0.001$). The Chi-square tests were used to detect the significant differences of PC-AKI and emergent hemodialysis within 30 dyas after CCT among all pairs of populations with different stages of chronic kidney disease, both $p < 0.001$. Result of post-hoc analyses are shown in Figure 2.

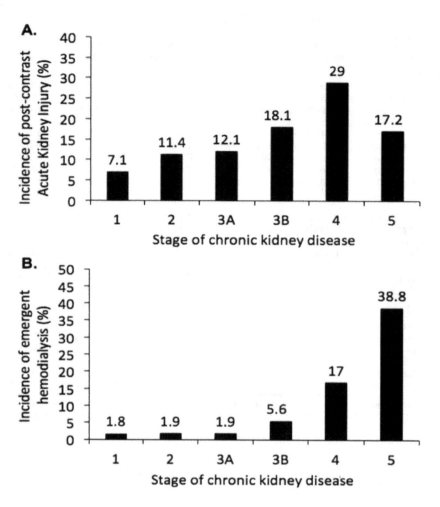

Figure 2. Renal outcome after contrast-enhanced computerized tomography (CCT) by the stage of chronic kidney disease: (**A**) Incidence of post-contrast acute kidney injury, defined by absolute increase of serum creatinine ≥ 0.3 mg/dL from baseline within 48 h or $\geq 50\%$ within seven days after CCT. Chi-square tests were used to detect the significant differences among all pairs of populations with different stages of chronic kidney disease, $p < 0.001$. Post-hoc analysis showed $p = 0.004$ in stage 1 vs. 3B, $p = 0.026$ in stage 1 vs. 4, $p = 0.001$ in stage 1 vs. 5, $p = 0.001$ in stage 2 vs. 4, $p = 0.006$ in stage 3A vs. 4. (**B**) Incidence of emergent hemodialysis within 30 days after CCT. Chi-square tests were used to to detect the significant differences among all pairs of populations with different stages of chronic kidney disease, $p < 0.001$. Post-hoc analysis showed $p < 0.001$ in stage 1 vs. 4, $p < 0.001$ in stage 1 vs. 5, $p < 0.001$ in stage 2 vs. 4, $p < 0.001$ in stage 2 vs. 5, $p < 0.001$ in stage 3A vs. 4, $p < 0.001$ in stage 3A vs. 5, $p < 0.001$ in stage 3B vs. 5, $p < 0.007$ in stage 4 vs. 5, respectively.

Moreover, the incidence of PC-AKI decreased in lower ranges of serum uric acid, from 17.8% in patients with serum uric acid ≥ 10 mg/dL to 8.1% in patients with serum uric acid 4–5.9 mg/dL (Figure 3A, $p < 0.001$), but increased to 12.2% in patients with serum uric acid ≤ 3.9 mg/dL. There was a J-shaped relationship between serum uric acid and PC-AKI after CCT. The incidence of emergent hemodialysis within 30 days after CCT increased from 2.2% in patients with serum uric acid <4 mg/dL to 15.5% in patients with serum uric acid ≥ 10 mg/dL (Figure 3B, $p < 0.001$). The Chi-square tests were used to detect the significant differences among all pairs of populations with different ranges of serum uric acid, both $p < 0.001$. Result of post-hoc analyses are shown in Figure 3.

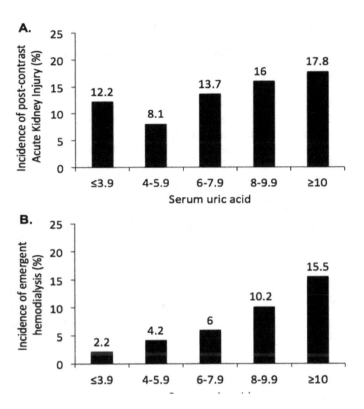

Figure 3. Renal outcome after contrast-enhanced computerized tomography stratified by baseline serum uric acid: **(A)** Incidence of post-contrast acute kidney injury, defined by absolute increase of serum creatinine ≥0.3 mg/dL from baseline within 48 h or ≥50% within seven days after CCT. Chi-square tests were used to detect the significant differences among all pairs of populations with different ranges of serum uric acid, $p < 0.001$. Post-hoc analysis showed $p = 0.033$ in sUA 4–5.9 vs. 8–9.9 mg/dL, $p = 0.028$ in sUA 4–5.9 vs. ≥10 mg/dL, respectively. **(B)** Incidence of emergent hemodialysis within 30 days after contrast enhanced computerized tomography. Chi-square tests were used to detect the significant differences among all pairs of populations with different ranges of serum uric acid, $p < 0.001$. Post-hoc analysis showed $p = 0.002$ in sUA ≤ 3.9 vs. 8–9.9 mg/dL, $p < 0.001$ in sUA ≤ 3.9 vs. ≥10 mg/dL, $p = 0.036$ in sUA ≤ 3.9 vs. 6–9.9 mg/dL, $p < 0.001$ in sUA 4–5.9 vs. ≥10 mg/dL, $p = 0.015$ in sUA 6–7.9 vs. ≥10 mg/dL, respectively.

3.3. Sensitivity Analysis: Impact of Serum Acid on Renal Outcome after CCT

Table 2 shows that the baseline serum uric acid ≥8.0 mg/dL was significantly associated with PC-AKI (OR, 1.54; 95% CI, 1.10~2.18, $p = 0.013$) and emergent hemodialysis within 30 days after CCT (OR, 2.93; 95% CI, 1.90~4.52, $p < 0.001$). Serum uric acid remained associated with PC-AKI (OR, 2.62, 95% CI, 1.27~5.38, $p = 0.009$) and emergent hemodialysis within 30 days after CCT (OR, 5.40, 95% CI, 1.39~21.04, $p = 0.015$) after adjustment for the age, gender, comorbidities (cancer, diabetic mellitus, hypertension, coronary arterial disease, heart failure, atrial fibrillation, cerebral vascular attack, chronic liver disease, peripheral arterial occlusive disease, gastrointestinal bleeding, and shock) and baseline laboratory data (serum albumin, hemoglobin) and medications (diuretics, ACEi/ARB, N-acetylcyestine, sodium bicarbonate, NSAID).

Table 2. Association between serum uric acid ≥8.0 mg/dL and the risk of acute kidney injury and dialysis within 30 days after contrast-enhanced computerized tomography.

	Odd Ratio	95% Confident Interval	p Value
Risk of acute kidney injury			
Unadjusted	1.54	1.10~2.18	0.013
Adjusted, model 1	2.40	1.31~4.42	0.005
Adjusted, model 2	2.62	1.27~5.38	0.009
Risk of dialysis within 30 days after CCT			
Unadjusted	2.93	1.90~4.52	<0.0001
Adjusted, model 1	6.42	1.91~21.56	0.003
Adjusted, model 2	5.40	1.39~21.04	0.015

Definition of acute kidney injury is absolute increase of serum creatinine ≥0.3 mg/dL from baseline within 48 h or ≥50% within seven days after contrast-enhanced computerized tomography. Model 1, adjusted by the comorbidities listed in Table 1. Model 2, adjusted by hemoglobin, serum albumin, bilirubin, uric acid, usage of diuretics, usage of ACE inhibitors/ARB, usage of N-acetylcysteine, usage of sodium bicarbonate, usage of non-steroidal anti-inflammatories, plus covariates listed in Model 1.

Incidence of serum uric acid ≥8.0 mg/dL significantly increased as the progression of renal function, from 6.2% in stage 1 CKD to 52% in stage 4 CKD, and decreased slightly to 41.4% in stage 5 CKD (Figure 4A, $p < 0.001$). Notably, in patients with stage 1 and 2 CKD, but not in patients with stage 3~5 CKD, serum uric acid ≥8.0 mg/dL was significantly associated with higher incidence of PC-AKI when comparing with serum uric acid < 8.0 mg/dL (Figure 4B, $p < 0.05$ in both stage 1 and stage 2 CKD). Patients with serum uric acid ≥ 8.0 mg/dL had higher incidence of emergent hemodialysis within 30 days after CCT in stage 2, 3A, and 3B CKD (Figure 4C). Overall, when comparing with serum uric acid < 8.0 mg/dL, patients with serum uric acid ≥ 8.0 mg/dL had higher incidence of PC-AKI (16.7% vs. 11.1%, $p = 0.012$, Figure 4D) and higher incidence of emergent hemodialysis within 30 days after CCT (12.1% vs. 4.3%, $p < 0.001$, Figure 4D). Compared to male patients, female patients had significantly higher risk to receive hemodialysis within 30 days after CCT (8.1% vs. 4.7%, $p = 0.012$), but not in PC-AKI (15.9% vs. 12.3%, $p = 0.075$). However, gender is not an independent risk factor when we perform regression analysis to detect the potential risk factor of post-contrast AKI.

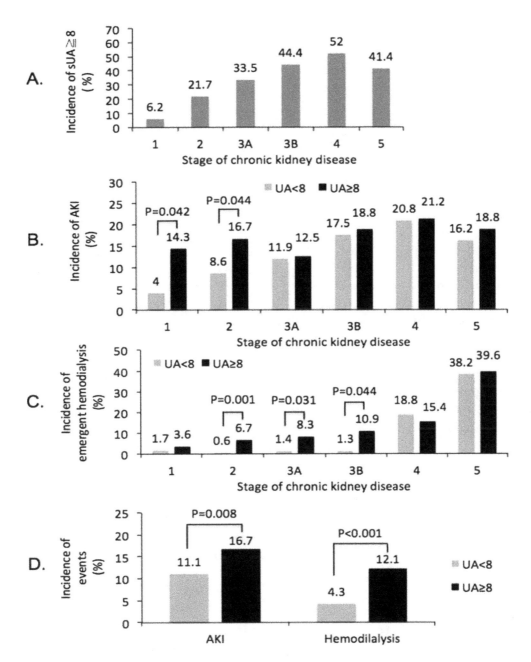

Figure 4. Impact of sUA ≥8.0 mg/dL on renal outcome after contrast-enhanced computerized tomography. (**A**) percentages of patients with sUA ≥ 8 mg/dL by stage of CKD, Chi-square tests were used to detect the significant differences among all pairs of populations with different stages of CKD, $p < 0.001$. (**B**) incidence of post-contrast AKI by stage of CKD. (**C**) Incidence of emergent hemodialysis within 30 days by stage of CKD. (**D**) difference of renal events, post-contrast AKI, and emergent hemodialysis with 30 days after contrast-enhanced computerized tomography, between patients with sUA <8 and ≥8 mg/dL. sUA = Serum uric acid. AKI = Acute kidney injury. CKD = Chronic kidney disease.

3.4. Analysis of Renal Outcome in three Months after CCT

We further collected renal function three months after CCT to compare the change of eGFR between AKI and non-AKI groups. The mean eGFR decreased 19.6 ± 37.4% in the AKI group and increased 1.3 ± 36.0% in the non-AKI group ($p < 0.001$, Figure 5A). Among them, 53.8% of patients with AKI had eGFR decreased by ≥20% compared to only 25.9% in patients without AKI ($p < 0.001$, Figure 5B).

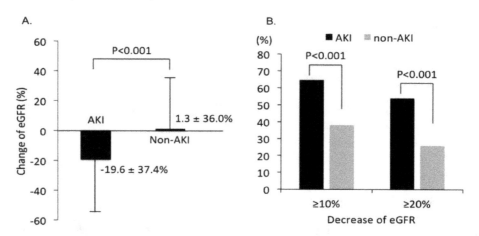

Figure 5. Impact of post-contrast acute kidney injury on renal outcome at three months after contrast-enhanced computerized tomography. (**A**) Change of eGFR at three months after contrast-enhanced computerized tomography. (**B**) Percentage of patients with eGFR decreased by ≥10% and ≥20% in patients with or without AKI, respectively. sUA = Serum uric acid. AKI = Acute kidney injury. eGFR = Estimated glomerular filtration rate.

3.5. Subgroups Analysis of Renal Outcome after CCT

In the subgroups analysis, we found the incidences of serum uric acid ≥ 8.0 mg/dL were 24.7% of 984 patients aged ≥60 years, 19.7% of 476 female patients, 26.4% of 870 hypertensive patients, and 24.3% of 452 patients with cancer. The odds ratios of serum uric acid ≥8.0 mg/dL for the predicting PC-AKI were 2.61 (95% CI = 1.02~2.24, $p = 0.040$) in patients aged ≥60 years, and 2.19 (95% CI = 1.21~3.94, $p = 0.009$) in female patients. The odds ratios of serum uric acid ≥8.0 mg/dL for the predicting emergent hemodialysis within 30 days after CCT were 2.07 (95% CI = 1.23~3.49, $p = 0.006$) in patients aged ≥60 years, 7.03 (95% CI = 3.01~16.44, $p < 0.0001$) in patients aged <60 years, 2.68 (95% CI = 1.02~5.89, $p = 0.014$) in female patients, 3.06 (95% CI = 1.81~5.17, $p < 0.0001$) in male patients, 3.00 (95% CI = 1.82~4.94, $p < 0.0001$) in hypertensive patients, 2.43 (95% CI = 1.34~4.41, $p = 0.003$) in diabetic patients, 3.49 (95% CI = 1.82~6.66, $p < 0.0001$) in non-diabetic patients, 2.73 (95% CI = 1.24~6.01, $p = 0.013$) in patients with coronary arterial disease, and 3.00 (95% CI = 1.78~5.05, $p < 0.0001$) in patients without coronary arterial disease.

4. Discussion

The primary finding of this study is the strong association between hyperuricemia and the risk of PC-AKI and the need of emergent hemodialysis within 30 days after CCT. Even after adjustment for patient characteristics, comorbidities, laboratory data, and medications, pre-contrast serum uric acid continued to be strongly associated with renal outcome after CCT. Our findings provide proof of concept that hyperuricemia, especially when serum uric acid is ≥8.0 mg/dL, was associated with higher risk of PC-AKI after CCT. The association between hyperuricemia and PC-AKI occurs more significantly in patients without advanced CKD stage 4 and 5.

The estimated GFR has been widely used to assess the risk of PC-AKI when patients need to receive contrast-enhanced image studies [2]. Regardless of the fact that hyperuricemia is more common in patients with advanced CKD, 11.6% of 865 patients with stage 1 and 2 CKD had serum uric acid ≥8.0 mg/dL in this study. These patients without advanced stage 3~5 CKD are generally considered to have relatively lower risk of PC-AKI. However, the incidence of PC-AKI and emergent hemodialysis within 30 days after CCT were 9.1% and 1.8%, respectively, in patients with eGFR ≥ 60 mL/min/1.73 m². In this study, we suggest that hyperuricemia could be one of the independent risk factors for the prediction of renal outcome after CCT. The impact of PC-AKI was further demonstrated by the fact that a significantly higher percentage of eGFR decreased ≥20% after three months of CCT.

The possible explanations for the increased risk of PC-AKI in patients with elevated serum uric acid include both crystal-dependent and crystal-independent mechanisms [8,24]. Elevated serum uric acid can induce renal vasoconstriction and impair auto-regulation, which leads to reduced renal blood flow and GFR [9,10]. A mild elevation of serum uric acid in rats could cause renal vasoconstriction in a crystal-independent pathway [11]. Several recent studies demonstrated that hyperuricemia could worsen the injury of the renal tubule via pro-inflammatory pathways involving activation of the renin-angiotensin system, chemokine expression, and endothelial dysfunction [8,9]. Importantly, contrast medium may increase the burden of hyperuricemia-induced kidney injury.

The association between hyperuricemia and an increased risk for developing AKI has been demonstrated in patients receiving cardiovascular surgery and percutaneous coronary interventions and acute paraquat intoxication [12–19]. Moreover, hyperuricemia has been proposed as a novel marker for early detection of AKI [25]. In this study, we demonstrate that hyperuricemia is an important predictor of developing PC-AKI and the need for emergent hemodialysis within 30 days after CCT.

Interestingly, the association between serum uric acid $\geq$ 8.0 mg/dL and PC-AKI was more significant in patients with stage 1 and 2 CKD, which accounts for 60.1% in this study cohort. Recently, Kuwabara and colleagues also reported that change in SUA is independently associated with change in eGFR over time in patients with eGFR $\geq$ 60 mL/min/1.73 m^2 [26]. These findings suggest that the impact of hyperuricemia, sUA $\geq$ 8.0 mg/dL, on PC-AKI is more prominent in early stage CKD patients. However, we do not have enough sUA after contrast CT to evaluate if the change of sUA will also impact on the development of PC-AKI.

On the other hand, female patients have significantly higher risk of receiving hemodialysis within 30 days after CCT, but not in PC-AKI. In general, the female population has lower average sUA than the male population. Although our results could not support the female gender as an independent risk factor to predict PC-AKI, more study is necessary to clarify the gender effect in the association of sUA and PC-AKI.

Even though increasing evidence support the idea that hyperuricemia may increase the risk of AKI development, interventions by lowering serum level of uric acid to prevent AKI remain scarce. A small-scale randomized control study showed that lowering serum uric acid by rasburicase, an urate oxidase, did not reduce the development of AKI after cardiac surgery by using traditional and non-traditional markers [27]. It is worth mentioning that hyperuricemia could be a reflection of diminished renal perfusion. Prerenal azotemia may lead to enhanced proximal tubular reabsorption of salt, water, urea, as well as uric acid [28].

In support of our findings, Lapsia and coworker demonstrated a J-shaped relationship between hyperuricemia and postoperative AKI [12]. An explanation for the higher risk of AKI in patients with lower serum levels of uric acid, <4 mg/dL for example, is due to oxidative stress, as uric acid can act as both an anti-oxidant and pro-oxidant agent [29,30]. Malnutrition and inflammation were also suggested to be important factors for lower serum levels of uric acid and a worse outcome [19]. Moreover, the systematic review and meta-analysis among the patients undergoing coronary angiography and/or percutaneous coronary intervention showed that hyperuricemia is independently associated with the occurrence of contrast–induced AKI and the risk of renal replacement therapy [31].

There are several important limitations in this study. This is a single-center historic cohort study. Out of 58,106 study subjects, only 1440 patients were included in analysis. The result is subject to selection bias and the finding might have limited generalizability. The statistical power was limited to detect the impact of hyperuricemia in AKI requiring dialysis in eGFR $\geq$ 60 mL/min/1.73 m^2 (n = 16, 1.8%) and serum uric acid < 4 mg/dL (n = 6, 2.2%), which is an important clinical end point. On the other hand, there is also no data available to evaluate if the intervention of lower serum uric acid will reduce the risk of PC-AKI. Since this study is an observational study in nature, it is difficult to show the causality. We do not have renal biopsy data to confirm the cause of PC-AKI. A multi-center, prospective large-scale study is eventually required to address these limitations.

5. Conclusions

Our findings provide additional evidence to demonstrate that elevated serum uric acid is an independent risk factor for AKI in patients undergoing contrast-enhanced image study PC-AKI. Moreover, we provide further evidence that PC-AKI is associated with the need of dialysis and long-term renal function progression. We suggest that serum level of uric acid, together with eGFR, is necessary for patients scheduled to receive CCT.

Author Contributions: Conceptualization, M.-J.W. and S.-F.T.; methodology, M.-J.W. and S.-F.T.; validation, M.-J.W., S.-F.T., C.-T.L. and C.-Y.W.; formal analysis, M.-J.W., S.-F.T. and C.-Y.W.; investigation, M.-J.W., S.-F.T., C.-T.L. and C.-Y.W.; resources, M.-J.W., S.-F.T. and C.-Y.W.; data curation, M.-J.W., S.-F.T. and C.-Y.W.; writing—original draft preparation, M.-J.W. and C.-Y.W..; writing—review and editing, M.-J.W. and C.-Y.W.; visualization, M.-J.W., C.-T.L. and C.-Y.W.; supervision, M.-J.W.; project administration, M.-J.W. and S.-F.T.

Acknowledgments: This work was funded in part by Taichung County Kidney Association. We thank the Clinical Informatics Research and Development Center of Taichung Veterans General Hospital for their assistance in collecting the data used in this study as well as Miss Fen-Yi Lin and Yi-Jyun Yeh for their assistance in data preparation and statistical analysis. The authors thank the Biostatistics Task Force of Taichung Veterans General Hospital and Mr. Chen, Jun-Peng for statistical analysis.

References

1.   Okusa, M.D.; Davenport, A. Reading between the (guide)lines—The KDIGO practice guideline on acute kidney injury in the individual patient. *Kidney Int.* **2014**, *85*, 39–48. [CrossRef] [PubMed]

2.   Khwaja, A. KDIGO clinical practice guidelines for acute kidney injury. *Nephron Clin. Pract.* **2012**, *120*, c179–c184. [CrossRef] [PubMed]

3.   Hsu, R.K.; McCulloch, C.E.; Heung, M. Exploring potential reasons for the temporal trend in dialysis-requiring AKI in the United States. *Clin. J. Am. Soc. Nephrol.* **2016**, *11*, 14–20. [CrossRef] [PubMed]

4.   McCullough, P.A. Contrast-induced acute kidney injury. *J. Am. Coll. Cardiol.* **2008**, *51*, 1419–1428. [CrossRef]

5.   Barrett, B.J. Contrast nephrotoxicity. *J. Am. Soc. Nephrol.* **1994**, *5*, 125–137. [PubMed]

6.   Weisbord, S.D.; Mor, M.K.; Resnick, A.L.; Hartwig, K.C.; Palevsky, P.M.; Fine, M.J. Incidence and outcomes of contrast-induced AKI following computed tomography. *Clin. J. Am. Soc. Nephrol.* **2008**, *3*, 1274–1281. [CrossRef] [PubMed]

7.   Horton, R.; Berman, P. Eliminating acute kidney injury by 2025: An achievable goal. *Lancet* **2015**, *385*, 2551–2552. [CrossRef]

8.   Shimada, M.; Johnson, R.J.; May, W.S.J.; Lingegowda, V.; Sood, P.; Nakagawa, T.; Van, Q.C.; Dass, B.; Ejaz, A.A. A novel role for uric acid in acute kidney injury associated with tumour lysis syndrome. *Nephrol. Dial. Transplant.* **2009**, *24*, 2960–2964. [CrossRef]

9.   Umekawa, T.; Chegini, N.; Khan, S.R. Increased expression of monocyte chemoattractant protein-1 (MCP-1) by renal epithelial cells in culture on exposure to calcium oxalate, phosphate and uric acid crystals. *Nephrol. Dial. Transplant.* **2003**, *18*, 664–669. [CrossRef]

10.   Devarajan, P. Update on mechanisms of ischemic acute kidney injury. *J. Am. Soc. Nephrol.* **2006**, *17*, 1503–1520. [CrossRef]

11.   Sánchez-Lozada, L.G.; Tapia, E.; Santamaría, J.; Avila-Casado, C.; Soto, V.; Nepomuceno, T.; Rodríguez-Iturbe, B.; Johnson, R.J.; Herrera-Acosta, J. Mild hyperuricemia induces vasoconstriction and maintains glomerular hypertension in normal and remnant kidney rats. *Kidney Int.* **2005**, *67*, 237–247. [CrossRef] [PubMed]

12.   Lapsia, V.; Johnson, R.J.; Dass, B.; Shimada, M.; Kambhampati, G.; Ejaz, N.I.; Arif, A.A.; Ejaz, A.A. Elevated uric acid increases the risk for acute kidney injury. *Am. J. Med.* **2012**, *125*, 9–17. [CrossRef] [PubMed]

13.   Lee, E.H.; Choi, J.H.; Joung, K.W.; Kim, J.Y.; Baek, S.H.; Ji, S.M.; Chin, J.H.; Choi, I.C. Relationship between serum uric acid concentration and acute kidney injury after coronary artery bypass surgery. *J. Korean Med. Sci.* **2015**, *30*, 1509–1516. [CrossRef] [PubMed]

14.   Durante, P.; Romero, F.; Pérez, M.; Chávez, M.; Parra, G. Effect of uric acid on nephrotoxicity induced by mercuric chloride in rats. *Toxicol. Ind. Health* **2010**, *26*, 163–174. [CrossRef] [PubMed]

15. Hillis, G.S.; Cuthbertson, B.H.; Gibson, P.H.; McNeilly, J.D.; Maclennan, G.S.; Jeffrey, R.R.; Buchan, K.G.; El-Shafei, H.; Gibson, G.; Croal, B.L. Uric acid levels and outcome from coronary artery bypass grafting. *J. Thorac. Cardiovasc. Surg.* **2009**, *138*, 200–205. [CrossRef]

16. Joung, K.W.; Jo, J.Y.; Kim, W.J.; Choi, D.K.; Chin, J.H.; Lee, E.H.; Choi, I.C. Association of preoperative uric acid and acute kidney injury following cardiovascular surgery. *J. Cardiothorac. Vasc. Anesth.* **2014**, *28*, 1440–1447. [CrossRef] [PubMed]

17. Liu, Y.; Tan, N.; Chen, J.; Zhou, Y.L.; Chen, L.L.; Chen, S.Q.; Chen, Z.J.; Li, L.W. The relationship between hyperuricemia and the risk of contrast-induced acute kidney injury after percutaneous coronary intervention in patients with relatively normal serum creatinine. *Clinics* **2013**, *68*, 19–25. [CrossRef]

18. Park, S.H.; Shin, W.Y.; Lee, E.Y.; Gil, H.W.; Lee, S.W.; Lee, S.J.; Jin, D.K.; Hong, S.Y. The impact of hyperuricemia on in-hospital mortality and incidence of acute kidney injury in patients undergoing percutaneous coronary intervention. *Circ. J.* **2011**, *75*, 692–697. [CrossRef]

19. Cheungpasitporn, W.; Thongprayoon, C.; Harrison, A.M.; Erickson, S.B. Admission hyperuricemia increases the risk of acute kidney injury in hospitalized patients. *Clin. Kidney J.* **2016**, *9*, 51–56. [CrossRef]

20. Mehran, R.; Dangas, G.D.; Weisbord, S.D. Contrast-Associated Acute Kidney Injury. *N. Engl. J. Med.* **2019**, *380*, 2146–2155. [CrossRef]

21. Silver, S.A.; Shah, P.M.; Chertow, G.M.; Harel, S.; Wald, R.; Harel, Z. Risk prediction models for contrast induced nephropathy: Systematic review. *BMJ* **2015**, *351*, h4395. [CrossRef] [PubMed]

22. Toprak, O. Conflicting and new risk factors for contrast induced nephropathy. *J. Urol.* **2007**, *178*, 2277–2283. [CrossRef] [PubMed]

23. Levey, A.S.; Stevens, L.A.; Schmid, C.H.; Zhang, Y.L.; Coresh, J.; Feldman, H.I.; Kusek, J.W.; Eggers, P.; Van Lente, F.; Greene, T.; et al. A new equation to estimate glomerular filtration rate. *Ann. Int. Med.* **2009**, *150*, 604–612. [CrossRef] [PubMed]

24. Ejaz, A.A.; Dass, B.; Kambhampati, G.; Ejaz, N.I.; Maroz, N.; Dhatt, G.S.; Arif, A.A.; Faldu, C.; Lanaspa, M.A.; Shah, G.; et al. Lowering serum uric acid to prevent acute kidney injury. *Med. Hypotheses* **2012**, *78*, 796–799. [CrossRef] [PubMed]

25. Ejaz, A.A.; Beaver, T.M.; Shimada, M.; Sood, P.; Lingegowda, V.; Schold, J.D.; Kim, T.; Johnson, R.J. Uric acid: A novel risk factor for acute kidney injury in high-risk cardiac surgery patients? *Am. J. Nephrol.* **2009**, *30*, 425–429. [CrossRef] [PubMed]

26. Kuwabara, M.; Bjounstad, P.; Hisatome, I.; Niwa, K.; Roncal-Jimenez, C.A.; Andres-Hernando, A.; Jensen, T.; Milagres, T.; Sato, Y.; Garcia, G.; et al. Elevated Serum Uric Acid Level Predicts Rapid Decline in Kidney Function. *Am. J. Nephrol.* **2017**, *45*, 330–337. [CrossRef] [PubMed]

27. Ejaz, A.A.; Dass, B.; Lingegowda, V.; Shimada, M.; Beaver, T.M.; Ejaz, N.I.; Abouhamze, A.S.; Johnson, R.J. Effect of uric acid lowering therapy on the prevention of acute kidney injury in cardiovascular surgery. *Int. Urol. Nephrol.* **2013**, *45*, 449–458. [CrossRef]

28. Steinhäuslin, F.; Burnier, M.; Magnin, J.L.; Munafo, A.; Buclin, T.; Diezi, J.; Biollaz, J. Fractional excretion of trace lithium and uric acid in acute renal failure. *J. Am. Soc. Nephrol.* **1994**, *4*, 1429–1437.

29. Kaneko, K.; Taniguchi, N.; Tanabe, Y.; Nakano, T.; Hasui, M.; Nozu, K. Oxidative imbalance in idiopathic renal hypouricemia. *Pediatr. Nephrol.* **2009**, *24*, 869–871. [CrossRef]

30. Sánchez-Lozada, L.G.; Soto, V.; Tapia, E.; Avila-Casado, C.; Sautin, Y.Y.; Nakagawa, T.; Franco, M.; Rodríguez-Iturbe, B.; Johnson, R.J. Role of oxidative stress in the renal abnormalities induced by experimental hyperuricemia. *Am. J. Physiol. Renal Physiol.* **2008**, *295*, F1134–F1141. [CrossRef]

31. Zuo, T.; Jiang, L.; Mao, S.; Liu, X.; Guo, L. Hyperuricemia and contrast-induced acute kidney injury: A systematic review and meta-analysis. *Int. J. Cardiol.* **2016**, *224*, 286–294. [CrossRef] [PubMed]

3

Meta-Analysis: Urinary Calprotectin for Discrimination of Intrinsic and Prerenal Acute Kidney Injury

Jia-Jin Chen [1], Pei-Chun Fan [1,2], George Kou [1], Su-Wei Chang [3,4], Yi-Ting Chen [1,5], Cheng-Chia Lee [1,2] and Chih-Hsiang Chang [1,2,*]

[1]   Department of Nephrology, Kidney Research Center, Chang Gung Memorial Hospital, Taoyuan 333, Taiwan; raymond110234@hotmail.com (J.-J.C.); franwis1023@gmail.com (P.-C.F.); b92401107@gmail.com (G.K.); ytchen@mail.cgu.edu.tw (Y.-T.C.); chia7181@gmail.com (C.-C.L.)

[2]   Graduate Institute of Clinical Medical Science, College of Medicine, Chang Gung University, Taoyuan 333, Taiwan

[3]   Clinical Informatics and Medical Statistics Research Center, College of Medicine, Chang Gung University, Taoyuan 333, Taiwan; shwchang@mail.cgu.edu.tw

[4]   Division of Allergy, Asthma, and Rheumatology, Department of Pediatrics, Chang Gung Memorial Hospital, Taoyuan 333, Taiwan

[5]   Department of Biomedical Sciences, College of Medicine, Chang Gung University, Taoyuan 333, Taiwan

*   Correspondence: franwisandsun@gmail.com or sunchang@cgmh.org.tw

Abstract: Background: Urinary calprotectin is a novel biomarker that distinguishes between intrinsic or prerenal acute kidney injury (AKI) in different studies. However, these studies were based on different populations and different AKI criteria. We evaluated the diagnostic accuracy of urinary calprotectin and compared its diagnostic performance in different AKI criteria and study populations. **Method:** In accordance with Preferred Reporting Items for Systematic Reviews and Meta-Analyses (PRISMA) guidelines, we searched PubMed, Embase, and the Cochrane database up to September 2018. The diagnostic performance of urinary calprotectin (sensitivity, specificity, predictive ratio, and cutoff point) was extracted and evaluated. **Result:** This study included six studies with a total of 502 patients. The pooled sensitivity and specificity were 0.90 and 0.93, respectively. The pooled positive likelihood ratio (LR) was 15.15, and the negative LR was 0.11. The symmetric summary receiver operating characteristic (symmetric SROC) with pooled diagnostic accuracy was 0.9667. The relative diagnostic odds ratio (RDOC) of the adult to pediatric population and RDOCs of different acute kidney injury criteria showed no significant difference in their diagnostic accuracy. **Conclusion:** Urinary calprotectin is a good diagnostic tool for the discrimination of intrinsic and prerenal AKI under careful inspection after exclusion of urinary tract infection and urogenital malignancies. Its performance is not affected by different AKI criteria and adult or pediatric populations.

Keywords: urine calprotectin; acute kidney injury; intrinsic renal injury

1. Introduction

Acute kidney injury (AKI) is a common and widespread problem with high mortality and morbidity. Despite understanding the pathogenesis of different etiologies, traditional diagnosis markers (including serum creatinine and urine output) are not a real-time, not a sensitive and specific renal marker for early diagnosis and interventions, not based on acute kidney etiology, and the differentiation of prerenal injury and intrinsic kidney injury is difficult. There are numerous causes of AKI, which are most commonly classified as prerenal, intrinsic (intrarenal), or postrenal kidney injury. To date, many studies have revealed that neutrophil gelatinase-associated lipocalin (NGAL) has shown promising results in the early diagnosis of AKI [1–4], distinguishing between prerenal and intrinsic kidney injury ([5–7], and predicting the need for renal replacement therapy and prognosis. [8,9]. Urinary calprotectin is a heterodimer protein involved in the immune system [10] and plays a role in the AKI pathophysiology. Early studies have shown that the release of urinary calprotectin from neutrophil and renal tubular epithelial cells also produces calprotectin in response to injury [10–12]. Calprotectin has been demonstrated to be similar to NGAL as a diagnostic marker for early diagnosis and to make a different diagnosis of AKI etiology [5,13–17]. This biomarker, which can early detect acute kidney injury and distinguish between prerenal and intrinsic AKI, can facilitate intervention, reduce the time to initiate therapy, and reduce the number of unnecessary renal biopsies. Nevertheless, these studies used different AKI criteria and were based on different populations. Therefore, we conducted a systemic review and meta-analysis for evaluating the differential diagnostic accuracy of urinary calprotectin between prerenal and intrinsic kidney injury.

2. Methods

2.1. Literature Search

Our two investigators (J.-J.C., C.-H.C.) systematically and independently conducted a review of the published data in accordance with Preferred Reporting Items for the Systematic Reviews and Meta-Analyses (PRISMA) guideline. A computerized search of the electronic databases of Pubmed, Embase, and the Cochrane database was performed to identify all relevant English-language studies up to September 2018 using the keywords and medical subject heading (MeSH) term: AKI, calprotectin, S100A8/A9 complex, and myeloid-related protein complex.

2.2. Study Selection

Two investigators independently determined the study eligibility based on an evaluation of the titles, abstracts, and subsequently, the full texts. Any difference in opinion regarding eligibility was resolved by consensus through discussion. Any article that was deemed potentially relevant was retrieved online for the full-text. Studies were included if they met the following criteria: full-length English original articles published and available, human studies, urinary calprotectin for distinguishing between intrinsic and pre-renal AKI, clear definition of AKI: (the Risk, Injury, Failure, Loss, End-Stage Kidney Disease (RIFLE), AKI Network (AKIN), Kidney Disease Improving Global Outcomes (KDIGO), or pediatric RIFLE criteria (pRIFLE)) and reported the definition/clinical criteria of intrinsic or prerenal AKI. Studies were excluded according to the following criteria: (1) focusing on chronic kidney disease, (2) duplicate cohort, (3) non-original studies (such as reviews, commentaries, letters), (4) studies with insufficient information, (5) studies that were not based on urinary calprotectin level, (6) studies with no reported intrinsic or prerenal AKI. Review articles or meta-analysis were not included in the analysis; however, their citations and references were searched for additional relevant studies. Full search strategies are available in Table S1.

2.3. Data Extraction

Two investigators (J.-J.C., C.-H.C.) independently extracted the relevant information from each study. Data elements related to the study level characteristics included first author, year of publication, study location, study design, definition of AKI, sample processing, method of storage, calprotectin measurement method, and test kit, see Table 1. As for patient characteristics, data included gender, age, diabetes, hypertension, urinary tract infection (UTI), creatinine on admission, creatinine prior to admission, C-reactive protein, urinary creatinine, urinary calprotectin, and urinary calprotectin to creatinine ratio and are summarized in Table 2. Items related to the diagnostic test performance were also extracted, including cutoff points based on the Youden index, sensitivity, specificity, and the number of intrinsic and prenatal kidney injuries, see Table 3.

2.4. Outcome Measures

The diagnostic criteria of AKI were different in the six enrolled studies. Four of which (Heller, 2011; Seibert, 2013; Seibert, 2016; Basiratnia, 2017) used AKIN criteria [18]. One (Chang, 2015) used KDIGO AKI criteria [19]. One (Westhoff, 2016) used the pRIFLE criteria modified by Ackan-Arikan et al. [20]. Two of which (Westhoff, 2016; Basiratnia, 2017) were pediatric population studies.

The reference test for differentiating intrinsic or prerenal acute kidney diagnosis was based on clinical criteria as mentioned below (most studies used predefined criteria). The histologic diagnosis of hepato-renal syndrome or cardio-renal syndrome was considered the golden standard. The response to volume repletion (return of creatinine to baseline within 48 to 72 h) was considered an obligatory diagnostic criterion for prerenal kidney injury. Other findings for the diagnosis of prerenal kidney injury included compatible history (dehydration, fluid loss, heart failure, liver cirrhosis), compatible physical examination (low blood pressure, low jugular pulse, tachycardia, orthostatic blood pressure changes, poor skin turgor), and compatible urine analysis (no proteinuria, no hematuria). UTI was classified as an intrinsic kidney injury in three enrolled studies (Heller, 2011; Seibert, 2013; Seibert, 2016).

2.5. Risk of Bias

We used the Quality Assessment of Diagnostic Accuracy Studies 2 (QUADAS-2) tool and Review Manager version 5.3 to assess the quality of the included studies [21]. The QUADAS-2 score is based on four domains (patient selection, index test, reference standard, and flow and timing) to judge the risk of bias. Each study was reviewed independently by J.-J.C., C.-H.C., and rated as high, low, or of unclear risk for all four domains. The judgment principle of "applicability" was the same as the bias section, but there were no signaling questions. Disagreements between the two reviewers were solved by consensus through discussion. If the answer to all signaling questions in each domain is "yes", the domain is considered as low risk. If any signaling question is answered "no", the domain is considered as having a high risk of bias.

2.6. Statistical Analysis

True positive (TP), true negative (TN), false positive (FP), and false negative (FN) rates for each study were calculated according to the reported sensitivity, specificity, and patient number of prerenal and intrinsic AKI. Based on these data, the positive likelihood ratio (+LR), negative likelihood ratio (−LR), and diagnostic odds ratio (DOR) could be obtained for each study. The summary measures were calculated using a random effects model (DerSimonian and Laird method). To assess the diagnostic performance of urinary calprotectin in predicting intrinsic AKI in AKI patients, a symmetric summary receiver operating characteristic (symmetric SROC) curve was constructed based on TP and FP rates. The threshold effect was detected using the Spearman correlation coefficient between the logit of sensitivity and logit of '1−specificity', where a non-significant threshold effect was warranted before performing further subgroup analysis or meta-regression [22]. The degree of heterogeneity among studies was evaluated using the I^2 index, with <25%, 25%–50%, and >50% indicating mild, moderate, and high heterogeneity, respectively. Likelihood ratios indicate that the accuracy of a particular test would be more accurate for patients with a disease than for subjects without disease. Two variables (adult vs. pediatric; AKI criteria) were performed as moderators in the meta-regression analyses to explore possible sources of heterogeneity. A sensitivity analysis was done to exclude patients with a UTI. All analyses were conducted by Meta-DiSc (version 1.4) software [23]. A two-sided p value of <0.05 was considered statistically significant.

Table 1. The characteristics of the six included studies.

Study/year	Location	Design	AKI Criteria	Population	Sample Time	Storage	Assay	Test Kit
Basiratnia/2017 [24]	Iran	PC	AKIN	Pediatric	Immediately at diagnosis of AKI	−20 °C, no centrifugation	ELISA	PhiCal® Calprotectin, catalogue number K 6928; Immundiagnostik AG, Bensheim, Germany
Chang/2015 [17]	Taiwan	PC	KDIGO	Adult CCU	Immediately at admission	−80 °C, centrifugation	ELISA	R&D Systems, DLCN20, McKinley Place NE Minneapolis; MPLS, USA and Phi Cal® Calprotectin, K 6935; and Immundiagnostik AG, Bensheim, Germany
Heller/2011 [13]	Germany	PC	AKIN	Adult	Within 3 days	−20 °C, no centrifugation	ELISA	PhiCal® Calprotectin, catalog number K 6935; Immundiagnostik AG, Bensheim, Germany
Seibert/2013 [5]	Germany	PC	AKIN	Adult	NR	−20 °C, no centrifugation	ELISA	PhiCal® Calprotectin, catalog number K 6935; Immundiagnostik AG, Bensheim, Germany
Seibert/2017 [14]	Germany	PC	AKIN	Adult transplant	At admission or on clinics	−20 °C, no centrifugation	ELISA	PhiCal® Calprotectin, catalogue number K 6928; Immundiagnostik AG, Bensheim, Germany
Westhoff/2016 [15]	Germany	PC	pRIFLE	Pediatric	Immediately at diagnosis or after admission with AKI.	−80 °C, centrifugation	ELISA	PhiCal® Calprotectin; Immundiagnostik AG, Bensheim, Germany

Abbreviation: AKI (acute kidney injury), AKIN (Acute Kidney Injury Network), CCU (coronary care unit), ELISA (enzyme linked immunosorbent assay), KDIGO (Kidney Disease Global Outcomes), NR (not reported), pRIFLE (pediatric Risk, Injury, Failure, Loss of kidney function and End stage kidney disease), PC (prospective cohort).

Table 2. Patient characteristics based on available data.

Variable	Adult			Pediatric		
	Prerenal (n = 116)	Intrinsic (n = 258)	p	Prerenal (n = 44)	Intrinsic (n = 84)	p
Male (%)	73.3	49.2	<0.001	54.6	40.5	<0.001
Age (years)	68 (66, 68)	68 (58, 71)	0.007	7.5 (2.6, 7.5)	6.0 (0.6, 6.0)	<0.001
Hypertension (%)	80.2	82.6	<0.001	NA	NA	NA
Diabetes (%)	28.5	30.6	<0.001	NA	NA	NA
Urinary tract infection (%)	0	41.1	<0.001	NA	NA	NA
Creatinine on admission or diagnosis (mg/dL)	3.1 (2.6, 4.4)	3.4 (3.1, 4.1)	0.054	1.1 (0.9, 1.1)	1.8 (1.8, 1.9)	<0.001
Creatinine at baseline (mg/dL)	1.4 (1.4, 1.7)	1.4 (1.4, 1.9)	0.023	NA	NA	NA
CRP (mg/dL)	5.2 (3.5, 5.3)	5.1 (0.7, 6.7)	0.412	NA	NA	NA
Urine creatinine (g/L)	0.7 (0.7, 0.8)	0.6 (0.5, 0.6)	<0.001	NA	NA	NA
Urinary calprotectin (ng/mL)	54 (28, 385)	1955 (1955, 2405)	<0.001	29 (19, 29)	1240 (427, 1240)	<0.001
Urinary calprotectin (ng/mL)/Cr (g/L) ratio	57 (52, 310)	2775 (2775, 3698)	<0.001	NA	NA	NA

CRP, C-reactive protein; NA, not applicable; Cr, creatinine; continuous variable was presented as median and interquartile range.

Table 3. Summary of diagnostic performance of the six included studies.

Study/Year	Sample Size	Event (Prerenal/Intrinsic)	Cufoff (ng/mL)	Sensitivity	Specificity	PPV	NPV
Basiratnia 2017	75	30/45	230	96.7	96.7	97.7	96.7
Chang 2015	74	31/43	314.6	88.4	96	NR	NR
Heller 2011	86	34/52	300	92.3	97.1	98	89.2
Seibert 2013	62	24/38	600	97.4	95.8	97.4	95.8
Seibert 2017	152	27/125	134.5	90.4	74.1	NR	NR
Westhoff 2016	53	14/39	76	77	93	97	60

PPV, positive predicted value; NPV, negative predicted value; NR, not reported.

3. Results

3.1. Literature Search

The initial search retrieved 83 records. After excluding duplicated articles and removing irrelevant articles, the remaining 30 articles were screened based on the title and abstract. Ten potentially relevant articles were identified and full-text articles were downloaded and accessed for eligibility. Of these 10 articles, one of which [16] was suspected of using a duplicate cohort to another study [15], two of which reported no data of intrinsic and prerenal AKI, and one of which had no data on urinary calprotectin. Finally, six studies were included in this meta-analytic study, see Figure 1.

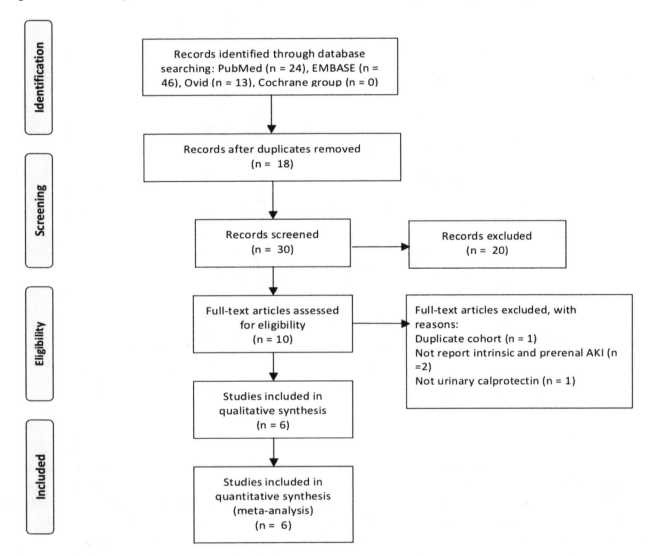

Figure 1. Preferred Reporting Items for Systematic Reviews and Meta-Analyses (PRISMA) flowchart.

3.2. Risk of Bias

With the QUADAS-2 tool, some study characteristics that might increase the risk of bias were identified. Domain 1 of QUADAS-2 focused on patient selection. Four of the included studies were based on an adult population and two on a pediatric population. One of the studies (Seibert, 2016) selected a population that was not a consecutive or random sample of patients but rather focused on post-kidney-transplant adults. Another study (Chang, 2015) selected a narrow spectrum population in the coronary care unit (CCU). Domain three addresses aspects of the reference standard. Inconsistent standard criteria of AKI (KDIGO, AKIN, or pRIFLE) and a lack of pathological evidence of intrinsic kidney injury were found in all studies. In addition, most studies used the clinical observation of a rapid decrease in serum creatinine with convergence to the baseline within 72 h after fluid repletion to diagnose prerenal AKI, except for one study (Basiratnia, 2017) that used 48 h as a time interval. Because there was one study (Seibert, 2016) with an adult kidney transplant population and two others (Basiratnia, 2017, Westhoff 2016) with pediatric populations, the answer regarding the applicability of the patient selection of these three studies was considered to be unclear. We summarized the risk of bias data for all the included studies in Figure 2.

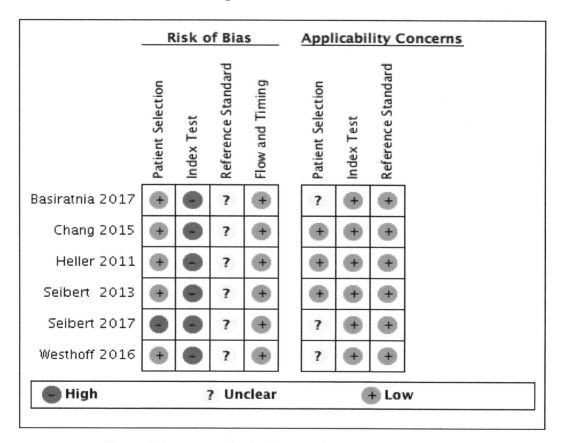

Figure 2. Summary of risk of bias and applicability concerns.

3.3. Study Characteristics

The characteristics of the six included studies are summarized in Table 1. Four of the studies were performed in Germany, one in Taiwan, and one in Iran. Sample sizes ranged from 53 to 152 patients. Two studies were conducted on pediatric populations, one on an adult kidney transplant population, and three on adult populations. Two studies excluded patients with UTI, two provided data for the entire cohort and data of excluded UTI patients, and three provided data of urinary calprotectin and normalization by urine creatinine. The optimal cutoffs were determined by the Youden index in three studies. These six studies adopted clinical diagnostic criteria for prerenal or intrinsic kidney injury, including rapid decreasing serum creatinine (Cr) (<72 h) after fluid repletion as prerenal AKI, physical examination finding, and urine examination. The detailed information of the reference test is described earlier in this article.

3.4. Patient's Characteristics

A total of 502 patients were included in these six studies. All studies were single-center trials. Study populations included adult and children populations, kidney transplant populations, and CCU patients. The mean age of the four adult AKI studies was 68 years, and there were more males with prerenal acute kidney than males with an intrinsic kidney injury ($p < 0.001$). The prevalence of hypertension, diabetes mellitus, and UTI was higher in the intrinsic kidney group. The level of serum creatinine on admission or AKI diagnosis was not significantly different ($p = 0.054$). The C-reactive protein level was also not significantly different ($p = 0.412$). Not surprisingly, the urinary calprotectin and urinary calprotectin to creatinine ration were higher in patients with an intrinsic kidney injury. Two pediatric AKI studies had a mean age of 7.5 and 6.0 years in the prerenal and intrinsic kidney injury groups, respectively. The level of serum creatinine on admission or AKI diagnosis was significantly higher in the pediatric intrinsic kidney injury group ($p < 0.001$). Detailed information is summarized in Table 2.

3.5. Urinary Calprotectin for Discriminating Prerenal and Intrinsic Acute Kidney Injuries

The diagnostic values, cutoffs, and key results are summarized in Table 3. The pooled sensitivity and specificity were 0.90 (95% CI: 0.87–0.93) and 0.93 (95% CI: 0.88–0.96), respectively. The pooled positive LR was 15.15 (95% CI: 4.45–51.55), and the negative LR was 0.11 (95% CI: 0.06–0.20), as shown in Figure 3. The symmetric SROC with pooled diagnostic accuracy was 0.9667, see Figure 4. The heterogeneity of the aforementioned four pooled indices was moderate to high (I^2 ranged from 55% to 68.9%).

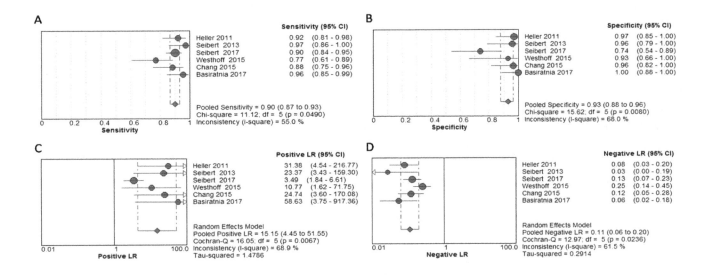

Figure 3. Diagnostic performance of urinary calprotectin on discriminating between intrinsic acute kidney injuries and prerenal acute kidney injury.

By using normalization according to urine creatinine, the data of three studies were pooled. The pooled sensitivity and specificity were 0.93 (95% CI: 0.87–0.97) and 0.95 (95% CI: 0.88–0.98), respectively. The pooled positive LR was 14.75 (95% CI: 5.54–39.3), and the negative LR was 0.08 (95% CI: 0.04–0.18), see Supplementary Information, Figure S1. The SROC with pooled diagnostic accuracy was 0.9840, see the Supplementary Information, Figure S2.

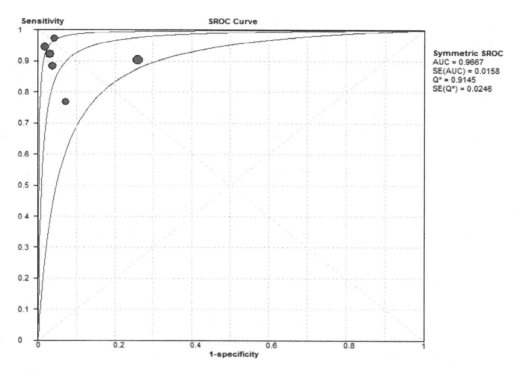

Figure 4. Symmetric summary receiver operating characteristic (symmetric SROC) according to the cutoffs of the six studies. Abbreviation: SROC, summary receiving operating characteristics; AUC, area under the curve; SE, standard error.

3.6. Subgroup Analysis

Due to the moderate to high heterogeneity, several study characteristics (population age and criteria of AKI) were used to explore the sources of heterogeneity. The analysis of the diagnosis threshold was performed with Spearman rank correlation ($\rho = -0.429$; $p = 0.397$), indicating no threshold effect and allowing for further subgroup analysis. The relative diagnostic odds ratio (RDOC) of the adult population relative to the pediatric population was 2.48 (95% CI: 0.01–737.91), indicating no significant difference in the diagnostic accuracy between adult and pediatric cohorts. The RDOCs of AKIN and KDIGO (both relative to RIFLE) were 25.13 (95% CI: 0.04–15927.64) and 5.38 (95% CI: 0.01–4757.39), respectively, indicating no significant difference in the diagnostic accuracy under different criteria of AKI (data not shown).

3.7. Sensitivity Analyses

There were three studies that provided data after excluding patients with a UTI. The pooled sensitivity and specificity of these two studies were 0.92 (95% CI: 0.85–0.96) and 0.98 (95% CI: 0.92–1.00), respectively. The pooled positive LR was 31.95 (95% CI: 9.40–108.54), and the negative LR was 0.10 (95% CI: 0.05–0.17), see the Supplementary Information, Figure S3. The symmetric SROC with pooled diagnostic accuracy was 0.9995, see the Supplementary Information, Figure S4.

4. Discussion

Calprotectin is a heterodimer protein (S100A8/S100A9) that plays a role in the innate immune system, acute kidney pathophysiology, and kidney repair processes as described below. Our findings can be summarized in the following points: (1) Urinary calprotectin is a good marker for differentiation of intrinsic and prerenal AKI; (2) the diagnostic performance of urinary calprotectin is not significantly different in different acute kidney diagnostic criteria and in adult or pediatric populations.

The urinary calprotectin is higher in intrinsic kidney injury than prerenal kidney injury. It may be reasonable to conclude that urinary calprotectin is a good diagnostic test in the discrimination of an intrinsic kidney injury with a pooled diagnostic accuracy of symmetric SROC of 0.9667.

It has been noted in earlier studies that calprotectin is released from the immune system cells (neutrophils and to lesser degree monocytes) and renal collecting duct epithelial cells [10,11,25,26]. It has also been demonstrated that renal tubular epithelial cells produce calprotectin in response to unilateral ureteral obstruction [11]. Calprotectin also increases expression after ischemia-reperfusion injury and plays a role in M2 macrophage-mediated renal repair [12]. It acts as a danger-associated molecular pattern protein that activates toll-like receptor 4 (TLR4). The available immunostainings of the clinical studies suggest that inflammatory infiltration rather than the tubular epithelial cells is the major source of urinary calprotectin in AKI [13,27]. Therefore, different etiologies of an intrinsic kidney injury which involved calprotectin, neutrophils infiltration, and TLR4 are expected to have higher urinary calprotectin. For example, in the leading causes of intrinsic kidney injury, renal epithelial tubular damage and inflammatory renal disease (including glomerulonephritis, tubular-interstitial nephritis and vasculitis, pyelonephritis) can lead to higher levels of urinary calprotectin. In contrast, in prerenal AKI, there is a functional deficit leading to low levels of urinary calprotectin. Elevated urinary calprotectin has been described in different diseases such as urinary bladder malignancies [28]. Gastroenterologists also used fecal calprotectin to distinguish between function disorder (irritable bowel syndrome) and inflammatory bowel diseases [29,30].

Heller (2011) has indicated that a UTI has a higher urinary calprotectin level than other intrinsic kidney injury causes. Pyuria is a potential confounder because it increases the calprotectin level in the urine, independent of renal function. Three above-mentioned studies (Heller, 2011; Seibert, 2013; Seibert, 2016) enrolled a UTI population as having intrinsic kidney injury. Three of the six enrolled studies (Heller, 2011; Chang 2015; Basiratnia, 2017) reported population or subgroup data showing an accuracy after exclusion of UTI and the symmetric SROC of pooled diagnostic accuracy was 0.9995. This might suggest that the diagnostic value of calprotectin is better if UTI can be excluded before examination.

Our research also supports the notion that the diagnostic accuracy of urinary calprotectin does not differ from different AKI criteria. The current AKI criteria are based on serum creatinine and urine output. It is widely noted that serum creatinine is not only a delayed but also a functional marker, rather than a damage marker to kidney injury. The novel biomarker was elevated earlier than serum Cr, and in a previous human renal ischemia-reperfusion study [26], calprotectin even increased earlier than NGAL (2 h and 8 h after injury, respectively). This may be an explanation for why we found that the accuracy of urinary calprotectin is not interfered by different AKI criteria.

Calprotectin has several characteristics that make it a promising novel marker and even a troponin for nephrologists [31]. First, as mentioned above, it rises earlier than NGAL. Second, according to Azimi [31], calprotectin combined with serum endocan may further differentiate pure tubular injury from glomerular-tubular injury. In addition, calprotectin has been reported to be associated with mortality and can predict the progression of kidney disease. In an AKI pediatric population, Westhoff et al. concluded that urinary calprotectin can predict the 30-day mortality and the need for renal replacement therapy [16]. Another kidney transplantation adult population study conducted by Tepel et al. revealed that urinary calprotectin levels on day 1 after operation predicted allograft injury and renal function decline after 1 month, 6 months, and 12 months after surgery [32].

The first limitation concerns the moderate to high heterogeneity of enrolled studies due to different study populations, even in adult patients (cardiac care unit and kidney transplant populations). As with other similar AKI biomarker systemic studies [33], different acute kidney definitions are also sources of heterogeneity. The second limitation is that our enrolled studies are all published online, the data may represent an optimistic estimate. In addition, few studies have addressed the role of calprotectin so far and only six articles were enrolled in our studies. Furthermore, to date, there is no clinical golden standard for the diagnosis of intrinsic AKI, and current studies are all based on history, clinical, and physical examination criteria. This may result in the misclassification of kidney injury etiology. Urogenital malignancies and UTI may increase urinary calprotectin concentrations independent of acute kidney injury. The careful inspection for urogenital malignancies and UTI is warranted before clinical application.

5. Conclusion

In conclusion, early diagnosis of acute kidney injury is of great significance to clinical practice and guides further therapy. Our study demonstrated that urinary calprotectin is a good diagnostic marker for discriminating intrinsic and prerenal AKI in adult or pediatric populations, and its performance was not interfered by different AKI criteria. Further large, multicenter trials may be needed to clarify and identify the possible role of urinary calprotectin in different populations. More efforts on developing biomarkers to guide therapy or treatment protocol and more rapid and accurate etiology diagnosis for AKI are still needed before before the troponin of nephrologist coming true.

Supplementary Materials:
Table S1: Primary reasons for exclusion of excluded studies, Figure S1. Diagnostic performance of the three studies providing data on urinary calprotectin with normalization to urine creatinine, Figure S2. Symmetric SROC according to the cutoffs of the three studies with urinary calprotectin with normalization to urine creatinine, Figure S3. Diagnostic performance of urinary calprotectin with three studies excluding patients with urinary tract infection, Figure S4. Symmetric SROC according to the cutoffs of the three studies excluding patients with urinary tract infection.

Author Contributions: J.-J.C. and C.-H.C. methodology; P.-C.F., G.K., S.-W.C., Y.-T.C., formal analysis; J.-J.C. and C.-H.C., data extraction; J.-J.C., writing—Original draft preparation; G.K., C.-C.L. and P.-C.F., writing—Review and editing; C.-H.C., project administration.

Abbreviations

AKI   acute kidney injury
Cr   creatinine
CCU   coronary care unit
CRP   C-reactive protein
ELISA   Enzyme linked immunosorbent assay
KDIGO   Kidney Disease Global outcomes
NGAL   Neutrophil gelatinase-associated lipocalin
NR   Not report
pRIFLE Pediatric Risk, Injury, Failure, Loss of kidney function and End stage kidney disease
PC   Prospective cohort

References

1.   Haase, M.; Devarajan, P.; Haase-Fielitz, A.; Bellomo, R.; Cruz, D.N.; Wagener, G.; Krawczeski, C.D.; Koyner, J.L.; Murray, P.; Zappitelli, M.; et al. The outcome of neutrophil gelatinase-associated lipocalin-positive subclinical acute kidney injury: A multicenter pooled analysis of prospective studies. *J. Am. Coll. Cardiol.* **2011**, *57*, 1752–1761. [CrossRef] [PubMed]

2.   Siew, E.D.; Ware, L.B.; Gebretsadik, T.; Shintani, A.; Moons, K.G.; Wickersham, N.; Bossert, F.; Ikizler, T.A. Urine neutrophil gelatinase-associated lipocalin moderately predicts acute kidney injury in critically ill adults. *J. Am. Soc. Nephrol.* **2009**, *20*, 1823–1832. [CrossRef] [PubMed]

3.   Koyner, J.L.; Vaidya, V.S.; Bennett, M.R.; Ma, Q.; Worcester, E.; Akhter, S.A.; Raman, J.; Jeevanandam, V.; O'Connor, M.F.; Devarajan, P.; et al. Urinary biomarkers in the clinical prognosis and early detection of acute kidney injury. *Clin. J. Am. Soc. Nephrol.* **2010**, *5*, 2154–2165. [CrossRef] [PubMed]

4.   Zelt, J.G.E.; Mielniczuk, L.M.; Liu, P.P.; Dupuis, J.Y.; Chih, S.; Akbari, A.; Sun, L.Y. Utility of Novel Cardiorenal Biomarkers in the Prediction and Early Detection of Congestive Kidney Injury Following Cardiac Surgery. *J. Clin. Med.* **2018**, *7*, 540. [CrossRef] [PubMed]

5. Seibert, F.S.; Pagonas, N.; Arndt, R.; Heller, F.; Dragun, D.; Persson, P.; Schmidt-Ott, K.; Zidek, W.; Westhoff, T.H. Calprotectin and neutrophil gelatinase-associated lipocalin in the differentiation of pre-renal and intrinsic acute kidney injury. *Acta Physiol. (Oxf.)* **2013**, *207*, 700–708. [CrossRef]

6. Singer, E.; Elger, A.; Elitok, S.; Kettritz, R.; Nickolas, T.L.; Barasch, J.; Luft, F.C.; Schmidt-Ott, K.M. Urinary neutrophil gelatinase-associated lipocalin distinguishes pre-renal from intrinsic renal failure and predicts outcomes. *Kidney Int.* **2011**, *80*, 405–414. [CrossRef] [PubMed]

7. Au, V.; Feit, J.; Barasch, J.; Sladen, R.N.; Wagener, G. Urinary neutrophil gelatinase-associated lipocalin (NGAL) distinguishes sustained from transient acute kidney injury after general surgery. *Kidney Int. Rep.* **2016**, *1*, 3–9. [CrossRef] [PubMed]

8. Zhang, A.; Cai, Y.; Wang, P.F.; Qu, J.N.; Luo, Z.C.; Chen, X.D.; Huang, B.; Liu, Y.; Huang, W.Q.; Wu, J.; et al. Diagnosis and prognosis of neutrophil gelatinase-associated lipocalin for acute kidney injury with sepsis: A systematic review and meta-analysis. *Crit. Care* **2016**, *20*, 41. [CrossRef] [PubMed]

9. Wu, V.C.; Shiao, C.C.; Chi, N.H.; Wang, C.H.; Chueh, S.J.; Liou, H.H.; Spapen, H.D.; Honore, P.M.; Chu, T.S. Outcome Prediction of Acute Kidney Injury Biomarkers at Initiation of Dialysis in Critical Units. *J. Clin. Med.* **2018**, *7*, 202. [CrossRef]

10. Striz, I.; Trebichavsky, I. Calprotectin—A pleiotropic molecule in acute and chronic inflammation. *Physiol. Res.* **2004**, *53*, 245–253.

11. Fujiu, K.; Manabe, I.; Nagai, R. Renal collecting duct epithelial cells regulate inflammation in tubulointerstitial damage in mice. *J. Clin. Investig.* **2011**, *121*, 3425–3441. [CrossRef] [PubMed]

12. Dessing, M.C.; Tammaro, A.; Pulskens, W.P.; Teske, G.J.; Butter, L.M.; Claessen, N.; van Eijk, M.; van der Poll, T.; Vogl, T.; Roth, J.; et al. The calcium-binding protein complex S100A8/A9 has a crucial role in controlling macrophage-mediated renal repair following ischemia/reperfusion. *Kidney Int.* **2015**, *87*, 85–94. [CrossRef] [PubMed]

13. Heller, F.; Frischmann, S.; Grunbaum, M.; Zidek, W.; Westhoff, T.H. Urinary calprotectin and the distinction between prerenal and intrinsic acute kidney injury. *Clin. J. Am. Soc. Nephrol.* **2011**, *6*, 2347–2355. [CrossRef] [PubMed]

14. Seibert, F.S.; Rosenberger, C.; Mathia, S.; Arndt, R.; Arns, W.; Andrea, H.; Pagonas, N.; Bauer, F.; Zidek, W.; Westhoff, T.H. Urinary Calprotectin Differentiates Between Prerenal and Intrinsic Acute Renal Allograft Failure. *Transplantation* **2017**, *101*, 387–394. [CrossRef]

15. Westhoff, J.H.; Fichtner, A.; Waldherr, S.; Pagonas, N.; Seibert, F.S.; Babel, N.; Tonshoff, B.; Bauer, F.; Westhoff, T.H. Urinary biomarkers for the differentiation of prerenal and intrinsic pediatric acute kidney injury. *Pediatr. Nephrol.* **2016**, *31*, 2353–2363. [CrossRef] [PubMed]

16. Westhoff, J.H.; Seibert, F.S.; Waldherr, S.; Bauer, F.; Tonshoff, B.; Fichtner, A.; Westhoff, T.H. Urinary calprotectin, kidney injury molecule-1, and neutrophil gelatinase-associated lipocalin for the prediction of adverse outcome in pediatric acute kidney injury. *Eur. J. Pediatr.* **2017**, *176*, 745–755. [CrossRef] [PubMed]

17. Chang, C.H.; Yang, C.H.; Yang, H.Y.; Chen, T.H.; Lin, C.Y.; Chang, S.W.; Chen, Y.T.; Hung, C.C.; Fang, J.T.; Yang, C.W.; et al. Urinary Biomarkers Improve the Diagnosis of Intrinsic Acute Kidney Injury in Coronary Care Units. *Medicine (Baltimore)* **2015**, *94*, e1703. [CrossRef]

18. Mehta, R.L.; Kellum, J.A.; Shah, S.V.; Molitoris, B.A.; Ronco, C.; Warnock, D.G.; Levin, A.; Acute Kidney Injury, N. Acute Kidney Injury Network: Report of an initiative to improve outcomes in acute kidney injury. *Crit. Care* **2007**, *11*, R31. [CrossRef]

19. Kidney Disease: Improving Global Outcomes (KDIGO) CKD Work Group. KDIGO 2012 clinical practice guideline for the evaluation and management of chronic kidney disease. *Kidney Int* **2012**, *2*, 19–36. [CrossRef]

20. Akcan-Arikan, A.; Zappitelli, M.; Loftis, L.L.; Washburn, K.K.; Jefferson, L.S.; Goldstein, S.L. Modified RIFLE criteria in critically ill children with acute kidney injury. *Kidney Int.* **2007**, *71*, 1028–1035. [CrossRef]

21. Whiting, P.F.; Rutjes, A.W.; Westwood, M.E.; Mallett, S.; Deeks, J.J.; Reitsma, J.B.; Leeflang, M.M.; Sterne, J.A.; Bossuyt, P.M.; QUADAS-2 Group. QUADAS-2: A revised tool for the quality assessment of diagnostic accuracy studies. *Ann. Intern. Med.* **2011**, *155*, 529–536. [CrossRef] [PubMed]

22. Arends, L.R.; Hamza, T.H.; van Houwelingen, J.C.; Heijenbrok-Kal, M.H.; Hunink, M.G.; Stijnen, T. Bivariate random effects meta-analysis of ROC curves. *Med. Decis. Making* **2008**, *28*, 621–638. [CrossRef] [PubMed]

23. Zamora, J.; Abraira, V.; Muriel, A.; Khan, K.; Coomarasamy, A. Meta-DiSc: A software for meta-analysis of test accuracy data. *BMC Med. Res. Methodol.* **2006**, *6*, 31. [CrossRef] [PubMed]

24. Basiratnia, M.; Kosimov, M.; Farhadi, P.; Azimi, A.; Hooman, N. Urinary calprotectin as marker to distinguish functional and structural acute kidney injury in pediatric population. *Iran. J. Pediatr.* **2017**, *27*, e9727. [CrossRef]

25. Vogl, T.; Tenbrock, K.; Ludwig, S.; Leukert, N.; Ehrhardt, C.; van Zoelen, M.A.; Nacken, W.; Foell, D.; van der Poll, T.; Sorg, C.; et al. Mrp8 and Mrp14 are endogenous activators of Toll-like receptor 4, promoting lethal, endotoxin-induced shock. *Nat. Med.* **2007**, *13*, 1042–1049. [CrossRef] [PubMed]

26. Ebbing, J.; Seibert, F.S.; Pagonas, N.; Bauer, F.; Miller, K.; Kempkensteffen, C.; Gunzel, K.; Bachmann, A.; Seifert, H.H.; Rentsch, C.A.; et al. Dynamics of Urinary Calprotectin after Renal Ischaemia. *PLoS One* **2016**, *11*, e0146395. [CrossRef] [PubMed]

27. Schrezenmeier, E.V.; Barasch, J.; Budde, K.; Westhoff, T.; Schmidt-Ott, K.M. Biomarkers in acute kidney injury—pathophysiological basis and clinical performance. *Acta Physiol. (Oxf.)* **2017**, *219*, 554–572. [CrossRef]

28. Ebbing, J.; Mathia, S.; Seibert, F.S.; Pagonas, N.; Bauer, F.; Erber, B.; Gunzel, K.; Kilic, E.; Kempkensteffen, C.; Miller, K.; et al. Urinary calprotectin: A new diagnostic marker in urothelial carcinoma of the bladder. *World J. Urol.* **2014**, *32*, 1485–1492. [CrossRef]

29. Langhorst, J.; Elsenbruch, S.; Koelzer, J.; Rueffer, A.; Michalsen, A.; Dobos, G.J. Noninvasive markers in the assessment of intestinal inflammation in inflammatory bowel diseases: Performance of fecal lactoferrin, calprotectin, and PMN-elastase, CRP, and clinical indices. *Am. J. Gastroenterol.* **2008**, *103*, 162–169. [CrossRef]

30. Gisbert, J.P.; McNicholl, A.G. Questions and answers on the role of faecal calprotectin as a biological marker in inflammatory bowel disease. *Dig. Liver Dis.* **2009**, *41*, 56–66. [CrossRef]

31. Azimi, A. Could "calprotectin" and "endocan" serve as "Troponin of Nephrologists"? *Med. Hypotheses* **2017**, *99*, 29–34. [CrossRef] [PubMed]

32. Tepel, M.; Borst, C.; Bistrup, C.; Marcussen, N.; Pagonas, N.; Seibert, F.S.; Arndt, R.; Zidek, W.; Westhoff, T.H. Urinary calprotectin and posttransplant renal allograft injury. *PLoS One* **2014**, *9*, e113006. [CrossRef] [PubMed]

33. Ho, J.; Tangri, N.; Komenda, P.; Kaushal, A.; Sood, M.; Brar, R.; Gill, K.; Walker, S.; MacDonald, K.; Hiebert, B.M.; et al. Urinary, Plasma, and Serum Biomarkers' Utility for Predicting Acute Kidney Injury Associated With Cardiac Surgery in Adults: A Meta-analysis. *Am. J. Kidney Dis.* **2015**, *66*, 993–1005. [CrossRef] [PubMed]

4

Does Beta-Trace Protein (BTP) Outperform Cystatin C as a Diagnostic Marker of Acute Kidney Injury Complicating the Early Phase of Acute Pancreatitis?

Justyna Wajda [1], Paulina Dumnicka [2,*], Mateusz Sporek [1,3], Barbara Maziarz [4], Witold Kolber [5], Anna Ząbek-Adamska [6], Piotr Ceranowicz [7,*], Marek Kuźniewski [7] and Beata Kuśnierz-Cabala [4]

[1] Department of Anatomy, Jagiellonian University Medical College, 31-034 Krakow, Poland; justynawajda87@tlen.pl (J.W.); msporek1983@gmail.com (M.S.)
[2] Department of Medical Diagnostics, Faculty of Pharmacy, Jagiellonian University Medical College, 30-688 Krakow, Poland
[3] Surgery Department, The District Hospital, 34-200 Sucha Beskidzka, Poland
[4] Department of Diagnostics, Chair of Clinical Biochemistry, Faculty of Medicine, Jagiellonian University Medical College, 31-501 Krakow, Poland; mbmaziar@cyf-kr.edu.pl (B.M.); mbkusnie@cyf-kr.edu.pl (B.K.-C.)
[5] Department of Surgery, Complex of Health Care Centers in Wadowice, 34-100 Wadowice, Poland; w.kolber@wp.pl
[6] Diagnostics Department of University Hospital in Krakow, 31-501 Krakow, Poland; azabek@su.krakow.pl
[7] Department of Nephrology, Jagiellonian University Medical College, 31-501 Kraków, Poland; marek.kuzniewski@uj.edu.pl
* Correspondence: paulina.dumnicka@uj.edu.pl (P.D.); piotr.ceranowicz@uj.edu.pl (P.C.)

Abstract: Acute pancreatitis (AP) belongs to the commonest acute gastrointestinal conditions requiring hospitalization. Acute kidney injury (AKI) often complicates moderately severe and severe AP, leading to increased mortality. Among the laboratory markers proposed for early diagnosis of AKI, few have been studied in AP, including cystatin C and neutrophil gelatinase-associated lipocalin (NGAL). Beta-trace protein (BTP), a low-molecular-weight glycoprotein proposed as an early marker of decreased glomerular filtration, has never been studied in AP. We investigated the diagnostic usefulness of serum BTP for early diagnosis of AKI complicating AP in comparison to previously studied markers. BTP was measured in serum samples collected over the first three days of hospital stay from 73 adult patients admitted within 24 h of mild to severe AP. Thirteen patients (18%) developed AKI in the early phase of AP. Serum BTP was higher in patients who developed AKI, starting from the first day of hospitalization. Strong correlations were observed between BTP and serum cystatin C but not serum or urine NGAL. On admission, BTP positively correlated with endothelial dysfunction. The diagnostic usefulness of BTP for AKI was similar to cystatin C and lower than NGAL. Increased BTP is an early predictor of AKI complicating AP. However, it does not outperform cystatin C or NGAL.

Keywords: beta-trace protein; cystatin C; acute pancreatitis; severity; acute kidney injury

---

1. Introduction

Beta-trace protein (BTP), also known as lipocalin-type prostaglandin D2 synthase, is a monomeric 168-aminoacid protein belonging to the lipocalin family. Its molecular weight varies according to glycosylation pattern and equals from 23 to 29 kDa [1]. BTP was initially detected in cerebrovascular fluid and was shown to be synthesized in the central nervous system. Currently, BTP serves as a laboratory marker of cerebrovascular fluid leakage, and, for that purpose, robust automated measurement method has been developed and is available in routine laboratories [2,3]. Further studies revealed BTP is expressed in other organs, e.g., heart, lungs or kidneys, and the protein is present in biological fluids such as blood and urine [4]. The low molecular weight allows for free glomerular filtration of BTP present in blood. These characteristics enabled the use of BTP as a laboratory marker of renal filtration [5].

Increased concentrations of BTP in serum or plasma and in urine correlate well with decreased glomerular filtration in patients with chronic kidney disease and the significant increase is observed in the early stages of the disease [5–9]. Moreover, increased BTP has been proposed as a marker of cardiovascular risk in patients with coronary artery disease and those with heart failure [1]. In patients with decompensated heart failure and after acute myocardial infarction, higher serum BTP was associated with long-term mortality [10,11].

Acute pancreatitis (AP) belongs to the most common acute gastrointestinal conditions requiring hospitalization [12]. Although the initial symptoms of acute abdominal pain, nausea and vomiting are serious, in most patients, the disease resolves without complications. Moderately severe or severe AP associated with local and/or systemic complications develops in approximately 20–30% of patients. The systemic complications, i.e., organ failure, including cardiovascular system, lungs or kidneys, may develop both in the early phase of AP (first 7–10 days) or later and lead to mortality in 20–30% of patients [13,14].

Acute kidney injury (AKI) is estimated to affect 7–20% of all in-hospital patients, and it is even more common in surgery and intensive care units [15,16]. The decline of renal function develops over several hours to several days. AKI is a heterogeneous syndrome, often caused by multiple insults [17]. However, in most patients, it is associated with hypoxia affecting renal medulla, caused by constriction or insufficient perfusion of renal arteries, leading to tubular necrosis and decreased glomerular filtration [18]. In severe acute pancreatitis (SAP), AKI is a common complication and may develop either in early phase in result of hypovolemia, systemic inflammation, and endothelial dysfunction, or in the late phase of AP, in association with sepsis [19–21]. The mortality of patients with SAP complicated with AP is twice as high as among those without AKI [13,19].

It is commonly recognized that early diagnosis of AKI may allow more efficient treatment and prevent the high mortality. Therefore, significant efforts are undertaken to find a laboratory marker (or a panel of markers) that would allow early diagnosis or prediction of AKI. Although several markers have been proposed [22,23], only few of them are currently available in routine laboratories and can be measured with short (2–3-h) turn-around times required for timely diagnosis. BTP is one of the markers that can be measured by fast automated immunonephelometric method that is available in most medical laboratories and is routinely used to measure such analytes as cystatin C, C-reactive protein, prealbumin or immunoglobulin chains. Moreover, the half-life of BTP in blood has been estimated to be shorter in comparison to other low-molecular-weight proteins [24]—in humans, it is estimated to be 1.2 h [25]. Thus, one may expect that the dynamic changes in renal function may be well reflected by serum BTP. However, studies evaluating BTP as a marker of AKI are scarce, and we were not able to identify any studies on BTP in AP.

The aim of the present study was the assessment of the diagnostic utility of serum BTP concentrations measured with automated immunonephelometric method for the prognosis of AKI in the early phase of AP. The diagnostic utility of serum BTP concentrations were compared with better characterized markers, i.e., serum cystatin C and serum and urine neutrophil gelatinase-associated lipocalin (NGAL).

2. Methods

2.1. Study Design and Patients

The retrospective study included two cohorts of patients admitted to hospital surgery departments with the diagnosis of AP. The first cohort was recruited at the Surgery Department, District Hospital in Sucha Beskidzka, Poland, between January and December 2014 [26]. The second cohort was recruited in the Department of Surgery, Complex of Health Care Centers in Wadowice, Poland, between March 2014 and December 2015 [27]. In July 2016, the available stored samples of serum collected from the patients were used to measure BTP. The Bioethical Committee of Jagiellonian University, Kraków, Poland (approval no KBET/247/B/2013) and the Bioethical Committee of the Beskidy Medical Chamber, Bielsko-Biała, Poland (2014/02/06/1) gave agreement for patients' recruitment and the use of patients' samples for the present study.

In both medical centers, patients were recruited according to following criteria:

- consecutive adult patients admitted to surgery department with symptoms of AP lasting no longer than 24 hours before admission were asked to join the study, and those who signed the informed consent were included in the study;
- the diagnosis of AP was based on revised 2012 Atlanta classification [28], i.e., AP was diagnosed when two of three diagnostic criteria were met, i.e., characteristic abdominal pain, characteristic signs in abdominal imaging (magnetic resonance imaging, contrast-enhanced computed tomography or ultrasonography); serum amylase or lipase exceeding the upper reference limit more than three times;
- patients with chronic pancreatitis, active cancer, or chronic liver diseases (viral hepatitis, liver cirrhosis) were excluded.

The collected demographic and clinical data included: age and sex; comorbidities including ischemic heart disease, diabetes, pulmonary and renal conditions, obesity defined as body mass index (BMI) >30 kg/m^2; etiology of AP, pancreatic necrosis or pleural effusions present in imaging, development of systemic inflammatory response syndrome (SIRS), transient or persistent organ failure, need for surgery or parenteral nutrition during the hospital stay, length of hospital stay, severity of AP, and outcome (discharge or death).

Based on clinical and laboratory data obtained on day 1 of the study, the bedside index of severity in AP (BISAP) was calculated [29]. The final severity of AP was defined according to the revised 2012 Atlanta classification [28], taking into account the persistent or transient cardiovascular, pulmonary, or renal failure as defined by modified Marshall scoring system (MMSS) [28], the systemic complications (exacerbation of comorbidities), and the local complications.

AKI was defined according to Kidney Disease Improving Global Outcomes (KDIGO) criteria [30] based on increase in serum creatinine of more than 50% or 26.5 μmol/L over 48 h. Renal failure was defined in agreement with MMSS [28] as serum creatinine concentration exceeding 170 μmol/L.

2.2. Laboratory Tests

In both centers, patients' blood samples were collected on admission (study day 1) and on two consecutive days (study days 2 and 3). A part of laboratory tests were performed on the day of collection in the centers recruiting the patients, these included complete blood counts with leukocyte differential counts, routine biochemistry (serum amylase, urea, creatinine, glucose, bilirubin, C-reactive protein), and coagulation tests (citrated plasma D-dimer). Moreover, urine samples were collected from patients treated in the District Hospital in Sucha Beskidzka on the three days of the study and the measurements of NGAL in urine were performed in the center's laboratory.

Excess serum samples collected on study days 1 to 3 were aliquoted and stored in −80 °C. BTP, cystatin C, soluble fms-like tyrosine kinase-1 (sFlt-1), and angiopoietin-2 were measured in samples from both study centers. Serum NGAL and uromodulin concentrations were only measured in samples collected in the District Hospital in Sucha Beskidzka.

BTP and cystatin C in sera were measured using immunonephelometric method on Nephelometer II analyzer (Siemens Healthcare, Erlangen, Germany). Serum sFlt-1 was measured by electrochemiluminescence immunoassay using the Cobas 8000 analyzer (Roche Diagnostics, Mannheim, Germany). The reference intervals for BTP and cystatin C in serum were <0.70 mg/L and 0.59–1.04 mg/L, respectively. The concentrations of sFlt-1 in healthy subjects were 63–108 pg/mL [31].

The measurements were performed in the Department of Diagnostics, University Hospital in Krakow. Serum angiopoietin 2 and NGAL were measured by enzyme immunoassays using commercially available kits: Quantikine ELISA Human Angiopoietin 2 Immunoassay (R&D Systems, McKinley Place, MN, USA), Human Uromodulin ELISA and Human Lipocalin-2/NGAL ELISA (BioVendor, Brno, Czech Republic). The reference values determined by the manufacturers of the kits were 1.065–8.907 ng/mL for serum angiopoietin 2 and 37.0–501.0 ng/mL for serum uromodulin. The readings were made with an automatic microplate reader Automatic Micro ELISA Reader ELX 808 (BIO-TEK® Instruments Inc., Winooski, VT, USA). The measurements were performed in the Department of Diagnostics, Chair of Clinical Biochemistry, Jagiellonian University Medical College, Kraków, Poland. Urine NGAL concentrations were measured with chemiluminescent microparticle immunoassay on Architect analyzer (Abbott Diagnostics, Lake Forest, IL, USA).

2.3. Statistical Analysis

Number of patients and percentage of appropriate group were reported for categories. The contingency tables were analyzed with Pearson's chi-squared test. Median (lower; upper quartiles) were reported for quantitative variables as most of the variables were non-normally distributed (the Shapiro–Wilk's test was used to assess normality). The differences between groups were assessed with Mann–Whitney's test or Kruskal–Wallis's analysis of variance. Spearman's rank coefficient was computed for simple correlations. Logistic regression analysis was used to check whether the differences between AKI and non-AKI subjects remain significant after adjustment for the confounders, i.e., age and prediagnosed renal comorbidity. Odds ratios (OR) for unit change were reported with 95% confidence intervals (95% CI). Receiver operating characteristic (ROC) curves were analyzed to compare the diagnostic accuracy of studied markers. The values of area under the ROC curve (AUC) were reported with 95% CI. The AUCs were compared using a method of Hanley et al. [32]. All statistical tests were two-tailed and the p-values of <0.05 indicated significant results. Statistica 12 (StatSoft, Tulsa, OK, USA) with Medical Bundle 3.0 (StatSoft, Kraków, Poland) was used for computation.

3. Results

Serum samples of 73 patients were available for the measurements of BTP, including 46 patients recruited in the Surgery Department, District Hospital in Sucha Beskidzka, Poland and 27 patients recruited in the Department of Surgery, Complex of Health Care Centers in Wadowice, Poland. In every case (73 patients), at least one sample was available of those collected within the first two days of the study (i.e., first 48 h of hospital stay). Therefore, we decided to report the maximum result of BTP obtained during the 48 h of hospital stay (or the only result, if only one sample from that time period was available) as our baseline measure.

Further, we also analyzed the BTP results obtained on separate study days. There were 65 samples available from day 1, 63 samples from day 2, and 45 samples from day 3. The whole set of samples (collected on days 1 to 3) allowing for the assessment of BTP changes over the study period was available in 33 patients.

Among 73 patients included in the study, 13 (18%) were diagnosed with AKI (Table 1). Patients with AKI were older and suffered from more severe AP, reflected by higher BISAP scores already on the day of admission, more common organ failure throughout the course of AP, a longer hospital stay and higher mortality (Table 1). A history of renal disease was significantly associated with AKI, although the number of patients with preexisting renal conditions was low (Table 1). The patients who developed AKI were characterized by more pronounced laboratory abnormalities during the first two days of hospital stay: lower hematocrit, higher CRP, higher D-dimer, angiopoietin-2 and sFlt-1 as well as higher results of laboratory tests associated with renal function (serum urea, creatinine, cystatin C and BTP, serum and urine NGAL) (Table 1). No difference was observed between AKI and non-AKI patients regarding minimum serum uromodulin (Table 1).

Table 1. Clinical characteristics of patients with acute pancreatitis (AP) and the maximum laboratory results obtained on first two days (48 h) of hospital stay (or minimum result in case of uromodulin). The quantitative data were presented as median (lower; upper quartile).

Characteristic	AKI ($n = 13$)	No AKI ($n = 60$)	p
Age, years	75 (67; 81)	56 (40; 72)	0.003
Male sex, n (%)	7 (54)	29 (48)	0.7
Preexisting comorbidities, n (%)	11 (85)	38 (63)	0.1
Ischemic heart disease, n (%)	6 (46)	16 (27)	0.2
Diabetes, n (%)	3 (23)	6 (10)	0.2
Pulmonary diseases, n (%)	1 (8)	5 (8)	0.9
Renal diseases, n (%)	3 (23)	1 (2)	0.002
BMI >30 kg/m^2, n (%)	0	9 (15)	0.2
AP etiology			
Billiary, n (%)	9 (69)	28 (47)	
Alcohol, n (%)	1 (8)	14 (23)	0.3
Hyperlipemia, n (%)	0	6 (10)	
Other or idiopathic, n (%)	3 (23)	12 (20)	
Pancreatic necrosis, n (%)	1 (8)	6 (10)	0.8
Pleural effusion, n (%)	8 (62)	27 (45)	0.3
SIRS, n (%)	8 (62)	23 (38)	0.1
BISAP score at 24 h, points	3 (2; 3)	1 (0; 2)	0.002
BISAP ≥3 points, n (%)	8 (62)	7 (12)	<0.001
Organ failure according to MMSS			
Transient, n (%)	8 (62)	15 (25)	0.010
Persistent, n (%)	4 (31)	3 (5)	0.004
AP severity			
MAP, n (%)	1 (8)	37 (62)	
MSAP, n (%)	8 (62)	20 (33)	<0.001
SAP, n (%)	4 (31)	3 (5)	
Surgery, n (%)	0	5 (8)	0.3
Parenteral nutrition, n (%)	2 (15)	3 (5)	0.2
Length of hospital stay, days	11 (8; 25)	7 (5; 11)	0.012
Mortality, n (%)	3 (23)	1 (2)	0.002
Amylase, U/L	829 (619; 1526)	1027 (537; 1897)	0.5
Hematocrit, %	37.4 (33.5; 45.2)	43.4 (41.0; 46.9)	0.011
Leukocyte count, ×10^3/μL	14.8 (12.3; 22.9)	12.1 (9.9; 16.2)	0.1
Neutrophil count, ×10^3/μL	11.4 (8.6; 19.6)	9.4 (7.5; 12.9)	0.2
CRP, mg/L	258 (182; 313)	104 (49; 229)	0.018
Glucose, mmol/L	8.93 (8.33; 12.25)	7.78 (6.56; 10.11)	0.06
Bilirubin, μmol/L	48.7 (36.4; 81.0)	35.5 (17.8; 65.1)	0.07
Urea, mmol/L	11.68 (6.72; 15.80)	5.83 (4.21; 6.57)	<0.001
Creatinine, μmol/L	120 (95; 207)	71 (61; 85)	<0.001
Cystatin C, mg/L	2.05 (0.84; 2.70)	0.86 (0.69; 1.13)	0.002
BTP, mg/L	0.897 (0.291; 1.470)	0.459 (0.254; 0.631)	0.019
Serum NGAL, ng/mL	313 (275; 489)	142 (101; 232)	<0.001
Urine NGAL, ng/mL	837 (551; 1252)	38 (20; 68)	0.002
Uromodulin, ng/mL	105 (90; 152)	146 (95; 205)	0.2
D-dimer, μg/mL	6.32 (3.82; 15.69)	2.90 (1.33; 4.20)	0.003
Angiopoietin 2, ng/mL	14.48 (5.77; 23.69)	3.25 (2.37; 5.33)	<0.001
sFlt-1, pg/mL	215 (192; 250)	140 (114; 173)	<0.001

AKI, acute kidney injury; AP, acute pancreatitis; BISAP, bedside index of severity in acute pancreatitis; BMI, body mass index; BTP, beta-trace protein; CRP, C-reactive protein; MAP, mild acute pancreatitis; MMSS, modified Marshall scoring system; MSAP, moderately severe acute pancreatitis; n, number of patients; NGAL, neutrophil gelatinase-associated lipocalin; SAP, severe acute pancreatitis; SIRS, systemic inflammatory response syndrome; sFlt-1, soluble fms-like tyrosine kinase-1.

As shown in Figure 1A–C, serum BTP concentrations on day 1 and day 3 of the study were also significantly higher in patients who developed AKI ($n = 12$ on day 1, $n = 13$ on day 2, and $n = 8$ on day 3) as compared to those who did not. Moreover, BTP concentrations on days 1 to 3 differed significantly between subjects who developed renal failure (diagnosed according to MMSS; $n = 6$ on day 1, $n = 6$ on day 2, and $n = 5$ on day 3) and those who did not (Figure 1D–F). In contrast, serum BTP did not differ significantly between patients with mild, moderately severe and severe AP (Figure 2). Only day 3

BTP concentrations significantly correlated with BISAP score (R = 0.60; $p < 0.001$) and the duration of hospital stay (R = 0.34; $p = 0.030$). No statistically significant changes in BTP concentrations over the three days of the study were observed.

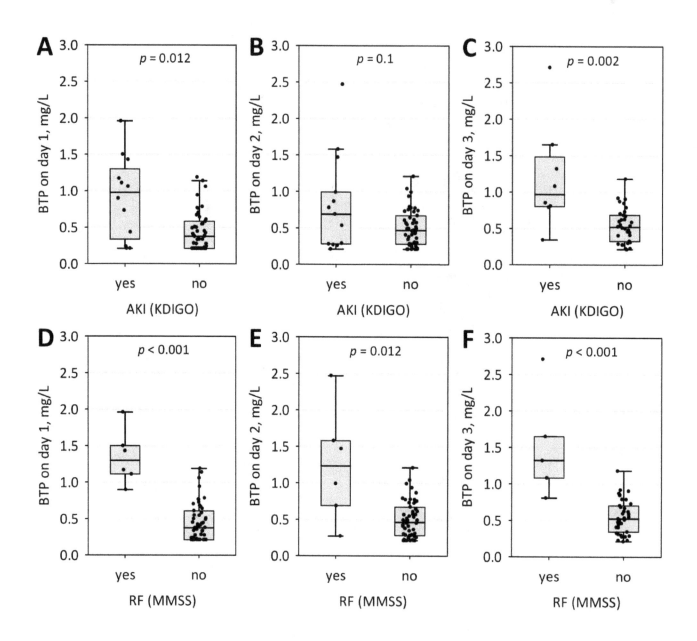

Figure 1. Serum beta-trace protein (BTP) concentrations on day 1 (**A,D**), 2 (**B,E**) and 3 (**C,F**) of hospital stay among patients with AP complicated with acute kidney injury (AKI) diagnosed according to Kidney Disease Improving Global Outcomes (KDIGO) guidelines (**A–C**) or renal failure (RF) diagnosed according to modified Marshall scoring system (MMSS) (**D–F**) versus patients without these complications. Data are shown as raw data (points), median (central line), interquartile range (box), and non-outlier range (whiskers).

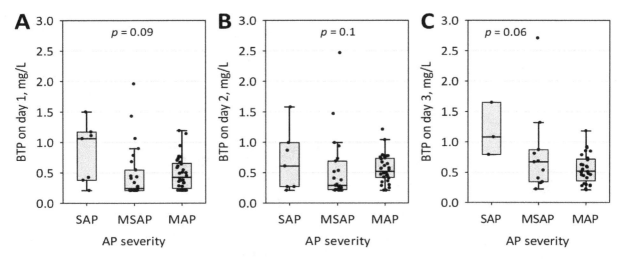

Figure 2. Serum BTP concentrations on day 1 (**A**), 2 (**B**) and 3 (**C**) of hospital stay among patients with acute pancreatitis (AP) of various severity (SAP, severe; MSAP, moderately severe; and MAP, mild) diagnosed according to the modified 2012 Atlanta classification. Data are shown as raw data (points), median (central line), interquartile range (box), and non-outlier range (whiskers).

Strong positive correlations were observed over the studied period between serum BTP and other studied laboratory markers increasing in result of impaired renal filtration, i.e., serum creatinine, cystatin C and urea (Table 2). Consequently, negative correlations were observed between serum BTP and serum uromodulin. In contrast, there was no significant correlation between BTP and the marker of tubular injury, i.e., urine NGAL, and the positive correlations between BTP and serum NGAL were not consistent throughout the study (Table 2). BTP measured on day 1 following admission as well as the maximum concentrations recorded on the first two days of hospital stay were also positively correlated with the studied markers of endothelial dysfunction: angiopoietin 2 and sFlt-1 (Table 2). No correlations were observed between BTP and the markers of inflammation: C-reactive protein, white blood cell and neutrophil counts (Table 2).

Table 2. Simple correlations between serum BTP concentrations in the whole studied group of AP patients and other markers of kidney dysfunction, epithelial dysfunction and inflammation measured at the specified time-points.

Variable	Serum BTP Concentrations			
	Maximum of Day 1 and 2* ($n = 73$)	Day 1 ($n = 65$)	Day 2 ($n = 63$)	Day 3 ($n = 45$)
Urea	R = 0.52; $p < 0.001$	R = 0.50; $p < 0.001$	R = 0.41; $p < 0.001$	R = 0.73; $p < 0.001$
Creatinine	R = 0.56; $p < 0.001$	R = 0.63; $p < 0.001$	R = 0.52; $p < 0.001$	R = 0.71; $p < 0.001$
Cystatin C	R = 0.60; $p < 0.001$	R = 0.68; $p < 0.001$	R = 0.63; $p < 0.001$	R = 0.91; $p < 0.001$
Serum NGAL	R = 0.17; $p = 0.3$	R = 0.43; $p = 0.007$	R = 0.22; $p = 0.2$	R = 0.35; $p = 0.023$
Urine NGAL	R = 0.23; $p = 0.3$	R = 0.17; $p = 0.38$	R = 0.30; $p = 0.1$	R = 0.37; $p = 0.07$
Uromodulin	R = −0.42; $p = 0.004$	R = −0.43; $p = 0.007$	R = −0.44; $p = 0.003$	R = −0.33; $p = 0.037$
D-dimer	R = 0.05; $p = 0.7$	R = 0.31; $p = 0.012$	R = −0.07; $p = 0.6$	R = −0.04; $p = 0.8$
Angiopoietin-2	R = 0.26; $p = 0.045$	R = 0.37; $p = 0.007$	R = 0.11; $p = 0.4$	R = 0.22; $p = 0.2$
sFlt-1	R = 0.25; $p = 0.044$	R = 0.34; $p = 0.011$	R = −0.03; $p = 0.8$	no data
Leukocytes	R = 0.11; $p = 0.4$	R = 0.07; $p = 0.6$	R = −0.02; $p = 0.9$	R = 0.05; $p = 0.8$
Neutrophils	R = 0.10; $p = 0.4$	R = −0.01; $p = 0.9$	R = −0.03; $p = 0.8$	R = 0.09; $p = 0.6$
CRP	R = −0.10; $p = 0.4$	R = 0.15; $p = 0.2$	R = −0.19; $p = 0.1$	R = −0.08; $p = 0.6$

* Minimum of day 1 and day 2 concentrations in case of uromodulin.

Serum BTP was highly correlated with patients' age (R = 0.65 for maximum BTP recorded during first two days of hospital stay; R from 0.65 on day 1 to 0.77 on day 3; $p < 0.001$ for all correlations). In logistic regression, the association between BTP and AKI became statistically insignificant after adjustment for age and preexisting renal pathology ($p > 0.05$ throughout the study), and only BTP concentrations on day 3 of hospital stay were significantly associated with AKI after adjustment for preexisting renal disease only (Table 3). This contrasts with cystatin C that proved a significant predictor of AKI after adjustment for renal comorbidity (Table 3).

Table 3. Odds ratios for the diagnosis of AKI according to KDIGO obtained in logistic regression adjusted for prediagnosed kidney comorbidity.

	BTP, per 1 mg/L		Cystatin C, per 1 mg/L	
	OR (95% CI)	p	OR (95% CI)	p
Maximum of day 1 and 2	1.29 (0.72–2.33)	0.4	2.10 (30.1–698)	0.002
Day 1	1.31 (0.72–2.37)	0.4	14.0 (2.34–83.6)	0.003
Day 2	1.15 (0.53–2.50)	0.7	5.12 (1.24–21.2)	0.021
Day 3	125 (2.7–5796)	0.001	33.2 (2.45–451)	0.006

OR, odds ratio; CI, confidence interval.

In ROC curve analysis, maximum BTP concentrations observed during the first two days of the study as well as BTP concentrations on day 1 and day 3 showed moderate diagnostic accuracy for AKI (AUC from 0.621 to 0.803; Figure 3A). For comparison, we presented the ROC curves for serum cystatin C, serum NGAL and urine NGAL in the diagnosis of AKI (Figure 3B–D). The values of AUC for these markers did not differ significantly from the AUCs of BTP at all the studied time-points ($p > 0.05$ for all comparisons). However, it should be noted that the diagnostic accuracy of serum BTP and cystatin C was very similar while the estimations of AUC for both serum and urine NGAL were consistently higher throughout the study.

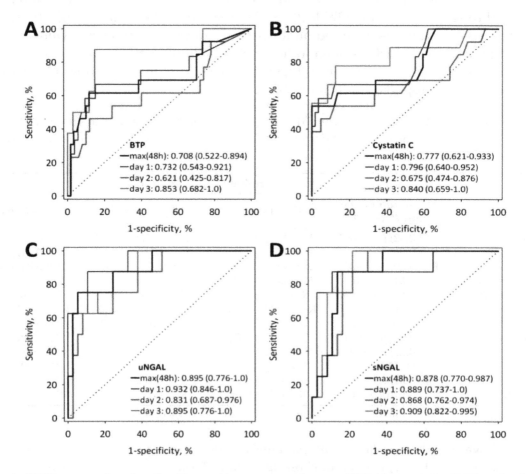

Figure 3. ROC curves showing the diagnostic accuracy of serum BTP (**A**), cystatin C (**B**), urine NGAL

(**C**) and serum NGAL (**D**) measured at the specified time-points for the diagnosis of AKI. The values of AUC with 95% CI are shown on the graphs; max(48h), maximum value observed during the first two days (or 48 h) of hospital stay.

4. Discussion

Most laboratory markers proposed for the fast prognosis or diagnosis of AKI have not been studied in AP [19]. Previously, serum cystatin C has been shown to predict AKI in AP with high diagnostic accuracy [33]. Our study shows for the first time that serum BTP, a marker of glomerular filtration, is increased early in patients with AP who develop AKI, in parallel to serum cystatin C. BTP concentrations were highly correlated with serum creatinine and cystatin C. The diagnostic accuracy of BTP for early diagnosis of AKI in the early phase of AP was comparable to that of serum cystatin C. However, it seemed lower than the diagnostic accuracy of serum and urine NGAL. Moreover, in logistic regression analysis, the association between increased BTP and AKI was dependent on previous renal disease, in contrast to what was found for serum cystatin C.

Although creatinine currently remains the main clinically used marker of glomerular filtration, and the only one acknowledged in clinical guidelines for the diagnosis of AKI [30], it is also commonly regarded the late marker of AKI. Significant increase in serum creatinine is not observed in mild renal impairment, in contrast to serum BTP and cystatin C [1,34]. Moreover, there are many non-renal factors associated with altered production of creatinine that affect serum creatinine concentrations, such as muscle mass, age, sex, race, or liver dysfunction [35,36]. Serum cystatin C and BTP seem less affected by non-renal determinants. However, the evidence is mostly based on the studies including patients with chronic kidney disease [35,36]. Of note, serum creatinine production is diminished in liver dysfunction, while BTP concentrations are not affected [37]. This is of importance, as hepatic dysfunction often accompanies SAP. As a marker of glomerular filtration, serum BTP may have an advantage over serum cystatin C in patients treated with glucocorticoids, including those after renal transplantation [1]. On the other hand, recent study that compared serum BTP with serum cystatin C in elderly patients showed better correlation of cystatin C based estimated glomerular filtration rate with measured filtration rate [38].

In AKI, there are very limited data on diagnostic accuracy of BTP. Recently, Saydam et al. [39] evaluated serum BTP, cystatin C and NGAL in comparison with serum creatinine in 57 patients after cardiopulmonary bypass of whom 24 developed AKI. Higher preoperative cystatin C and BTP were associated with AKI, reflecting higher risk for AKI in patients with chronic kidney impairment. Postoperative increase in cystatin C was better predictive marker of AKI than BTP. In our study, serum BTP and cystatin C measured on first three days of AP had similar diagnostic accuracy for AKI (similar areas under the ROC curves). However, the association between BTP and the development of AKI was more affected by kidney disease preceding AP and became insignificant after adjustment for age. Older age is associated with a decrease in glomerular filtration rate, and this decrease results in chronically increased serum concentrations of BTP [38]. Kidney disease preceding the development of AP in our patients could also be a cause of chronically decreased glomerular filtration and increased BTP. We may hypothesize that the increase in BTP associated with the development of AKI is less dynamic in such patients as compared with the increase in cystatin C. However, this interpretation needs to be tested in larger study as the numbers of patients with AKI in our study is low, adversely affecting the power of multiple statistical models, and the number of patients with prediagnosed renal disease in our study is very low.

Serum cystatin C has been evaluated as a marker of AKI in various settings, including sepsis [40,41] and AP [33]. Recent study in over 200 patients with AP reported excellent diagnostic accuracy for AKI (area under ROC curve of 0.948) [33]. In our study, the diagnostic accuracy of cystatin C was lower. However, both SAP and AKI were more prevalent in our study group (9.6% and 18% versus 5% and 7.6%, respectively). Our study included patients admitted within 24 h from the onset of AP symptoms; this time-period was not defined in the study of Chai et al. [33] and might be longer. Moreover, Chai et al. [33]

excluded patients with prediagnosed renal disease, whereas in our group four patients had kidney disease diagnosed before the onset of AP.

Serum and urine NGAL are known markers of AKI [23]. In AP, good diagnostic accuracy for AKI of both serum and urine NGAL was previously reported by Siddappa et al. [42] (AUCs of 0.8 to 0.9), comparable with our present results. To our knowledge, there is no published evidence comparing the accuracy of NGAL and BTP in the diagnosis of AKI. Our findings suggest that in AP, the decrease in glomerular filtration reflected by increased BTP is not strictly accompanied by simultaneous increase in NGAL (we did not observe consistent correlations between the markers over the study period). Moreover, the diagnostic accuracy of both serum and urine NGAL for AKI was better than observed for BTP, although it must be remembered that NGAL measurements were available only in patients from one study center.

Cystatin C and BTP are both the low-molecular-weight proteins, easily filtered in renal glomeruli. Increased serum concentrations of both proteins reflect decreased renal function (decreased glomerular filtration rate). Both proteins may be easily measured in serum with automated laboratory methods. However, an international standard is only available for cystatin C, allowing the standardization of the assays [43]. In contrast, the measurements of serum NGAL have not been automated. Moreover, neutrophils are important source of NGAL in serum of patients with acute inflammation, which may decrease the diagnostic accuracy of this marker for AKI as has been shown in septic patients [44]. Urinary NGAL may be measured with an automated laboratory method. However, the sample—urine—may not be available in some patients with AKI. Increased NGAL reflects the injury to proximal and distal renal tubules, irrespective of glomerular function. A combination of a functional marker, i.e., serum BTP or cystatin C with the marker of tubular injury, i.e., serum or preferably urine NGAL might be proposed for the diagnosis of AKI in AP, to be verified in a larger, prospective study.

AP is associated an acute inflammation, which influences the concentrations of many serum proteins. We have not found significant correlations between serum BTP and the inflammatory markers (C-reactive protein, white blood cell and neutrophil count), even though higher CRP was observed in patients with AKI. BTP concentrations did not differ significantly between patients with severe, moderately severe and mild AP. The finding is in line with the evidence regarding patients with chronic kidney disease [25]. However, BTP has been assigned proinflammatory role in allergies and ulcerative colitis and immunomodulatory role has been suggested in bacterial infections [4]. Thus, larger studies are needed to exclude the weak association between serum BTP and acute systemic inflammation.

On day 1 following patients' admission, we have found significant positive correlations between serum BTP and the markers of endothelial dysfunction or injury, i.e., serum angiopoietin-2 and sFlt-1. Both these endothelial markers have been shown to predict the severity of AP [26,31,45,46] and have increased in patients with kidney injury complicating AP [26] or have correlated with impaired renal function [46]. Angiopoietin-2 has also been shown to predict AKI in other patient populations, e.g., after myocardial infarction [47], after cardiopulmonary bypass [48], with acute respiratory distress syndrome [49], or among patients of intensive care unit [50]. Endothelial injury and vascular leak syndrome are important pathophysiological factors of organ (including kidney) injury and failure in SAP [51]. BTP synthesis is induced in endothelial cells under shear stress. Through prostaglandin D2 synthesis, BTP exerts vasodilating effects [52]. However, the role of BTP in endothelial dysfunction associated with systemic inflammation or sepsis remains to be elucidated.

Our study has several limitations. It was a post-hoc analysis of a small number of patients recruited in two centers. Although the percentage of patients with AKI was within the range previously reported in AP [19], the number of patients with AKI was low, which must be acknowledged as the main limitation of the study. Larger prospective studies are needed to confirm our preliminary results. We measured BTP in available samples stored frozen in −80 °C for a period of one–two years. However,

BTP concentrations have been shown to remain stable over long periods in frozen serum samples [53].

In conclusion, our study showed for the first time that serum BTP increases in the early phase of AP in patients who develop AKI in parallel with serum cystatin C and creatinine. Increased BTP is an early predictor of AKI complicating AP.However, its diagnostic accuracy does not seem better as compared to serum cystatin C or serum and urine NGAL. Serum BTP concentrations in the early phase of AP are not affected by the severity of inflammation but correlates with endothelial dysfunction.

Author Contributions: Conceptualization: J.W., P.D, P.C. and B.K-C.; methodology: B.K.-C., B.M. and A.Z.-A.; validation: J.W., P.D., P.C. and B.K.-C.; formal analysis: P.D., B.K.-C. and P.C., investigation: J.W., B.K.-C., B.M. and A.Z.-A., resources: M.S. and W.K., data curation: M.S., W.K. and B.K.-C., writing – original draft preparation: J.W., P.D. and B.K.-C., writing – review and editing: P.D., J.W., B.K.-C., M.K. and P.C., supervision: B.K.-C. and P.D., project administration: B.K.-C. and P.C., funding acquisition: B.K.-C. and P.C. J.W. and P.D. have contributed equally to this work. All authors have read and agreed to the published version of the manuscript.

References

1.　Orenes-Piñero, E.; Manzano-Fernández, S.; López-Cuenca, Á.; Marín, F.; Valdés, M.; Januzzi, J.L. β-Trace protein: From GFR marker to cardiovascular risk predictor. *Clin. J. Am. Soc. Nephrol.* **2013**, *8*, 873–881. [CrossRef]

2.　Meco, C.; Oberascher, G.; Arrer, E.; Moser, G.; Albegger, K. β-trace protein test: New guidelines for the reliable diagnosis of cerebrospinal fluid fistula. *Otolaryngol.-Head Neck. Surg.* **2003**, *129*, 508–517. [CrossRef]

3.　Bachmann, G.; Petereit, H.; Djenabi, U.; Michel, O. Predictive Values of β-Trace Protein (Prostaglandin D Synthase) by Use of Laser-Nephelometry Assay for the Identification of Cerebrospinal Fluid. *Neurosurgery* **2002**, *50*, 571–577.

4.　Joo, M.; Sadikot, R.T. PGD Synthase and PGD 2 in Immune Response. *Mediators Inflamm.* **2012**, *2012*, 1–6. [CrossRef]

5.　Donadio, C.; Lucchesi, A.; Ardini, M.; Donadio, E.; Giordani, R. Serum levels of beta-trace protein and glomerular filtration rate–preliminary results. *J. Pharm. Biomed. Anal.* **2003**, *32*, 1099–1104. [CrossRef]

6.　Donadio, C. Serum and urinary markers of early impairment of GFR in chronic kidney disease patients: Diagnostic accuracy of urinary β-trace protein. *Am. J. Physiol. Renal Physiol.* **2010**, *299*, F1407–F1423. [CrossRef] [PubMed]

7.　Spanaus, K.S.; Kollerits, B.; Ritz, E.; Hersberger, M.; Kronenberg, F.; Von Eckardstein, A. Serum creatinine, cystatin C, and β-trace protein in diagnostic staging and predicting progression of primary nondiabetic chronic kidney disease. *Clin. Chem.* **2010**, *56*, 740–749. [CrossRef] [PubMed]

8.　Donadio, C.; Bozzoli, L. Urinary β-trace protein. A unique biomarker to screen early glomerular filtration rate impairment. *Medicine* **2016**, *95*, e5553. [CrossRef] [PubMed]

9.　Bacci, M.R.; Cavallari, M.R.; de Rozier-Alves, R.M.; Alves, B.D.C.A.; Fonseca, F.L.A. The impact of lipocalin-type-prostaglandin-D-synthase as a predictor of kidney disease in patients with type 2 diabetes. *Drug Des. Devel. Ther.* **2015**, *9*, 3179–3182. [PubMed]

10.　Manzano-Fernández, S.; López-Cuenca, Á.; Januzzi, J.L.; Parra-Pallares, S.; Mateo-Martínez, A.; Sánchez-Martínez, M.; Pérez-Berbel, P.; Orenes-Piñero, E.; Romero-Aniorte, A.I.; Avilés-Plaza, F.; et al. Usefulness of β-trace protein and cystatin C for the prediction of mortality in non ST segment elevation acute coronary syndromes. *Am. J. Cardiol.* **2012**, *110*, 1240–1248. [CrossRef] [PubMed]

11.　Manzano-Fernández, S.; Januzzi, J.L.; Boronat-Garcia, M.; Bonaque-González, J.C.; Truong, Q.A.; Pastor-Pérez, F.J.; Muñoz-Esparza, C.; Pastor, P.; Albaladejo-Otón, M.D.; Casas, T.; et al. β-trace protein and cystatin C as predictors of long-term outcomes in patients with acute heart failure. *J. Am. Coll. Cardiol.* **2011**, *57*, 849–858. [CrossRef] [PubMed]

12.　Peery, A.F.; Dellon, E.S.; Lund, J.; Crockett, S.D.; McGowan, C.E.; Bulsiewicz, W.J.; Gangarosa, L.M.; Thiny, M.T.; Stizenberg, K.; Morgan, D.R.; et al. Burden of gastrointestinal disease in the United States: 2012 update. *Gastroenterology* **2012**, *143*, 1179–1187. [CrossRef] [PubMed]

13.　Párniczky, A.; Kui, B.; Szentesi, A.; Balázs, A.; Szűcs, Á.; Mosztbacher, D.; Czimmer, J.; Sarlós, P.; Bajor, J.; Gódi, S.; et al. Prospective, multicentre, nationwide clinical data from 600 cases of acute pancreatitis. *PLoS ONE* **2016**, *11*, e0165309. [CrossRef] [PubMed]

14.　Lankisch, P.G.; Apte, M.; Banks, P.A. Acute pancreatitis. *Lancet* **2015**, *386*, 85–96. [CrossRef]

15. Susantitaphong, P.; Cruz, D.N.; Cerda, J.; Abulfaraj, M.; Alqahtani, F.; Koulouridis, I.; Jaber, B.L. Acute Kidney Injury Advisory Group of the American Society of Nephrology World incidence of AKI: A meta-analysis. *Clin. J. Am. Soc. Nephrol.* **2013**, *8*, 1482–1493. [CrossRef]

16. Hoste, E.A.J.; Bagshaw, S.M.; Bellomo, R.; Cely, C.M.; Colman, R.; Cruz, D.N.; Edipidis, K.; Forni, L.G.; Gomersall, C.D.; Govil, D.; et al. Epidemiology of acute kidney injury in critically ill patients: the multinational AKI-EPI study. *Intensive Care Med.* **2015**, *41*, 1411–1423. [CrossRef]

17. Druml, W.; Lenz, K.; Laggner, A.N. Our paper 20 years later: From acute renal failure to acute kidney injury—The metamorphosis of a syndrome. *Intensive Care Med.* **2015**, *41*, 1941–1949. [CrossRef]

18. Ostermann, M.; Liu, K. Pathophysiology of AKI. *Best Pract. Res. Clin. Anaesthesiol.* **2017**, *31*, 305–314. [CrossRef]

19. Wajda, J.; Dumnicka, P.; Maraj, M.; Ceranowicz, P.; Kuźniewski, M.; Kuśnierz-Cabala, B. Potential prognostic markers of acute kidney injury in the early phase of acute pancreatitis. *Int. J. Mol. Sci.* **2019**, *20*, 3714. [CrossRef]

20. Lin, H.-Y.; Lai, J.-I.; Lai, Y.-C.; Lin, P.-C.; Chang, S.-C.; Tang, G.-J. Acute renal failure in severe pancreatitis: A population-based study. *Ups. J. Med. Sci.* **2011**, *116*, 155–159. [CrossRef]

21. Nassar, T.I.; Qunibi, W.Y. AKI Associated with Acute Pancreatitis. *Clin. J. Am. Soc. Nephrol.* **2019**, *14*, 106–1115. [CrossRef] [PubMed]

22. Beker, B.M.; Corleto, M.G.; Fieiras, C.; Musso, C.G. Novel acute kidney injury biomarkers: Their characteristics, utility and concerns. *Int. Urol. Nephrol.* **2018**, *50*, 705–713. [CrossRef] [PubMed]

23. Schrezenmeier, E.V.; Barasch, J.; Budde, K.; Westhoff, T.; Schmidt-Ott, K.M. Biomarkers in acute kidney injury—Pathophysiological basis and clinical performance. *Acta Physiol.* **2017**, *219*, 554–572. [CrossRef] [PubMed]

24. Li, W.; Mase, M.; Inui, T.; Shimoda, M.; Isomura, K.; Oda, H.; Yamada, K.; Urade, Y. Pharmacokinetics of recombinant human lipocalin-type prostaglandin D synthase/β-trace in canine. *Neurosci. Res.* **2008**, *61*, 289–293. [CrossRef]

25. Chen, H.H. β-trace protein versus cystatin C: which is a better surrogate marker of renal function versus prognostic indicator in cardiovascular diseases? *J. Am. Coll. Cardiol.* **2011**, *57*, 859–860. [CrossRef] [PubMed]

26. Sporek, M.; Dumnicka, P.; Gala-Błądzińska, A.; Ceranowicz, P.; Warzecha, Z.; Dembiński, A.; Stępień, E.; Walocha, J.; Drożdż, R.; Kuźniewski, M.; et al. Angiopoietin-2 is an early indicator of acute pancreatic-renal syndrome in patients with acute pancreatitis. *Mediators Inflamm.* **2016**, *5780903*, 1–7. [CrossRef] [PubMed]

27. Kolber, W.; Kuśnierz-Cabala, B.; Dumnicka, P.; Maraj, M.; Mazur-Laskowska, M.; Pędziwiatr, M.; Ceranowicz, P. Serum Urokinase-Type Plasminogen Activator Receptor Does Not Outperform C-Reactive Protein and Procalcitonin as an Early Marker of Severity of Acute Pancreatitis. *J. Clin. Med.* **2018**, *7*, 305. [CrossRef]

28. Banks, P.A.; Bollen, T.L.; Dervenis, C.; Gooszen, H.G.; Johnson, C.D.; Sarr, M.G.; Tsiotos, G.G.; Vege, S.S. Classification of acute pancreatitis-2012: revision of the Atlanta classification and definitions by international consensus. *Gut* **2013**, *62*, 102–111. [CrossRef]

29. Wu, B.U.; Johannes, R.S.; Sun, X.; Tabak, Y.; Conwell, D.L.; Banks, P. The early prediction of mortality in acute pancreatitis: a large population-based study. *Gut* **2008**, *57*, 1698–1703. [CrossRef]

30. Kellum, J.A.; Lameire, N.; Aspelin, P.; Barsoum, R.S.; Burdmann, E.A.; Goldstein, S.L.; Herzog, C.A.; Joannidis, M.; Kribben, A.; Levey, A.S.; et al. KDIGO Clinical Practice Guideline for Acute Kidney Injury. *Kidney Int. Suppl.* **2012**, *2*, 1–138.

31. Dumnicka, P.; Kuśnierz-Cabala, B.; Sporek, M.; Mazur-Laskowska, M.; Gil, K.; Kuźniewski, M.; Ceranowicz, P.; Warzecha, Z.; Dembiński, A.; Bonior, J.; et al. Serum concentrations of angiopoietin-2 and soluble fms-like tyrosine kinase 1 (sFlt-1) are associated with coagulopathy among patients with acute pancreatitis. *Int. J. Mol. Sci.* **2017**, *18*, 735. [CrossRef] [PubMed]

32. Hanley, J.A.; Hajian-Tilaki, K.O. Sampling variability of nonparametric estimates of the areas under receiver operating characteristic curves: An update. *Acad. Radiol.* **1997**, *4*, 49–58. [CrossRef]

33. Chai, X.; Huang, H.-B.; Feng, G.; Cao, Y.-H.; Cheng, Q.-S.; Li, S.-H.; He, C.-Y.; Lu, W.-H.; Qin, M.-M. Baseline Serum Cystatin C Is a Potential Predictor for Acute Kidney Injury in Patients with Acute Pancreatitis. *Dis. Markers* **2018**, *2018*, 1–7. [CrossRef] [PubMed]

34. Basu, R.K.; Wong, H.R.; Krawczeski, C.D.; Wheeler, D.S.; Manning, P.B.; Chawla, L.S.; Devarajan, P.; Goldstein, S.L. Combining functional and tubular damage biomarkers improves diagnostic precision for acute kidney injury after cardiac surgery. *J. Am. Coll. Cardiol.* **2014**, *64*, 2753–2762. [CrossRef]

35. Juraschek, S.P.; Coresh, J.; Inker, L.A.; Levey, A.S.; Köttgen, A.; Foster, M.C.; Astor, B.C.; Eckfeldt, J.H.; Selvin, E. Comparison of serum concentrations of β-trace protein, β2-microglobulin, cystatin C, and creatinine in the US population. *Clin. J. Am. Soc. Nephrol.* **2013**, *8*, 584–592. [CrossRef]

36. Liu, X.; Foster, M.C.; Tighiouart, H.; Anderson, A.H.; Beck, G.J.; Contreras, G.; Coresh, J.; Eckfeldt, J.H.; Feldman, H.I.; Greene, T.; et al. Non-GFR Determinants of Low-Molecular-Weight Serum Protein Filtration Markers in CKD. *Am. J. Kidney Dis.* **2016**, *68*, 892–900. [CrossRef]

37. Chakraborty, D.; Akbari, A.; Knoll, G.A.; Flemming, J.A.; Lowe, C.; Akbari, S.; White, C.A. Serum BTP concentrations are not affected by hepatic dysfunction. *BMC Nephrol.* **2018**, *19*, 87. [CrossRef]

38. Werner, K.; Pihlsgård, M.; Elmståhl, S.; Legrand, H.; Nyman, U.; Christensson, A. Combining Cystatin C and Creatinine Yields a Reliable Glomerular Filtration Rate Estimation in Older Adults in Contrast to β-Trace Protein and β2-Microglobulin. *Nephron* **2017**, *137*, 29–37. [CrossRef]

39. Saydam, O.; Türkmen, E.; Portakal, O.; Arici, M.; Doğan, R.; Demircin, M.; Paşaoğlu, İ.; Yilmaz, M. Emerging biomarker for predicting acute kidney injury after cardiac surgery: Cystatin C. *Turkish J. Med. Sci.* **2018**, *48*, 1096–1103. [CrossRef]

40. Dai, X.; Zeng, Z.; Fu, C.; Zhang, S.; Cai, Y.; Chen, Z. Diagnostic value of neutrophil gelatinase-associated lipocalin, cystatin C, and soluble triggering receptor expressed on myeloid cells-1 in critically ill patients with sepsis-associated acute kidney injury. *Crit. Care* **2015**, *19*, 223. [CrossRef]

41. Leem, A.Y.; Park, M.S.; Park, B.H.; Jung, W.J.; Chung, K.S.; Kim, S.Y.; Kim, E.Y.; Jung, J.Y.; Kang, Y.A.; Kim, Y.S.; et al. Value of Serum Cystatin C Measurement in the Diagnosis of Sepsis-Induced Kidney Injury and Prediction of Renal Function Recovery. *Yonsei Med. J.* **2017**, *58*, 604. [CrossRef] [PubMed]

42. Siddappa, P.K.; Kochhar, R.; Sarotra, P.; Medhi, B.; Jha, V.; Gupta, V. Neutrophil gelatinase-associated lipocalin: An early biomarker for predicting acute kidney injury and severity in patients with acute pancreatitis. *JGH Open* **2018**, *3*, 105–110. [CrossRef] [PubMed]

43. Ebert, N.; Delanaye, P.; Shlipak, M.; Jakob, O.; Martus, P.; Bartel, J.; Gaedeke, J.; van der Giet, M.; Schuchardt, M.; Cavalier, E.; et al. Cystatin C standardization decreases assay variation and improves assessment of glomerular filtration rate. *Clin. Chim. Acta.* **2016**, *456*, 115–121. [CrossRef] [PubMed]

44. Aydoğdu, M.; Gürsel, G.; Sancak, B.; Yeni, S.; Sari, G.; Taşyürek, S.; Türk, M.; Yüksel, S.; Senes, M.; Özis, T.N. The use of plasma and urine neutrophil gelatinase associated lipocalin (NGAL) and Cystatin C in early diagnosis of septic acute kidney injury in critically ill patients. *Dis. Markers* **2013**, *34*, 237–246. [CrossRef]

45. Buddingh, K.T.; Koudstaal, L.G.; van Santvoort, H.C.; Besselink, M.G.; Timmer, R.; Rosman, C.; van Goor, H.; Nijmeijer, R.M.; Gooszen, H.; Leuvenink, H.G.D.; et al. Early angiopoietin-2 levels after onset predict the advent of severe pancreatitis, multiple organ failure, and infectious complications in patients with acute pancreatitis. *J. Am. Coll. Surg.* **2014**, *218*, 26–32. [CrossRef]

46. Dumnicka, P.; Sporek, M.; Mazur-Laskowska, M.; Ceranowicz, P.; Kuźniewski, M.; Drożdż, R.; Ambroży, T.; Olszanecki, R.; Kuśnierz-Cabala, B. Serum soluble fms-Like tyrosine kinase 1 (sFlt-1) predicts the severity of acute pancreatitis. *Int. J. Mol. Sci.* **2016**, *17*, 2038. [CrossRef]

47. Liu, K.L.; Lee, K.T.; Chang, C.H.; Chen, Y.C.; Lin, S.M.; Chu, P.H. Elevated plasma thrombomodulin and angiopoietin-2 predict the development of acute kidney injury in patients with acute myocardial infarction. *Crit. Care* **2014**, *18*, R100. [CrossRef]

48. Jongman, R.M.; Van Klarenbosch, J.; Molema, G.; Zijlstra, J.G.; De Vries, A.J.; Van Meurs, M.; Long, D. Angiopoietin/Tie2 dysbalance is associated with acute kidney injury after cardiac surgery assisted by cardiopulmonary bypass. *PLoS ONE* **2015**, *10*, e0136205. [CrossRef]

49. Araújo, C.B.; de Oliveira Neves, F.M.; de Freitas, D.F.; Arruda, B.F.T.; de Macêdo Filho, L.J.M.; Salles, V.B.; Meneses, G.C.; Martins, A.M.C.; Libório, A.B. Angiopoietin-2 as a predictor of acute kidney injury in critically ill patients and association with ARDS. *Respirology* **2019**, *24*, 345–351. [CrossRef]

50. Robinson-Cohen, C.; Katz, R.; Price, B.L.; Harju-Baker, S.; Mikacenic, C.; Himmelfarb, J.; Liles, W.C.; Wurfel, M.M. Association of markers of endothelial dysregulation Ang1 and Ang2 with acute kidney injury in critically ill patients. *Crit. Care* **2016**, *20*, 1–8. [CrossRef]

51. Dumnicka, P.; Maduzia, D.; Ceranowicz, P.; Olszanecki, R.; Drożdż, R.; Kuśnierz-Cabala, B. The interplay between inflammation, coagulation and endothelial injury in the early phase of acute pancreatitis: Clinical implications. *Int. J. Mol. Sci.* **2017**, *18*, 354. [CrossRef] [PubMed]

52. Song, W.L.; Ricciotti, E.; Liang, X.; Grosser, T.; Grant, G.R.; FitzGerald, G.A. Lipocalin-like prostaglandin D synthase but not hemopoietic prostaglandin D synthase deletion causes hypertension and accelerates thrombogenesis in mice. *J. Pharmacol. Exp. Ther.* **2018**, *367*, 425–432. [CrossRef] [PubMed]

53. Juraschek, S.P.; Coresh, J.; Inker, L.A.; Rynders, G.P.; Eckfeldt, J.H.; Selvin, E. The effects of freeze–thaw on β-trace protein and β2-microglobulin assays after long-term sample storage. *Clin. Biochem.* **2012**, *45*, 694–696. [CrossRef] [PubMed]

5

Does the Implementation of a Quality Improvement Care Bundle Reduce the Incidence of Acute Kidney Injury in Patients Undergoing Emergency Laparotomy?

James F. Doyle [1,2], Alexander Sarnowski [1], Farzad Saadat [1], Theophilus L. Samuels [3], Sam Huddart [1], Nial Quiney [1], Matthew C. Dickinson [1], Bruce McCormick [4], Robert deBrunner [4], Jeremy Preece [4], Michael Swart [5], Carol J. Peden [6], Sarah Richards [7] and Lui G. Forni [1,8,*]

[1]   Department of Intensive Care Medicine and Surrey Peri-Operative Anaesthesia and Critical Care Collaborative Research Group (SPACER), Royal Surrey County Hospital NHS Foundation Trust, Guildford, Surrey GU2 7XX, UK

[2]   Department of Intensive Care Medicine, Royal Brompton & Harefield NHS Foundation Trust, London SW3 6NP, UK

[3]   Department of Anaesthesia and Intensive Care Medicine, Surrey & Sussex Healthcare NHS Trust, Redhill RH1 5RH, UK

[4]   Department of Anaesthesia, Royal Devon & Exeter NHS Foundation Trust, Exeter EX2 5DW, UK

[5]   Department of Anaesthesia, Torbay & South Devon NHS Foundation Trust, Torquay TQ2 7AA, UK

[6]   Department of Anaesthesia, Royal United Hospitals Bath NHS Foundation Trust, Avon BA1 3NG, UK

[7]   Department of Surgery, Royal United Hospitals Bath NHS Foundation Trust, Avon BA1 3NG, UK

[8]   Department of Clinical & Experimental Medicine, Faculty of Health and Medical Sciences, University of Surrey, Guildford Guildford, GU2 7YS, UK

*   Correspondence: luiforni@nhs.net

Abstract: Purpose: Previous work has demonstrated a survival improvement following the introduction of an enhanced recovery protocol in patients undergoing emergency laparotomy (the emergency laparotomy pathway quality improvement care (ELPQuiC) bundle). Implementation of this bundle increased the use of intra-operative goal directed fluid therapy and ICU admission, both evidence-based strategies recommended to improve kidney outcomes. The aim of this study was to determine if the observed mortality benefit could be explained by a difference in the incidence of AKI pre- and post-implementation of the protocol. Method: The primary outcome was the incidence of AKI in the pre- and post-ELPQuiC bundle patient population in four acute trusts in the United Kingdom. Secondary outcomes included the KDIGO stage specific incidence of AKI. Serum creatinine values were obtained retrospectively at baseline, in the post-operative period and the maximum recorded creatinine between day 1 and day 30 were obtained. Results: A total of 303 patients pre-ELPQuiC bundle and 426 patients post-ELPQuiC bundle implementation were identified across the four centres. The overall AKI incidence was 18.4% in the pre-bundle group versus 19.8% in the post bundle group $p = 0.653$. No significant differences were observed between the groups. Conclusions: Despite this multi-centre cohort study demonstrating an overall survival benefit, implementation of the quality improvement care bundle did not affect the incidence of AKI.

Keywords: post-operative complications; acute kidney injury; enhanced recovery; goal directed therapy; emergency surgery; laparotomy

1. Introduction

Enhanced recovery pathways are now integral in many surgical pathways in order to optimize patient care, with the aim of reducing both post-operative morbidity and mortality [1]. The application of standardized pathways has been shown to reduce both post-operative complications and length of stay in elective surgery [2]. The adoption of care bundles in order to improve outcomes has been applied to both scheduled non-emergent surgery and also to emergency surgery. Recently published data reported a significant case mix-adjusted risk of death reduction from 15.6% to 9.6% at 30 days following the implementation of the emergency laparotomy pathway quality improvement care (ELPQuiC) bundle [3]. This pathway is comprised of the following steps:

1. All emergency surgical admissions risk assessed using the M(EWS) score [4]. Those with M(EWS) ≥4 reviewed by critical care outreach team.
2. Broad spectrum antibiotics given to all patients with suspicion of peritoneal soiling or with sepsis.
3. Once the decision is made for a laparotomy then next available theatre slot is used (or within 6 h) with senior clinical input (consultant anaesthetist and surgeon).
4. Resuscitation commenced using goal-directed techniques and continued for a minimum of six hours post-operatively.
5. All patients admitted to critical care when possible after surgery or held in a post anaesthetic care unit for at least six hours.

The need for such an integrated approach was highlighted in the UK when the Emergency Laparotomy Network group published data on 1800 patients showing a 30 day mortality of 14.9%, which rose to 24.4% in patients aged 80 and over [5]. This high mortality was also demonstrated in other countries with differing healthcare systems [6,7]. Following the evidence of such high mortality, standards of care were developed in the UK which recommended defined pathways with evidence-based interventions for all high risk and emergency surgical patients [8]. The use of a care-bundle concept is not new in critical care with several successful examples in current practice, such as the Surviving Sepsis Campaign with substantial morbidity and mortality improvements observed through the global implementation of this care bundle [9].

The observed mortality and morbidity in high risk groups of patients admitted to intensive care, including patients undergoing emergency surgery, remains significant with acute kidney injury (AKI) being a major factor complicating critical illness. AKI is associated with a mortality rate of up to 60% [10]. The relevance of AKI in emergency surgery is reflected in the results from the AKI EPI study where AKI complicated 51% of elective surgical patients admitted to ICU, and increased further to 56% in those undergoing emergency surgery [11]. This is further compounded in elderly patients with higher rates of AKI and worse mortality [12]. Furthermore, the long term sequelae after an episode of AKI are substantial, with a single episode of AKI independently associated with an increase in 10-year mortality [13]. Currently available treatment strategies have the potential to improve patient outcome and provide considerable health savings if implemented early [14]. The implementation of the ELPQuiC bundle was associated with significant increase in the use of goal directed fluid therapy and admission to ICU across the participating sites. These interventions form part of the KDIGO (Kidney Disease Improving Global Outcomes) clinical practice guidelines for the management of AKI, which recommend maintenance of perfusion pressure, functional haemodynamic monitoring and ICU admission [15]. It is unclear whether the adoption of such a goal directed approach in high risk patients may result in a reduction in AKI or indeed whether the development of AKI in this group is specifically associated with worse outcomes [16]. Given the observed risk-adjusted mortality improvement seen in the ELPQuiC study, we examined the data to see if this effect could be explained by a reduction in AKI translating into a survival benefit.

2. Methods

Development and components of the care bundle are described elsewhere [3,17]. The ELPQUiC study was conducted in 4 acute hospital trusts in the United Kingdom, with an intervention period from December 2012 to July 2013 after a baseline monitoring period. A multi-centre cohort subgroup analysis was performed with data gathered from the original ELPQuiC study. Colleagues in the ELPQuiC collaborator group accessed the relevant components of their ELPQuiC raw data. Where needed, additional biochemical data was obtained from the hospital's electronic pathology system. All data was reviewed by a second investigator.

AKI was defined as described by the KDIGO serum creatinine thresholds only. Urine output thresholds were not used, as data for this was not complete. We defined the reference or baseline creatinine as the lowest preoperative serum creatinine from the 12 months prior to admission. Serum creatinine values at baseline, immediately post-operatively (within the first 24 h but usually within hours of surgery completion), on day 30 and the maximum recorded creatinine between day 1 and day 30 were taken. P-POSSUM (Physiological and Operative Severity Score for the enumeration of Mortality and morbidity) and 30-day mortality data were also collected [18]. CKD stage was identified via the MDRD (Modification of Diet in Renal Disease study) equation with age, gender and baseline creatinine [19].

The primary outcome was the incidence of AKI in the pre- and post-ELPQuiC bundle patient population. Secondary outcomes included the KDIGO stage specific incidence of AKI.

As this project was an assessment of current practice and implementation of best-practice guidelines, it was confirmed by the National Research Ethics service that formal ethical approval was not required [3].

Statistical Analysis

For discrete data, we used Pearson's chi-squared test, Fisher's exact test, Wilcoxon rank sum test and the Mantel-Haenszel odds ratio (stratifying for centre), along with the φ-coefficient or Goodman-Kruskal γ statistic where appropriate. In addition, we used four-fold plots to provide a visual representation of the odds ratios, which align the vertical and horizontal quadrants with an odds ratio equal to 1. This also permits the use of confidence rings that provide a visual indication for the test of no association; they will only overlap if and only if the observed counts are consistent with the null hypothesis. Furthermore, the width of the confidence rings provides a visual guide to the precision of the data. All analyses were carried using the open source statistical package R (Foundation for Statistical Computing, Vienna, Austria) [20], along with ggplot2 [21], Forest plot [22] and vcd packages [23].

3. Results

Table 1 shows the baseline demographics and outcomes obtained from the four centres. A total of 292 patients pre-ELPQuiC bundle and 424 patients post-ELPQuiC were identified across the four centres with no significant differences observed between the groups. Ten patients from the initial ELPQuiC study were excluded due to incomplete data on renal function. There was no significant difference in P-POSSUM scores pre- or post-ELPQuiC implementation: the pre-ELPQuiC median was 9.0% (IQR 2.9–27.0%) versus the post-ELPQuiC median of 8.6% (IQR 3.5–31.4%) (Wilcoxon rank sum test $p = 0.5842$; Figure 1). However, although the baseline CKD rates in the pooled post-ELPQuiC group were significantly higher than in the pre-ELPQuiC group, $p = 0.01961$, the Goodman and Kruskal γ statistic of 0.036 suggests this is a very weak association. Moreover, this is for all CKD, if one considers only CKD stages 3 to 5 (the highest risk of AKI) then there is no difference ($p = 0.19$).

Table 1. Demographics and outcomes of patients before and after implementation of the emergency laparotomy pathway quality improvement care bundle.

	Site 1		Site 2		Site 3		Site 4		All Patients	
	Before ELPQuiC (n = 51)	After ELPQuiC (n = 109)	Before ELPQuiC (n = 144)	After ELPQuiC (n = 144)	Before ELPQuiC (n = 44)	After ELPQuiC (n = 97)	Before ELPQuiC (n = 60)	After ELPQuiC (n = 77)	Before ELPQuiC (n = 299)	After ELPQuiC (n = 427)
Age (years) *	66.6 (16.6)	65.3 (17.7)	65.1 (16.6)	63.7 (17.5)	65.7 (13.9)	69.3 (14.0)	66.2 (15.0)	66.0 (15.5)	65.6 (15.8)	65.8 (16.5)
Sex										
F	38 (75)	56 (51.4)	73 (50.7)	79 (54.9)	19 (43)	49 (51)	31 (52)	41 (53)	161 (53.8)	225 (52.7)
M	13 (25)	53 (48.6)	71 (49.3)	65 (45.1)	25 (57)	48 (49)	29 (48)	36 (47)	138 (46.2)	202 (47.3)
Outcomes at 30 days										
alive	42 (82)	96 (88.1)	123 (85.4)	126 (87.5)	39 (89)	89 (92)	53 (88)	71 (92)	257 (86.0)	382 (89.5)
dead	9 (18)	13 (11.9)	21 (14.6)	18 (12.5)	5 (11)	8 (8)	7 (12)	6 (8)	42 (14.0)	45 (10.5)
Died in hospital										
no	41 (80)	96 (88.1)	122 (84.7)	125 (86.8)	37 (84)	89 (92)	52 (87)	70 (91)	252 (84.3)	380 (89.0)
yes	10 (20)	13 (11.9)	22 (15.3)	19 (13.2)	7 (16)	8 (8)	8 (13)	7 (9)	47 (15.7)	47 (11.0)
ASA fitness grade										
I	5 (10)	14 (12.8)	12 (8.3)	16 (11.1)	4 (9)	8 (8)	6 (10)	7 (9)	27 (9.0)	45 (10.5)
II	10 (20)	36 (33.0)	48 (33.3)	52 (36.1)	9 (21)	32 (33)	28 (47)	27 (35)	95 (31.8)	147 (34.4)
III	19 (37)	40 (36.7)	46 (31.9)	44 (30.6)	18 (41)	40 (41)	20 (33)	32 (42)	103 (34.5)	156 (36.5)
IV	16 (31)	18 (16.5)	31 (21.5)	26 (18.1)	12 (27)	12 (12)	5 (8)	10 (13)	64 (21.4)	66 (15.5)
V	1 (2)	1 (0.9)	7 (4.9)	6 (4.2)	1 (2)	5 (5)	1 (2)	1 (1)	10 (3.3)	13 (3.0)
Length of hospital stay (days) †	11 (7–24)	11 (7–21)	12 (7–23)	10 (6–18)	12 (8–21)	12 (8–19)	10 (7–21)	13 (6–32)	11 (7–23)	11 (6–21)
P-POSSUM risk score *	0.226 (0.282)	0.251 (0.298)	0.193 (0.234)	0.267 (0.307)	0.200 (0.207)	0.179 (0.241)	0.179 (0.237)	0.159 (0.212)	0.197 (0.239)	0.223 (0.278)
p ‡	0.730		0.140		0.764		0.755		0.395	

Values in parentheses are percentages unless indicated otherwise; * values are mean (s.d.) and † median (i.q.r.) for survivors. ELPQuiC, emergency laparotomy pathway quality improvement care; ASA, American Society of Anesthesiologists; P-POSSUM, Portsmouth modification of Physiological and Operative Severity Score for the enumeration of Mortality and morbidity; ‡, test for proportions.

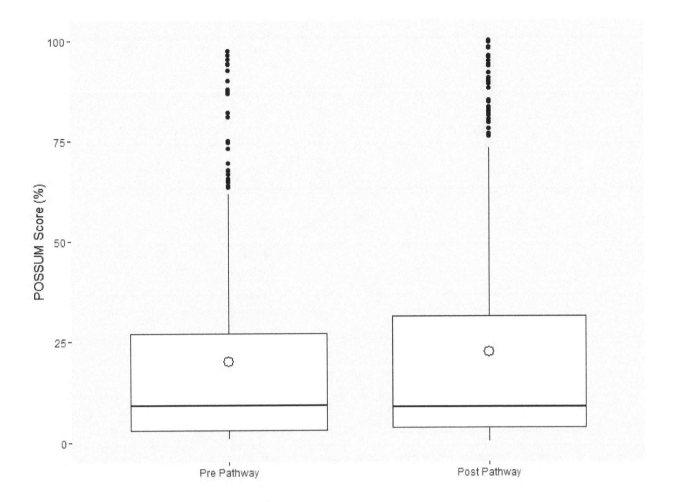

Figure 1. Cumulative P-POSSUM scores pre- and post-ELPQuiC implementation—circle represents the mean value.

3.1. Day 1 AKI

For our primary outcome; incidence of AKI between pre- and post-ELPQuiC implementation on day 1 post-op, the Mantel-Haenszel odds ratio (95% CI) for the four centres was 0.93 (0.72, 1.61). Using four-fold plots, crude numbers for day 1 incidence of AKI for each centre demonstrate that the odds ratios do not significantly differ from 1, but that the precision of the data is low (Figures and 2). Additionally, the cumulative rates of AKI for day 1 post-surgery were 18.4% versus 19.8% (pre- and post-pathway, respectively), with the data for each centre and combined data for all 4 centres showing no statistical significance (Centre 1; $p = 0.460$, Centre 2; $p = 0.346$, Centre 3; $p = 0.319$, Centre 4; $p = 0.817$, pooled $p = 0.686$).

There was no significant association between the incidence of KDIGO defined AKI and the use of the pathway on the first post-operative day for each individual centre or when the data was merged.

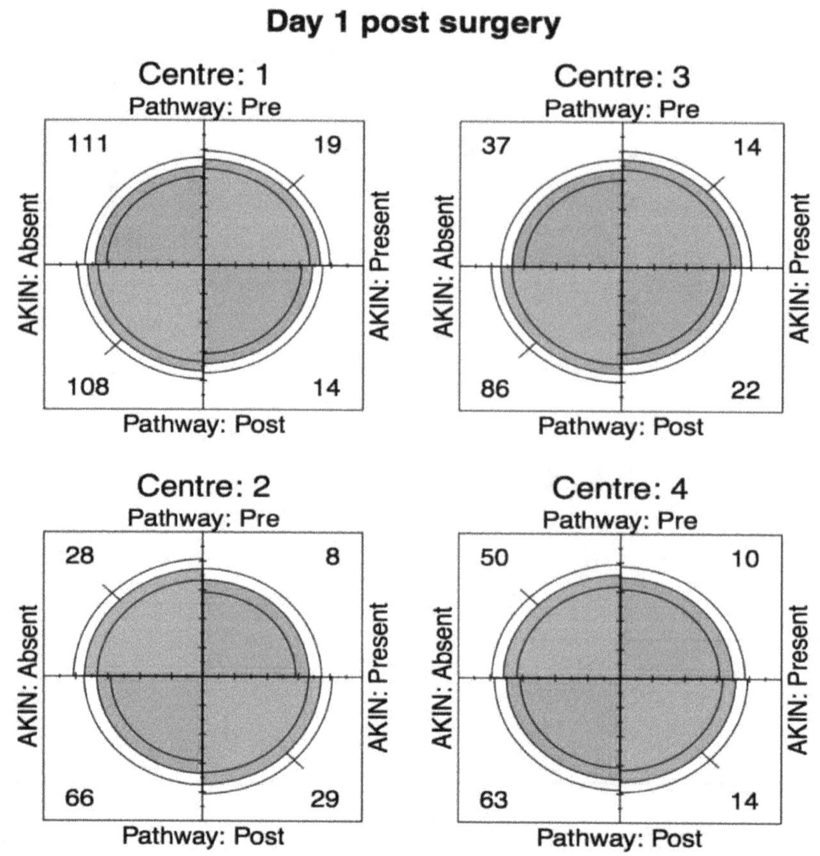

Day 1 post surgery

Figure 2. Four-fold Plot. Incidence of AKI day 1 post-op.

3.2. Maximum AKI Day 1–30

Using the maximum creatinine level and associated AKI incidence between days 1 and 30 post-surgery, the Mantel-Haenszel odds ratio (95% CI) for the 4 centres was 0.87 (0.61, 1.24) (Figure 3). There was no significant association between the incidence of AKI and the use of the pathway (Centre 1; $p = 0.137$, Centre 2; $p = 0.501$, Centre 3; $p = 0.388$, Centre 4; $p = 0.680$) or when the data was pooled ($p = 0.740$) (Figure 4B). For the maximum creatinine levels (when assessed using KDIGO criteria) there was no significant association demonstrated for each individual centre or when the data was merged.

3.3. Day 30 AKI

On day 30 after surgery, the Mantel-Haenszel odds ratio (95% CI) for the 4 centres was 0.56 (0.31, 1.00) (Figure 3). Using four-fold plots, crude numbers demonstrate that the day 30 incidence of AKI does not significantly differ from day 1, but the precision of the data is very low and varied across the centres (Figure 4).

There was no significant association between the incidence of AKI and the implementation of ELPQuiC at day 30 post-operatively for each individual centre (Centre 1 $p = 1.00$, Centre 2 $p = 1.00$, Centre 3 $p = 0.077$, Centre 4 $p = 0.241$). However, a small and weak association was observed when the data was pooled (Figure 4C) $p = 0.069$, phi-coefficient 0.09).

In a comparison of KDIGO AKI subgroups, again no significant difference was found on either day 1 ($p = 0.5321$) or day 30 ($p = 0.1516$) using crude data.

However, when correcting for rates of AKI for pre-existing CKD the Mantel-Haenzel Chi Squared test confirmed that the incidence of AKI relating to ELPQuiC implementation is not statistically associated with pre-existing CKD (Day 1 AKI $p = 0.771$, Max day 1–30 AKI $p = 0.929$, Day 30 AKI $p = 0.087$).

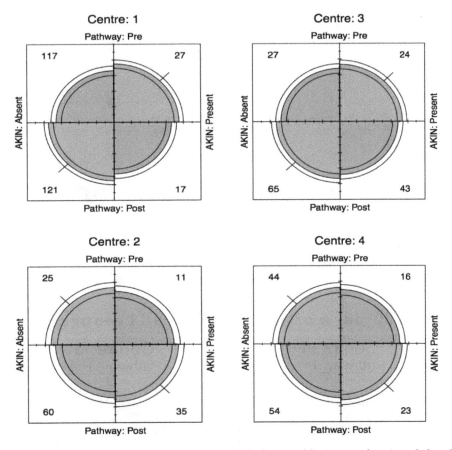

Figure 3. Four-fold Pl–t. Incidence of maximum AKI obtained between day 1 and day 30 post-op.

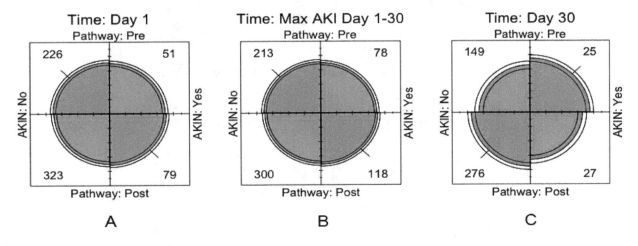

Figure 4. Cumulative AKI incidence (**A**) Day 1, (**B**) Max (day1-day30) and (**C**) Day 30 post-op pre and post-ELPQuiC implementation:

3.4. Mortality

Mortality incidence at 30 days was reported by the original ELPQuiC study and there was no significant association between the incidence of unadjusted 30-day mortality and the implementation of ELPQuiC for each individual centre (Figures 5 and 6, respectively) or when the data was pooled ($p = 0.08$) (Figure 7), this is in keeping with the original ELPQuiC paper [3], which then identified the risk-adjusted survival benefit.

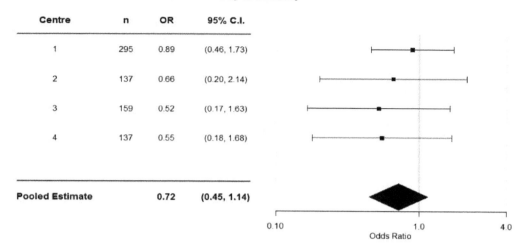

Figure 5. Incidence of 30-day mortality.

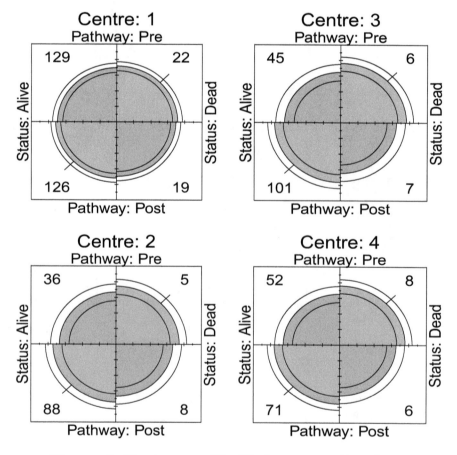

Figure 6. Centre specific 30-day mortality data.

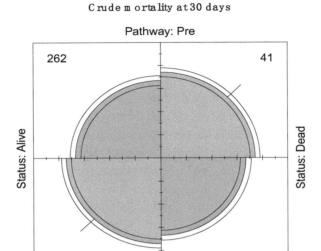

Crude mortality at 30 days

Pathway: Pre

262   41

Status: Alive   Status: Dead

386   40

Pathway: Post

Figure 7. Cumulative 30-day mortality data.

4. Discussion

Our results suggest that the implementation of a quality improvement care bundle, although conferring a survival benefit, does not affect the incidence of AKI in the immediate post-operative period or in the 30 days after surgery. This is true for both the individual institutions and the cumulative data from all four centres. Therefore, it is reasonable to conclude that the survival benefit seen in the original study is not related to a reduction in AKI, as defined by changes in serum creatinine. This is in keeping with studies on goal-directed therapy in surgery, where a benefit in terms of renal outcomes tends to be observed mainly where vasopressors are employed together with goal directed fluid therapy. The effects of goal-directed fluid therapy have been examined in major gastrointestinal surgery. The OPTIMISE trial randomised 734 high risk patients across 17 UK centres who were undergoing major gastrointestinal surgery to receive usual care or goal-directed fluid therapy and inotropy (dopexamine) to achieve stroke volume targets. Observer blinding was used. Primary outcomes included moderate or major complications and mortality. These outcomes occurred in 36.6% of patients in the intervention group and 43.4% in the usual care group giving a relative risk of 0.84 (95% CI 0.71–1.01; $p = 0.07$), which failed to reach statistical significance. Secondary outcomes, including infection, length of stay, mortality at 30 and 180 days, and morbidity at day 7 were also no different between the cohorts [24]. However, meta-analyses and systematic reviews have suggested some benefits of peri-operative goal directed therapy. A 2014 Cochrane review by Grocott et al. of 31 studies with 5292 patients showed reductions in renal failure, respiratory failure and wound infections in intervention groups. Fewer patients suffered complications in the intervention groups and on average their hospital length of stay was 1.16 days shorter. Mortality and total time in critical care was no different. However, the review was limited by a single large study that exerted a sizeable influence on the overall data pool and this must be considered when interpreting the results. It was noted that there seemed to be no harm associated with the use of goal-directed therapy; and therefore, with some putative benefits it may be a reasonable peri-operative strategy [25].

In the ELPQuiC study, commencement, dosing or timing of vasopressor use was not protocolised in either group. This may be of relevance given that vasopressin, for example, has achieved popularity as the vasopressor of choice in terms of limiting the degree of AKI, notably most recently in the VANISH trial for sepsis associated AKI [26]. It is unknown whether unit preferences for vasopressors affected the incidence of AKI in this study or affected the observed mortality benefit. Interestingly the incidence of overall AKI at day one post-surgery is about 50% of that reported in AKI-EPI, although this probably reflects the fact that all comers were admitted to ICU or held in a post-anaesthesia recovery area for an extended period, where the incidence of AKI would be expected to be less. Furthermore, given that 25% of patients had AKI at day 1 this almost certainly implies that the AKI was present prior to surgery given the creatinine kinetics following AKI. This gives further support to the importance of caring for these patients in a critical care setting where renal function and fluid balance can be closely monitored. The use of vasopressors may limit intra-operative hypotension (a risk factor for AKI), the extent and duration of which relate to the severity of the renal insult. Sun et al. conducted a retrospective analysis of 5127 patients undergoing elective non-cardiac surgery to delineate the relationship of intra-operative hypotension with renal outcomes. Mean arterial pressures of less than 60 mmHg for more than 20 min or less than 55 mmHg for more than 10 min were associated with increased risk of acute kidney injury [27]. This is unsurprising given the findings in both animal and human studies, which have demonstrated that renal blood flow becomes pressure-dependent when mean arterial pressure falls below the level at which the kidneys can autoregulate. Outside this window, renal blood flow declines with reductions in mean arterial pressure. Renal perfusion is also dependent on an adequate cardiac output in addition to a sufficient mean arterial pressure [28,29]. We did not stratify according to the presence of intra-operative hypotension, or additional risk factors for AKI, including use of nephrotoxic drugs, sepsis or volume depletion in the pre-operative period. These risk factors may be particularly relevant to the population undergoing emergency laparotomy. Moreover, we have defined AKI solely by serum creatinine, which is relevant in that several studies that have demonstrated a reduction in AKI post operatively with the use of a care bundle, principally observed an increase in urine output and hence a reduction in AKI using this criteria [30,31]. Given the heterogeneity in terms of AKI, it is unlikely that such an approach would influence AKI rates, but this provides further support for the observed mortality benefit being a product of global improvement in care rather than one aspect.

Consensus in terms of the nomenclature of AKI [32,33], has allowed a considerable body of evidence to accumulate regarding the epidemiology and pathophysiology of this syndrome. However, the methods of assessing renal function remain limited. For this study, creatinine was used as the renal biomarker, which has significant limitations outside steady state conditions [34]. Utilising more specific renal biomarkers may unmask "sub clinical AKI" and improved renal recovery with the implementation of a quality improvement care bundle, which may yet explain the survival improvement, particularly if sustained. Moreover, given the data on long term morbidity and mortality following an episode of AKI, any possibility of significantly reducing AKI after emergency laparotomy would be expected to see improved long term benefits.

Since the ELPQuIC project was published, the National Emergency Laparotomy Audit data has documented outcome data on almost 24,000 cases [35]. The 30 day mortality across all English and Welsh hospitals appears to have decreased from the 14.9% previously described in the US and UK [3,6] to 9.5%, according to the fourth NELA report on 2017 data. It is likely that the increased focus on patients undergoing emergency surgery and the quality improvement approach used in the ELPQuIC study and the larger EPOCH and Emergency Laparotomy Collaborative studies [36] are helping to improve outcomes in this high risk group of patients.

Limitations of this study include the lack of urinary output data for AKI classification and assessment of fluid balance. Using serum creatinine alone in such a heterogenous group may lead to inaccuracies in GFR estimation given changes in creatinine metabolism as well as the effects of administered drugs, although it seems unlikely that this was different in the two groups. Data was also lacking on the rates and duration of any renal replacement therapy (RRT) provided to those patients with an AKI 3. However, in the initial post-operative period the rate of RRT in one of the four centres was 22% amongst those patients classified as having AKI 3. Given a larger number of study participants it is possible that the strength of the association for ELPQuIC implementation and a reduction of AKI by day 30 would improve, however, the aim of this subgroup analysis was not to consider the power to detect AKI but rather, the reason for the identified risk-adjusted survival benefit.

5. Conclusions

This multi-centre cohort subgroup analysis suggests that the implementation of a quality improvement care bundle did not affect the incidence of AKI. This is in contrast to the survival benefit demonstrated using a care bundle and provides the stimulus to clarify the factors that may yet improve AKI in this high-risk patient group.

Author Contributions: J.F.D., A.S., F.S. and L.G.F.: Writing, original draft, review and editing and formal analysis; T.L.S.: statistical analysis; S.H., N.Q., M.C.D., B.M., R.d., J.P., M.S., C.J.P. and S.R.: Data acquisition.

Acknowledgments: The ELPQuiC Collaborator Group was formed from four acute hospital trusts in England. The group is grateful to the hard-working staff in all these hospitals who were able to implement the ELPQuiC bundle so effectively. Funding from the Health Foundation was provided to all hospitals (Shine Grant 2012). Baseline data collection at the Royal United Hospital Bath was funded by an Innovation grant from the South West Strategic Health Authority. LiDCO Group (London, UK) provided LiDCO rapid cardiac output monitors, consumables and education at all sites, depending on local experience and requirements. LiDCO Group was not involved in any project discussions, protocol design, meetings or data analysis.

Abbreviations

AKI   Acute kidney injury
ELPQuiC   Emergency laparotomy pathway quality improvement care bundle

References

1. Gustafsson, U.O.; Scott, M.J.; Schwenk, W.; Demartines, N.; Roulin, D.; Francis, N.; McNaught, C.E.; Macfie, J.; Liberman, A.S.; Soop, M.; et al. Guidelines for perioperative care in elective colonic surgery: Enhanced Recovery After Surgery (ERAS) Society recommendations. *World J. Surg.* **2013**, *37*, 259–284. [CrossRef] [PubMed]

2. Nicholson, A.; Lowe, M.C.; Parker, J.; Lewis, S.R.; Alderson, P.; Smith, A.F. Systematic review and meta-analysis of enhanced recoveryprogrammes in surgical patients. *Br. J. Surg.* **2014**, *101*, 172–188. [CrossRef] [PubMed]

3. Huddart, S.; Peden, C.J.; Swart, M.; McCormick, B.; Dickinson, M.; Mohammed, M.A.; Quiney, N.; Group, E.L.C. Use of a pathway quality improvement care bundle to reduce mortality after emergency laparotomy. *Br. J. Surg.* **2015**, *102*, 57–66. [CrossRef]

4. Subbe, C.P.; Kruger, M.; Rutherford, P.; Gemmel, L. Validation of a modified Early Warning Score in medical admissions. *QJM* **2001**, *94*, 521–526. [CrossRef] [PubMed]

5. NELA Project Team. *The First Patient Report of the National Emergency Laparotomy Audit*; RCoA: London, UK, 2015.

6. Al-Temimi, M.H.; Griffee, M.; Enniss, T.M.; Preston, R.; Vargo, D.; Overton, S.; Kimball, E.; Barton, R.; Nirula, R. When is death inevitable after emergency laparotomy? Analysis of the American College of Surgeons National Surgical Quality Improvement Program database. *J. Am. Coll. Surg.* **2012**, *215*, 503–511. [CrossRef]

7. Vester-Andersen, M.; Lundstrøm, L.H.; Møller, M.H.; Waldau, T.; Rosenberg, J.; Møller, A.M. Mortality and postoperative care pathways after emergency gastrointestinal surgery in 2904 patients: A population-based cohort study. *Br. J. Anaesth.* **2014**, *112*, 860–870. [CrossRef]

8. The Royal College of Surgeons of England. *The Higher Risk General Surgical Patient: Towards Improved Care for a Forgotten Group*; RCSENG: London, UK, 2011.

9. Chang, C.H.; Fan, P.C.; Chang, M.Y.; Tian, Y.C.; Hung, C.C.; Fang, J.T.; Yang, C.W.; Chen, Y.C. Acute kidney injury enhances outcome prediction ability of sequential organ failure assessment score in critically ill patients. *PLoS ONE* **2014**, *9*, e109649. [CrossRef] [PubMed]

10. Hoste, E.A.; Bagshaw, S.M.; Bellomo, R.; Cely, C.M.; Colman, R.; Cruz, D.N.; Edipidis, K.; Forni, L.G.; Gomersall, C.D.; Govil, D.; et al. Epidemiology of acute kidney injury in critically ill patients: The multinational AKI-EPI study. *Intensive Care Med.* **2015**, *41*, 1411–1423. [CrossRef] [PubMed]

11. Howes, T.E.; Cook, T.M.; Corrigan, L.J.; Dalton, S.J.; Richards, S.K.; Peden, C.J. Postoperative morbidity survey, mortality and length of stay following emergency laparotomy. *Anaesthesia* **2015**, *70*, 1020–1027. [CrossRef]

12. Linder, A.; Fjell, C.; Levin, A.; Walley, K.R.; Russell, J.A.; Boyd, J.H. Small acute increases in serum creatinine are associated with decreased long-term survival in the critically ill. *Am. J. Respir. Crit. Care Med.* **2014**, *189*, 1075–1081. [CrossRef] [PubMed]

13. Doyle, J.F.; Forni, L.G. Acute kidney injury: Short-term and long-term effects. *Crit. Care* **2016**, *20*, 188. [CrossRef]

14. Khwaja, A. KDIGO Clinical Practice Guideline for Acute Kidney Injury. *Nephron Clin. Pract.* **2012**, *120*, 179–184. [CrossRef] [PubMed]

15. O'Connor, M.E.; Kirwan, C.J.; Pearse, R.M.; Prowle, J.R. Incidence and associations of acute kidney injury after major abdominal surgery. *Intensive Care Med.* **2016**, *42*, 521–530. [CrossRef]

16. Quiney, N.H.S.; Peden, C.; Dickinson, M. Use of a care bundle to reduce mortality following emergency laparotomy. *Br. J. Hosp. Med.* **2015**, *76*, 358–362. [CrossRef]

17. Prytherch, D.R.; Whiteley, M.S.; Higgins, B.; Weaver, P.C.; Prout, W.G.; Powell, S.J. POSSUM and Portsmouth POSSUM for predicting mortality. Physiological and Operative Severity Score for the enUmeration of Mortality and morbidity. *Br. J. Surg.* **1998**, *85*, 1217–1220. [CrossRef] [PubMed]

18. Levey, A.S.; Coresh, J.; Greene, T.; Stevens, L.A.; Zhang, Y.L.; Hendriksen, S.; Kusek, J.W.; Van Lente, F. Using standardized serum creatinine values in the modification of diet in renal disease study equation for estimating glomerular filtration rate. *Ann. Intern. Med.* **2006**, *145*, 247–254. [CrossRef] [PubMed]

19. The R Development Core Team. *R: A Language and Environment for Statistical Computing*; R Foundation for Statistical Computing: Vienna, Austria, 2015.

20. Wickham, H. *Ggplot2: Elegant Graphics for Data Analysis*; Springer: New York, NY, USA, 2009.

21. Gordon, M.L.T. Advanced Forest Plot Using 'grid' Graphics. Available online: https://cran.r-project.org/web/packages/forestplot/forestplot.pdf (accessed on 20 August 2019).

22. Meyer, D.Z.A.; Hornik, A. Vcd: Visualizing Categorical Data. Available online: https://cran.r-project.org/web/packages/vcd/vcd.pdf (accessed on 20 August 2019).

23. Pearse, R.M.; Harrison, D.A.; MacDonald, N.; Gillies, M.A.; Blunt, M.; Ackland, G.; Grocott, M.P.; Ahern, A.; Griggs, K.; Scott, R.; et al. Effect of a perioperative, cardiac output-guided hemodynamic therapy algorithm on outcomes following major gastrointestinal surgery: A randomized clinical trial and systematic review. *JAMA* **2014**, *311*, 2181–2190. [CrossRef] [PubMed]

24. Grocott, M.P.; Dushianthan, A.; Hamilton, M.A.; Mythen, M.G.; Harrison, D.; Rowan, K. Perioperative increase in global blood flow to explicit defined goals and outcomes after surgery: A Cochrane Systematic Review. *Br. J. Anaesth.* **2013**, *111*, 535–548. [CrossRef]

25. Russell, J.A.; Walley, K.R.; Singer, J.; Gordon, A.C.; Hébert, P.C.; Cooper, D.J.; Holmes, C.L.; Mehta, S.; Granton, J.T.; Storms, M.M.; et al. Investigators TV: Vasopressin versus Norepinephrine Infusion in Patients with Septic Shock. *N. Eng. J. Med.* **2008**, *358*, 877–887. [CrossRef]

26. Sun, L.Y.; Wijeysundera, D.N.; Tait, G.A.; Beattie, W.S. Association of intraoperative hypotension with acute kidney injury after elective noncardiac surgery. *Anesthesiology* **2015**, *123*, 515–523. [CrossRef]

27. Rhee, C.J.; Kibler, K.K.; Easley, R.B.; Andropoulos, D.B.; Czosnyka, M.; Smielewski, P.; Brady, K.M. Renovascular reactivity measured by near-infrared spectroscopy. *J. Appl. Physiol.* **2012**, *113*, 307–314. [CrossRef] [PubMed]

28. Bayliss, W.M. On the local reactions of the arterial wall to changes of internal pressure. *J. Physiol.* **1902**, *28*, 220–231. [CrossRef] [PubMed]

29. Meersch, M.; Schmidt, C.; Hoffmeier, A.; Van Aken, H.; Wempe, C.; Gerss, J.; Zarbock, A. Prevention of cardiac surgery-associated AKI by implementing the KDIGO guidelines in high risk patients identified by biomarkers: The PrevAKI randomized controlled trial. *Intensive Care Med.* **2017**, *43*, 1551–1561. [CrossRef] [PubMed]

30. Gocze, I.; Jauch, D.; Gotz, M.; Kennedy, P.; Jung, B.; Zeman, F.; Gnewuch, C.; Graf, B.M.; Gnann, W.; Banas, B.; et al. Biomarker-guided Intervention to Prevent Acute Kidney Injury After Major Surgery: The Prospective Randomized BigpAK Study. *Ann. Surg.* **2017**, *267*, 1013–1020. [CrossRef]

31. Eknoyan, G.; Lameire, N.; Eckardt, K.; Kasiske, B.; Wheeler, D.; Levin, A.; Stevens, P.E.; Bilous, R.W.; Lamb, E.J.; Coresh, J.; et al. KDIGO 2012 Clinical Practice Guideline for the Evaluation and Management of Chronic Kidney Disease. *Kidney Int.* **2013**, *3*, 5–14.

32. Bellomo, R.; Ronco, C.; Kellum, J.A.; Mehta, R.L.; Palevsky, P. Acute renal failure—Definition, outcome measures, animal models, fluid therapy and information technology needs: The Second International Consensus Conference of the Acute Dialysis Quality Initiative (ADQI) Group. *Crit. Care* **2007**, *11*, 411.

33. Ye, M.; Dai, Q.; Zheng, J.; Jiang, X.; Wang, H.; Lou, S.; Yu, K. The significance of post-operative creatinine in predicting prognosis in cardiac surgery patients. *Cell Biochem. Biophys.* **2014**, *70*, 587–591. [CrossRef]

34. Pearse, R. *Enhanced Peri-Operative Care for High-risk patients (EPOCH) Trial: A stepped Wedge Cluster Randomised Trial of a Quality Improvement Intervention for Patients Undergoing Emergency Laparotomy*; Queen Mary University of London: London, UK, 2014.

35. Dellinger, R.P.; Levy, M.M.; Rhodes, A.; Annane, D.; Gerlach, H.; Opal, S.M.; Sevransky, J.E.; Sprung, C.L.; Douglas, I.S.; Jaeschke, R.; et al. Surviving Sepsis Campaign: International Guidelines for Management of Severe Sepsis and Septic Shock: 2012. *Crit. Care Med.* **2013**, *41*, 580–637.

36. Aggarwal, G.; Peden, C.J.; Mohammed, M.A.; Pullyblank, A.; Williams, B.; Stephens, T.; Kellett, S.; Kirkby-Bott, J.; Quiney, N.; Emergency Laparotomy, C. Evaluation of the Collaborative Use of an Evidence-Based Care Bundle in Emergency Laparotomy. *JAMA Surg.* **2019**, *154*, e190145. [CrossRef]

6

Urinary NMR Profiling in Pediatric Acute Kidney Injury

Claudia Muhle-Goll [1,2,*]**, Philipp Eisenmann** [2]**, Burkhard Luy** [1,2]**, Stefan Kölker** [3]**, Burkhard Tönshoff** [4]**, Alexander Fichtner** [4] **and Jens H. Westhoff** [4,*]

[1] Karlsruhe Institute of Technology, Institute for Biological Interfaces 4, P.O. Box 3640, 76021 Karlsruhe, Germany; burkhard.luy@kit.edu

[2] Karlsruhe Institute of Technology, Institute of Organic Chemistry, Fritz-Haber-Weg 6, 76131 Karlsruhe, Germany; philipp-michael.eisenmann@kit.edu

[3] Division of Pediatric Neurology and Metabolic Medicine, University Children's Hospital Heidelberg, Im Neuenheimer Feld 430, 69120 Heidelberg, Germany; stefan.koelker@med.uni-heidelberg.de

[4] Department of Pediatrics I, University Children's Hospital Heidelberg, Im Neuenheimer Feld 430, 69120 Heidelberg, Germany; burkhard.toenshoff@med.uni-heidelberg.de (B.T.); alexander.fichtner@med.uni-heidelberg.de (A.F.)

* Correspondence: claudia.muhle-goll@kit.edu (C.M.-G.); jens.westhoff@med.uni-heidelberg.de (J.H.W.)

Abstract: Acute kidney injury (AKI) in critically ill children and adults is associated with significant short- and long-term morbidity and mortality. As serum creatinine- and urine output-based definitions of AKI have relevant limitations, there is a persistent need for better diagnostics of AKI. Nuclear magnetic resonance (NMR) spectroscopy allows for analysis of metabolic profiles without extensive sample manipulations. In the study reported here, we examined the diagnostic accuracy of NMR urine metabolite patterns for the diagnosis of neonatal and pediatric AKI according to the Kidney Disease: Improving Global Outcomes (KDIGO) definition. A cohort of 65 neonatal and pediatric patients (0–18 years) with established AKI of heterogeneous etiology was compared to both a group of apparently healthy children ($n = 53$) and a group of critically ill children without AKI ($n = 31$). Multivariate analysis identified a panel of four metabolites that allowed diagnosis of AKI with an area under the receiver operating characteristics curve (AUC-ROC) of 0.95 (95% confidence interval 0.86–1.00). Especially urinary citrate levels were significantly reduced whereas leucine and valine levels were elevated. Metabolomic differentiation of AKI causes appeared promising but these results need to be validated in larger studies. In conclusion, this study shows that NMR spectroscopy yields high diagnostic accuracy for AKI in pediatric patients.

Keywords: acute kidney injury; metabolomics; urine; NMR spectroscopy; multivariate analysis

---

1. Introduction

Acute kidney injury (AKI) is associated with poor outcomes, including increased morbidity (e.g., days on ventilator, length of hospital and intensive care unit stay) and mortality, and an increased risk for the development of chronic kidney disease [1–3]. The prevalence of neonatal and pediatric AKI among critically ill and high-risk cohorts is high, and AKI incidence is still increasing. Based on recent consensus definitions, AKI occurs in 27% and 29.9% of patients of the pediatric (PICU) and neonatal intensive care unit (NICU), respectively [4,5]. Remarkably, in non-critically ill hospitalized children and adolescents, AKI incidence is still as high as 5% [6]. The current gold standard for the diagnosis of AKI relies upon serum creatinine and urine output measurements, both of which, however, reveal relevant drawbacks. As such, serum creatinine is a late and indirect marker of reduced glomerular filtration rate that does not allow for differentiation of the specific cause of renal impairment. Urine output measurements, on the other hand, demand longer-term evaluations and are influenced, e.g., by diuretic medication. Of note, an earlier and more specific identification of patients with AKI and especially of those who are at highest risk for adverse outcome can influence physicians' decision-making and medical treatment and may ultimately improve patient outcome.

In recent years, several urinary proteins including neutrophil gelatinase-associated lipocalin (NGAL), kidney injury molecule-1 (KIM-1), tissue inhibitor of metalloprotease-2 (TIMP-2), insulin-like growth factor-binding protein 7 (IGFBP7), and others have been proposed as useful biomarkers for early diagnosis, differentiation, and/or prediction of patient outcome in adult and pediatric AKI [7–10]. Unfortunately, the specificity of the above protein biomarkers for kidney injury and their clinical performance are insufficient for clinical implementation [11,12]. Hence, there is an unmet need for novel markers of AKI alone or in combination that i) improve patient risk stratification, ii) optimize early and precise detection of renal damage, iii) enable an early etiological classification of AKI, iv) monitor and target clinical management, and v) predict clinical outcome following AKI.

Untargeted metabolomics provides a functional fingerprint of the physiological and pathophysiological state of an organism and can be used both for pattern recognition and metabolite identification [13]. Nuclear magnetic resonance (NMR) and gas chromatography or liquid chromatography, together with mass spectrometry, are generally used to separate and identify metabolites. Metabolic approaches, i.e., by mass spectrometry, have been adopted to uncover new small molecule biomarkers or biochemical mechanisms as well as signaling pathways in chronic kidney disease, diabetic nephropathy, AKI, renal cancer, kidney transplantation, and polycystic kidney diseases [14,15]. These studies were performed in either rodents or humans and investigated blood, urine, or kidney tissue samples. In an experimental pig model of sepsis-induced AKI, NMR-based metabolomics was a potentially useful tool for biomarker identification [16]. Characteristic urine NMR spectra were also demonstrated in murine renal ischemia-reperfusion injury models [17,18]. Archdekin et al. using mass spectrometry of urine samples demonstrated the potential of a urine metabolite classifier to detect non-rejection kidney injury in pediatric kidney transplant patients and non-invasively discriminated non-rejection kidney injury from rejection [19]. While metabolomic profiles have been investigated in prematurity, low birth weight neonates, perinatal asphyxia, pediatric respiratory and neurological diseases, gastrointestinal diseases and inborn errors of metabolism, only very few clinical studies have been published that investigated the application of a metabolomic approach in pediatric AKI [20,21].

This prompted us to investigate the accuracy of NMR-based urine metabolomics for the diagnosis of AKI in a pilot cohort study of neonates and children with established Kidney Disease: Improving Global Outcomes (KDIGO) AKI of heterogeneous etiology. We further aimed to investigate if metabolomic fingerprints and biomarkers allow for a differentiation of specific AKI subtypes.

2. Results

2.1. Characteristics of the Study Population

Subject characteristics are shown in Table 1. As the urine heavily reflects environmental influences, two different control groups were included into the study in order to reduce the risk of a selection bias. While the first control group consisted of apparently healthy children ("healthy controls"), the second control group comprised neonatal and pediatric ICU patients without AKI ("non-AKI patients"). In brief, there was no significant difference regarding age, gender, proportion of neonates, and body mass index (BMI) standard deviation score (SDS) between AKI patients, non-AKI patients, and healthy controls. The etiology of AKI was heterogeneous including both prerenal and intrinsic causes. The more frequent AKI etiologies included dehydration ($n = 15$), hemolytic uremic syndrome ($n = 13$), septic shock ($n = 12$), perinatal asphyxia ($n = 7$), hemodynamic instability ($n = 4$), and interstitial nephritis ($n = 4$). Serum creatinine on study enrollment was significantly ($p < 0.001$) higher in AKI patients compared to non-AKI patients and, accordingly, estimated creatinine clearance (eCCl) was significantly reduced ($p < 0.001$).

Table 1. Characteristics of the study population. Numeric data are presented as median with interquartile range (IQR) in parenthesis. Categorical data are presented as a number with the percentage in parenthesis. Statistical tests used for the individual parameters are described in the section Statistical Analysis. $p < 0.05$ was regarded as statistically significant. Abbreviations: AKI, acute kidney injury; BMI, body mass index; eCCl, estimated creatinine clearance; KDIGO, Kidney Disease: Improving Global Outcomes; SDS, standard deviation score.

Characteristic	AKI Patients ($n = 65$)	Non-AKI Patients ($n = 31$)	Healthy Controls ($n = 53$)	p-Value
Age (years)	3.0 (0.6 to 13.5)	1.0 (0.4 to 7.4)	6.0 (1.0 to 10.0)	0.21
Male	30 (46.2%)	15 (48.4%)	26 (49.1%)	0.57
Female	35 (53.8%)	16 (51.6%)	27 (50.9%)	
Neonates	12 (18.5%)	6 (19.4%)	11 (20.8%)	0.95
BMI SDS	−0.5 (−1.2 to 0.5)	−0.8 (−1.9 to 0.6)		0.25
AKI etiology				
Dehydration	15 (23.0%)			
Hemolytic uremic syndrome	13 (20.0%)			
Septic shock	12 (18.5%)			
Perinatal asphyxia	7 (10.8%)			
Hemodynamic	4 (6.2%)			
Interstitial nephritis	4 (6.2%)			
Other	10 (15.4%)			
Serum creatinine on study enrollment (mg/dL)	1.60 (0.9 to 3.5)	0.3 (0.2 to 0.5)		<0.001
eCCl on study enrollment (mL/min per 1.73 m^2)	19.2 (11.0 to 42.0)	123.0 (80.9 to 170)		<0.001
KDIGO staging of AKI				
Stage 1	5 (7.7%)			
Stage 2	9 (13.8%)			
Stage 3	51 (78.5%)			
Proteinuria (g/L)	0.6 (0.2 to 1.5)	0.1 (0.0 to 0.1)		<0.001
Urinary protein-to-creatinine ratio (mg/g)	239 (48.6 to 955)	34.6 (24.6 to 49.3)		<0.001
Urinary leukocytes (per μL)	22.0 (4.5 to 93.0)	5.0 (0.0 to 26.5)		<0.01
Urinary erythrocytes (per μL)	15.0 (2.0 to 136.0)	5.0 (2.0 to 37.3)		<0.05
Squamous epithelium (per μL)	0.0 (0.0 to 1.5)	0.0 (0.0 to 0.0)		0.074
C-reactive protein (mg/L)	30.9 (7.5 to 98.8)	2.4 (0.0 to 19.0)		0.001
Renal replacement therapy	27 (41.5%)	0 (0%)	0 (0%)	<0.001
3-month mortality	11 (16.9%)	0 (0%)	0 (0%)	<0.05

Maximum KDIGO stage during the clinical course was Stage 3 in 51 patients (78,5%), Stage 2 in nine patients (13.8%), and Stage 1 in five patients (7.7%). Proteinuria ($p < 0.001$), urinary protein-to-creatinine-ratio ($p < 0.001$), urinary leukocytes ($p = 0.002$), urinary erythrocytes ($p < 0.05$), and C-reactive protein ($p = 0.001$) were significantly increased in AKI patients compared to non-AKI patients. Twenty-seven AKI patients (41.5%) required renal replacement therapy during the clinical course, 11 AKI patients (16.9%) deceased within 3 months following study enrollment.

2.2. Nuclear Magnetic Resonance (NMR) Spectroscopy Analysis

Ten typical spectra of the urines of AKI patients, non-AKI patients, and healthy controls, respectively, are shown in Supplemental Figure S1. Whereas spectra of healthy children had a uniform appearance, corresponding to the typical urine spectra of healthy people [22], AKI spectra revealed a different picture. Not only did the spectra show increased intensities due to the reduced urine volume, but metabolite composition varied between the different individuals. In addition, some AKI spectra revealed a background of broad unresolved resonances most likely originating from large protein or lipid/steroid signals. Non-AKI patient spectra were in-between the two other groups, showing variation in their metabolite composition, but not to the same extent as the AKI spectra. Because of the observed spectral diversity, we performed variable bucketing and selected preferably those peaks that were common among all three groups.

2.3. Multivariate Analysis

When performing a principle component analysis (PCA), the AKI group could be clearly separated from the healthy control group (Figure 1A). However, the separation between the AKI and the non-AKI group was less apparent. Principal components 1 (PC1) and 2 (PC2) explained 13.4% and 12.4% of the variation. Quality control (QC) samples clustered tightly within the healthy control group and showed that measurements were highly reproducible. Neonatal spectra appeared to have more negative PC1 values. Especially among the healthy control group, neonatal spectra clustered in the upper left corner. Thus, the subsequent analyses were performed twice, with neonates either included or excluded. When neonates were excluded from the analysis (12 AKI patients, 11 healthy control subjects, six non-AKI control patients), separation was more pronounced (Figure 1B).

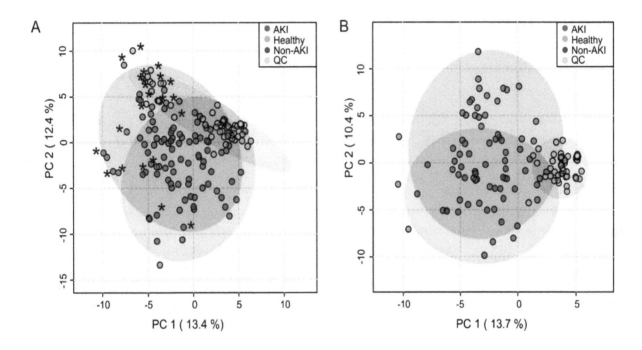

Figure 1. Principle component analysis of the urine spectral bucket table. Variable bucketing was employed leading to 129 buckets. Metabolites were assigned, whenever possible, based on comparison with database entries or literature and were confirmed by spiking experiments. (**A**) All spectra (AKI patients, $n = 65$; healthy controls, $n = 53$; non-AKI patients, $n = 31$; QC, $n = 15$), * denotes neonatal spectra, (**B**) neonatal spectra excluded (AKI patients, $n = 53$; healthy controls, $n = 42$; non-AKI patients, $n = 25$; QC, $n = 15$). Outliers were not detectable. AKI, acute kidney injury; QC, quality control.

Partial least squares discriminant analysis (PLS-DA) was performed to separate within group variation from class-related differentiation (Figure 2A). Quality control parameters showed that AKI patients could be reliably separated from the control group (quality of prediction Q^2: 0.55, explained variance R^2: 0.76). Omitting neonatal samples (Figure 2B) only slightly improved the separation and predictive power (Q^2: 0.64, R^2: 0.82). A 1000-fold permutation analysis confirmed that this result was not fortuitous in both cases ($p < 0.001$). Separation into prerenal and intrinsic causes of AKI based on previously published criteria [23] was explored, but did not lead to improved clustering in the PCA or PLS-DA (Supplemental Figure S2) and was consequently abandoned.

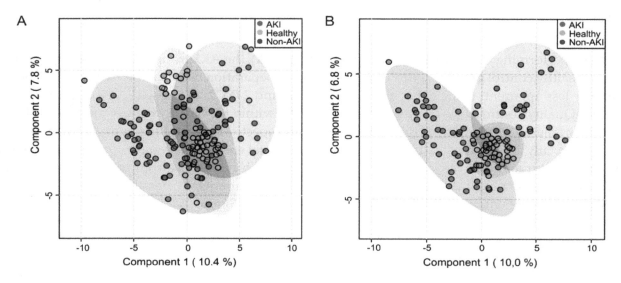

Figure 2. Partial least squares discriminant analysis of the urine spectral bucket table. Neonatal spectra (**A**) included (AKI patients, $n = 65$; healthy controls, $n = 53$; non-AKI patients, $n = 31$), (**B**) excluded (AKI patients, $n = 53$; healthy controls, $n = 42$; non-AKI patients, $n = 25$). AKI, acute kidney injury.

As mentioned before, non-AKI patient spectra separated less well from AKI spectra than healthy control spectra. We questioned whether the analysis preferentially selected general traits of morbidity like markers of increased catabolic pathways or drug metabolism. To rule out this argument, we performed both PCA and PLS-DA in healthy controls and non-AKI controls (Supplemental Figure S3). Metabolites that separated the two groups were identified in a PLS-DA (Supplemental Table S1) and those with variable importance in projection (VIP) values higher than 1.5 were excluded in the following analyses. For further analyses, the healthy control group and the non-AKI patient group were combined. This led to a visibly better separation already in a PCA (Supplemental Figure S4A). A PLS-DA model could be obtained with three components and quality parameters Q^2 of 0.66 and R^2 of 0.79 (Supplemental Figure S4B, Table 2). Omitting neonates further improved the separation between the groups to a Q^2 value of 0.73 and a R^2 value of 0.89 (Supplemental Figure S5A and S5B, Table 2). The VIP plot (Supplemental Figures S4C and S5C) revealed that citrate, bile acid signals, leucine, valine, general lipid signals, cis-aconitic acid, formate, as well as non-assigned aliphatic (unk_al/x) compounds were mainly responsible for the separation.

Table 2. Explained variance and predictability for AKI and subgroups when compared to the combined control group (non-AKI patients plus healthy control subjects).

Group	No. of Components	PLS-DA Parameters		
		Q^2	R^2	Permutation *: Empirical p-Value
AKI (total)	3	0.63	0.78	< 0.001
AKI (neonates excluded in AKI and CTL)	4	0.73	0.89	< 0.001
Dehydration	3	0.44	0.80	< 0.001
Perinatal asphyxia	2	0.26	0.61	0.159
Septic shock	4	0.73	0.95	< 0.001
Hemolytic uremic syndrome	4	0.69	0.90	< 0.001

* resulting from 1000 times permutation analysis.

2.4. Biomarker Analysis

To analyze whether the spectral information or a combination of several metabolites could be used as biomarker, 20% of randomly selected spectra (11 AKI, six non-AKI, and eight healthy control spectra) were not used for initial analysis and served as validation cohort. Neonates were excluded as the previous analysis had shown that their spectral characteristics differ to a certain degree. We developed a diagnostic model based on the metabolites with the highest VIP values in the PLS-DA analysis (Supplemental Figure S5C, Table 3). They all demonstrated AUC-ROC values > 0.70 and confidence intervals that did not cross 0.5. Yet a logistic regression model with these 15 markers did not converge. Thus, we successively reduced the number of potential markers based on the calculated z values and Pr(>|z|) to a set of four markers: Citrate with its resonance at 2.69 ppm, leucine (0.96 ppm), valine with its resonance at 1.00 ppm, and bile acid (0.69–0.81 ppm).

Table 3. Top 15 metabolites according to PLS-DA of AKI compared to the combined control group (non-AKI patients plus healthy control subjects), neonatal spectra excluded. AKI, acute kidney injury; PLS-DA, partial least squares discriminant analysis.

Metabolite Importance Number	Metabolite	VIP Score	AUC *	95% CI **
1	Citrate1 ***	2.73	0.94	0.88–0.98
2	Bile acid	2.52	0.91	0.84–0.97
3	Citrate2 ***	2.50	0.92	0.85–0.96
4	Unk_al1	2.49	0.90	0.83–0.96
5	unk_al28	2.19	0.84	0.75–0.91
6	Leucine	2.13	0.83	0.73–0.90
7	unk_al24	2.07	0.83	0.74–0.92
8	unk_al26	2.07	0.82	0.73–0.91
9	Valine	1.89	0.79	0.70–0.89
10	unk_al10	1.86	0.80	0.70–0.89
11	cis-Aconitic acid	1.86	0.79	0.69–0.88
12	Formate	1.80	0.84	0.75–0.91
13	LipidCH$_2$	1.65	0.82	0.72–0.90
14	Glycine	1.50	0.71	0.61–0.81
15	Asparagine	1.48	0.76	0.65–0.85

* ROC AUC values from univariate testing. ** 95% confidence interval was calculated using 500 bootstrappings. *** Citrate is characterized by two separate buckets, one for each proton of the degenerate CH$_2$ group.

We obtained a regression equation with a best threshold (or cut-off) for the predicted p (= Pr(y=1|x)) of 0.34 (Table 4A).

Table 4. Logistic regression model—summary of each feature: (**A**) With four, (**B**) with six features.

(A) logit(p) = log(p/(1 − P)) = −0.667 − 2.723 citrate + 2.538 leucine − 3.42 valine + 3.164 bile acid

	Estimate	Std. Error	z Value	Pr(>|z|)	Odds
(Intercept)	−0.667	0.571	−1.167	0.243	-
citrate (2.69 ppm)	−2.723	0.83	−3.281	0.001	0.07
leucine	2.538	1.089	2.33	0.02	12.65
valine	−3.42	1.374	−2.489	0.013	0.03
bile acid	3.164	1.096	2.887	0.004	23.67

(B) logit(P) = log(P/(1 − P)) = 0.034 − 3.193 citrate + 4.859 leucine − 6.191 valine + 4.207 bile acid - 2.694 unk_al1 − 2.489 unk_al28

	Estimate	Std. Error	z value	Pr(>|z|)	Odds
(Intercept)	0.034	0.998	0.034	0.973	-
citrate (2.69 ppm)	−3.193	1.682	−1.898	0.058	0.04
leucine	4.859	2.182	2.227	0.026	128.88
valine	−6.191	2.617	−2.366	0.018	0
bile acid	4.207	1.774	2.372	0.018	67.18
unk_al1/3.16 ppm	2.694	1.414	−1.906	0.057	0.07
unk_al28/2.15 ppm	−2.489	1.093	−2.278	0.023	0.08

p-values above this threshold classified samples as AKI. The area under the receiver operating characteristics curve (AUC-ROC) was 0.95 with a 95% confidence interval of 0.86–1.00 (Figure 3A). When the classification performance was tested on the validation cohort, one AKI test sample (out of 11) was wrongly classified, but no control spectra. A modified marker set including two additional unidentified aliphatic compounds, one with a resonance at 3.16 ppm (unk_al1) and one overlapping with glutamine (2.12–2.17 ppm, unk_al28), classified all spectra of the validation set correctly, but had a slightly lower AUC-ROC value of 0.93 (95% CI: 0.82–0.99) (Table 4B and Figure 3B). Details about each feature are listed in Table 4A,B.

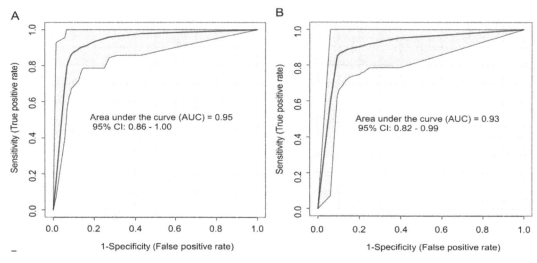

Figure 3. ROC curve for the diagnostic accuracy of selected metabolites from NMR spectroscopy for the diagnosis of KDIGO AKI obtained from a linear regression analysis using (**A**) four selected features (citrate (2.69 ppm), leucine (0.96 ppm), valine (1.00 ppm), and bile acid (0.69–0.81 ppm)) and (**B**) six selected features (citrate (2.69 ppm), leucine (0.96 ppm), valine (1.00 ppm), bile acid (0.69–0.81 ppm), unk_al1 (3.16 ppm), and unk_al28 (2.12–2.17 ppm)). AKI, acute kidney injury; KDIGO, Kidney Disease: Improving Global Outcomes; NMR, nuclear magnetic resonance; ROC, receiver operating characteristic.

2.5. Differentiation of Acute Kidney Injury (AKI) Etiologies

We next analyzed whether NMR spectroscopy allows for etiologic differentiation of underlying AKI causes (Figure 4). Four AKI subgroups had sufficient patient numbers for statistical analysis ($n > 5$). Here we used a reduced set of buckets and excluded all buckets of the original set that had variable importance in projection (VIP) values < 1.1 when the AKI group was compared against the combined control group. This led to a reduced set of 48 buckets. The logic behind this choice was to remove potential noise as the number of variables by far exceeded the number of spectra.

We performed PLS-DA with each of the subgroups (i.e., dehydration, hemolytic uremic syndrome, septic shock, perinatal asphyxia) against the combined control group to search for distinct group specific patterns. Quality control values were good for two subgroups (septic shock and hemolytic uremic syndrome) and acceptable for the dehydration subgroup (Table 2). A moderate Q^2-value and a high empirical p-value for a 1000-fold permutation test showed that the subgroup perinatal asphyxia was less well identifiable with the employed metabolite set.

Figure 4 displays the VIP values of the most important metabolites (VIP > 1.1 in at least one group) together with their fold change calculated for each subgroup. The VIP patterns (Figure 4A) showed that in addition to metabolite buckets that were important for general AKI identification in all AKI subjects, AKI subtype-specific metabolite buckets appeared to be identifiable. Fold changes analysis displayed an even more distinct picture (Figure 4B). A fold change in citrate was common in all groups. Others seemed to be specific for the underlying AKI etiology. For example, gluconate and lactate-to-threonine ratio had large fold changes in perinatal asphyxia and septic shock, but were less informative for dehydration and hemolytic uremic syndrome.

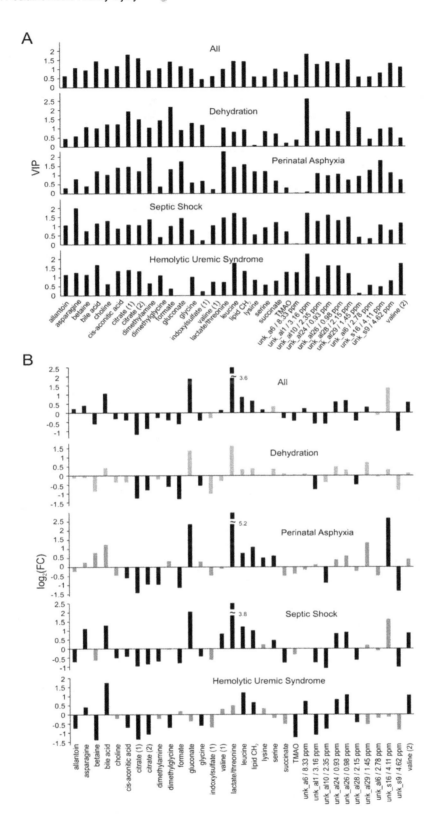

Figure 4. (**A**) Overview of discriminant identified metabolites according to variable importance in projection (VIP) values analyzed separately for each etiology. VIP values were obtained from a PLS-DA analysis. Only metabolite buckets are shown that had VIP values > 1.1 for at least one of the different groups. (**B**) The respective fold changes (log₂(FC)) for the same metabolites are given for comparison. Black bars denote fold changes with an associated *p*-value < 0.01, grey bars those with a *p*-value > 0.01. PLS-DA, partial least squares discriminant analysis.

3. Discussion

Several metabolomic studies investigating various renal diseases have been published in the past decade, however, metabolomics data on pediatric AKI is scarce (for an overview see [14,15,24]). In the present study, ^{1}H-NMR profiling was applied to urinary samples of neonatal and pediatric patients with established AKI and compared to healthy children and to hospitalized children without AKI. By multivariate analysis, we identified a panel of metabolites that enabled AKI diagnosis by yielding an AUC-ROC of 0.95. The identified metabolites that enabled the diagnosis of AKI (KDIGO) included, among several unknown compounds, increases in leucine, valine, bile acid and decreases in citrate (Figure 4B). In addition, in our rather small pilot study population NMR-fingerprints seemed to allow for differentiation between different AKI etiologies.

A crucial point in our analysis was the selection of the control group. The AKI cohort was very heterogeneous with respect to the underlying cause of AKI, and patients were treated with a variety of medications. As urine reflects all these impacts as well as nutritional influences, comparing the AKI children only to a healthy control cohort would enhance the risk for the selection of markers not related to AKI but rather to general morbidity. Creatinine may be such an example, as it is not only used to determine renal clearance but is also a marker of muscle mass. For that reason, we decided to further include a control group of critically ill ICU patients without AKI that were also exposed to diverse medical treatments. PCA and PLS-DA analysis proved that this grouping was possible and that AKI spectra showed their own distinct pattern. Moreover, in this way we identified metabolites like mannitol, lactose, and creatinine as crucial for the general distinction between healthy children and hospitalized patients without AKI. Mannitol and lactose are applied as additive drug components, whereas creatinine may be a common sign of catabolic metabolism or a sign of a minor reduction in renal clearance (Supplemental Table S1). By omitting these metabolites, we are confident that the distinction of AKI from non-AKI patients was not based on common medication or general signs of morbidity. Strikingly, some markers that were excluded from analysis after comparison of healthy control and non-AKI patient control spectra (hippurate, indoxylsulfate, creatinine) were among those that were previously classified as markers for AKI in animal models [25–27]. However, in animal models, only healthy untreated animals served as control. This does not allow a distinction between general signs of morbidity and specific ones for AKI.

Previous human AKI studies resulted in the identification of a variety of potential metabolite biomarkers [14,24]. Interestingly, almost no overlap exists between the respective metabolites [28–34] and the metabolites identified in our study. For example, Beger et al. identified homovanillinic acid sulfate, a dopamine metabolite as the most important marker in the urine of children who developed AKI after cardiac surgery [21]. This finding was confirmed by Mercier et al. investigating the urine of neonates with AKI [29]. By contrast, aromatic compounds other than 3-indoxylsulfate and hippurate are not among the important metabolites in our study.

Animal studies present a somewhat more homogeneous picture of putative biomarkers. In the majority, AKI was induced in healthy animals through application of drugs or surgery [25–27,34–38]. Although the identified biomarkers rarely fully matched between the different studies, metabolites of the citric acid cycle (TCA) cycle, branched-chain amino acids, creatinine, hippurate, and 3-indoxylsulfate emerged as common markers of drug-induced AKI [25–27,34–38]. Some prospective markers in rodent models of drug-induced AKI (e.g., by cisplatin or gentamicin) were already altered in early phases of drug-induced nephrotoxicity [25]. Strikingly though, the metabolite selection mentioned above overlaps with the markers identified in our study. Especially citrate, leucine, and valine were among the most relevant metabolites responsible for AKI diagnosis and were main components of our developed logistic regression model.

Why do our results match better to studies on animals than on humans? Previous human studies generally examined very homogeneous groups of patients with respect to AKI etiology. In our study, AKI patients comprised a broad etiologic spectrum of AKI which is reflected by the diverse peak patterns in the aromatic area (Figure 1). This diversity may have helped in identifying a robust common denominator. Enhanced branched-chain amino acids and a reduction in citrate excretion has been reported previously, but for other nephropathies including chronic kidney disease, [39,40], diabetic nephropathy [41] and polycystic kidney disease [42]. They may be signs of early kidney damage, as a reduction of citrate can be a sign for mitochondrial dysfunction of the proximal tubular cell [24].

In fact, a reduction of TCA cycle metabolites as reflected in our study presumably mirrors tubular dysfunction due to inadequate energy supply. This dysfunction might originate from missing driving forces of the tubular cell membrane due to a lack of adenosine triphosphate (ATP) that ultimately impairs transcellular transport of dicarbonic acids by organic anion transporters (OAT), i.e., OAT4 [43]. The reason for the reduction of urinary formic acid in pediatric AKI patients can only be speculated on. Energy deficiency might cause a reduced outwardly directed electrochemical gradient for formate, a metabolite that was also significantly reduced in AKI patients. This, in consequence, is a driving force for tertiary active Cl- absorption via the Cl-/formate anion exchange transporter [44].

In our study, the percentage of spectra originating from neonates was 18.5% in the AKI group, 19.4% in the non-AKI patient group, and 20.8% in the healthy control group. Omitting these from the statistical analyses further improved the separation between the AKI group and the combined control group comprising both healthy children and critically ill ICU patients without AKI. Similar observations were made previously when investigating novel protein biomarkers of renal damage in mixed neonatal and pediatric cohorts [23]. This observation might be attributed, at least in part, to the relatively high percentage of low KDIGO AKI stages in neonates. As such, four neonates (33.3%) were classified as Stage 1 KDIGO AKI, three neonates (25%) were classified as Stage 2 and only five patients (41.7%) were classified as Stage 3 AKI. By contrast, 46 (86.8%) pediatric AKI patients fulfilled Stage 3 KDIGO AKI criteria, six (11.3%) fulfilled Stage 2 criteria and only one pediatric AKI patient (1.9%) fulfilled Stage 1 criteria. In addition, several metabolomics studies demonstrated that the urine of neonates shows characteristic differences compared to older children. Scalabre et al. stressed the differential impact of age, height, and weight in metabolomic studies on urinary metabolic profiles in children aged < 1 year [45]. Among the metabolites identified as markers of age, they also identified citrate as an important marker. In that study, it was correlated with an increase in weight and height, and showed a negative correlation with age like succinate, which was confirmed in two other studies [20,46,47]. In comparison, in our study AKI patients of all ages showed a decrease of citrate levels compared to non-AKI subjects. Other age-related metabolites identified in these studies showed no significant effect in our analysis. Thus, we are confident that in our study age-related effects were marginal compared to the metabolic changes caused by AKI.

There are several limitations to our study. First, the number of patients participating in our single-center pilot study was low, hence requiring larger population studies. Nevertheless, robust identification of AKI patients by ^{1}H-NMR spectroscopy was feasible despite the wide variety of AKI etiologies. Second, due to the low number of study participants investigated, this study was not appropriate for analyzing the impact of AKI severity as reflected by KDIGO stage on NMR spectra. Third, the presented study primarily focuses on the diagnosis of established AKI using the serum creatinine- and urine output-based KDIGO AKI criteria as gold standard. However, due to a variety of reasons both parameters can be problematic for AKI diagnosis, especially in children. Future studies will have to deal with the implementation of ^{1}H-NMR spectroscopy for early detection of imminent AKI, for differentiation of varying AKI subtypes and for therapy monitoring and prognosis of AKI outcome. In fact, early identification of patients at highest risk for AKI and for adverse outcome can help physicians in early decision-making, e.g., with respect to the timely insertion of dialysis catheters and initiation of renal replacement therapy.

4. Materials and Methods

4.1. Ethics Statement

The study was conducted in accordance with the Declaration of Helsinki and approved by the ethics committee of the Heidelberg Medical Faculty (Protocol S-133/2011, permission: 15 July 2011, amendment: 13 June 2016). Legal guardian of each patient gave written informed consent and, when appropriate, assent from the patient was obtained as well.

4.2. Study Design and Participants

A prospective pilot cohort study was conducted at the University Children's Hospital Heidelberg. Patients aged 0 to 18 years who developed AKI during their hospital stay and patients who were referred to our Children's Hospital with established AKI were enrolled in the study from October 2011 to March 2019. Of note, the study population has partly been published before [23,48,49]. Criteria for study exclusion were (i) prematurity, (ii) postrenal AKI as examined by initial renal ultrasound, and (iii) children undergoing cardiac surgery. AKI was classified either according to the Kidney Disease: Improving Global Outcomes (KDIGO) AKI definition [50] for pediatric patients or according to the modified KDIGO definition for neonatal patients aged ≤ 28 days of life [51]. When serum creatinine and urine output criteria resulted in different KDIGO stages, the higher stage was chosen. The revised Schwartz formula (k = 0.413 × height / serum creatinine) was used for calculation of eCCl [52]. Baseline serum creatinine was defined as last value within the previous three months before study enrollment. In the case of missing baseline data, the eCCl was assumed to be 120 mL per minute per 1.73 m^2 in pediatric patients and 40 mL per minute per 1.73 m^2 in neonates [4,48]. Control subjects without AKI were taken from two different cohorts [23]. While the "non-AKI patients" group ($n = 31$) consisted of neonatal and pediatric ICU patients without AKI, the "healthy controls" group ($n = 53$) comprised apparently healthy neonates, children, and adolescents aged 0–18 years. Diagnoses of inpatients without AKI were postoperative care ($n = 25$ including neurosurgery, $n = 11$; pediatric surgery, $n = 6$; maxillofacial surgery, $n = 6$; orthopedics, $n = 1$; otorhinolaryngology, $n = 1$), seizures ($n = 1$), respiratory diseases ($n = 1$), perinatal asphyxia ($n = 1$), infectious diseases ($n = 2$), and cardiovascular diseases ($n = 1$). Exclusion criteria for the healthy control group have been previously published [48]. Patients' characteristics are given in Table 1.

4.3. Sample and Data Collection

Urine samples were collected immediately following KDIGO AKI diagnosis or after admission to our hospital. In case of anuria, urine samples were obtained after restoration of diuresis. Following centrifugation, the supernatants of the urine samples were frozen, stored at −80 °C and thawed prior to analysis. After thawing urine samples were centrifuged for 10 min at 15,871 g. A total of 500 μL of samples were mixed with 100 μL sodium phosphate buffer (150 mM final concentration in D_2O, pH 7.2) containing 2 mM trimethylsilylpropanoic acid for spectral referencing. D_2O was used as lock substance. Measurement of SCr was performed using an IDMS-traceable enzymatic method.

4.4. ^{1}H-NMR Spectroscopy of Urine Samples

A 600 MHz Avance II spectrometer (Bruker Biospin, Rheinstetten, Germany) with a double resonance 5-mm BBI probe was used to acquire the ^{1}H NMR spectra at 300 K. Temperature calibration was performed on a daily basis. Quality control (QC) samples consisting of urine aliquots of a healthy male volunteer were included every 10 h of measurement. One-dimensional spectra were acquired with the Bruker pulse sequence noesygppr1D using a relaxation delay of 10 s, 32 transients of 64 K data points, and a spectral width of 20 ppm. Water suppression was achieved through presaturation with a bandwidth of 25 Hz. Automatic phase- and baseline-correction was employed. Spectra were calibrated to the signal of TSP. Prior to Fourier transformation, spectra were multiplied with an exponential function with a 0.3 Hz line broadening factor. Topspin3.2 (Bruker Biospin, Rheinstetten, Germany) was used for data acquisition and processing.

Variable bucketing was employed leading to 129 buckets. Metabolites were assigned on the basis of comparison with data bases entries or literature whenever possible. Spiking experiments, where specific metabolites were added to a representative, already measured sample, were used to confirm the assignments in cases of doubt. Two windows were excluded: 4.74–4.84 ppm and 6.0–5.56 ppm, where water or urea resonances, respectively, appear. Missing values did not occur.

4.5. Statistical Analysis

As clinical data was non-normally distributed, median and interquartile range are presented. For statistical analysis of intergroup differences of numeric parameters, the Kruskal–Wallis test with post hoc Dunn's test or the Mann–Whitney U-test were used. Categorical parameters were compared by Pearson's Chi-squared test. For age-independent estimates, BMI was converted to SDS values, related to age- and gender-specific means and SD of European reference populations.

PCA and PLS-DA were performed with R (version 3.5.3) using the package MetaboanalystR and default parameters [53]. Probabilistic quotient normalization [54] was employed prior to statistical analysis using the healthy control samples as reference to take into account that the urine of AKI patients is as such more often concentrated leading to higher peak intensities. Data distribution showed that the data were skewed. To take this into account, data were log transformed and scaled to unit variance. To assess the quality of the resulting statistical models, 10-fold internal cross-validation as well as permutation tests were performed. To judge the predictive power of PLS-DA, quality parameters Q^2 (quality of prediction) and R^2 (explained variance) were calculated. In a second round, metabolites that separated healthy controls and non-AKI controls were identified in a PLS-DA (Supplemental Table S1) and those with VIP values higher than 1.5 (18 buckets) were excluded from the subsequent analyses.

Biomarker analysis was performed with the respective module of MetaboanalystR using PLS-DA for identification of a set of marker peaks, support vector machines, and logistic regression to assess the suitability of a reduced set for class prediction of unknown spectra and univariate ROC curve analysis for the calculation of individual metabolite AUC values.

For etiological analysis a reduced set of metabolites was used. All buckets were taken out that had variable importance in projection (VIP) values < 1.1 when the AKI group was compared against the combined control group. This led to a reduced set of 48 buckets. Metabolite fold changes between the groups were assessed with the non-parametric Mann-Whitney U-test using the Fold-Change Analysis Module of MetaboanalystR.

5. Conclusions

In conclusion, the present study underlines the value of 1H-NMR spectroscopy for the identification of novel biomarkers of renal damage in pediatric AKI. By use of this elegant technique, we were able to identify a panel of four metabolites that in linear regression analysis yielded an excellent accuracy for the diagnosis of AKI. In addition, detailed breakdown of signaling pathways being involved in the AKI cascade might further pave the way for the development of new therapeutic options for AKI.

Supplementary Materials:
Figure S1: Ten representative spectra of each group, Figure S2: PCA of AKI classified into prerenal (AKI-pre) and intrinsic (AKI-intrin), Figure S3: PCA and PLS-DA of healthy control group vs. hospitalized patients without AKI (Non-AKI), Figure S4: PCA and PLS-DA after taking out buckets separating healthy control group from hospitalized patients without AKI, Figure S5: Same as Figure S4, with neonatal spectra excluded. Table S1: Variable importance in projection (VIP) –Values from PLS-DA of healthy control group vs. hospitalized patients without AKI (Non-AKI).

Author Contributions: All authors have read and agreed to the published version of the manuscript. Conceptualization, C.M.-G., P.E., B.T. and J.H.W.; methodology, C.M.-G., P.E., A.F. and J.H.W.; validation, C.M.-G. and J.H.W.; formal analysis, C.M.-G., P.E. and J.H.W.; data curation, C.M.-G., P.E. and J.H.W.; writing—original draft preparation, C.M.-G. and J.H.W.; writing—review and editing, B.L., S.K., B.T., A.F.

Acknowledgments: The authors would like to thank Miriam Himmelsbach and Anne Mayer for help with spectra acquisition and spiking of metabolites. Pavleta Tzvetkova has been invaluable in help with spectrometer and many discussions. C.M.-G. acknowledges support by the Helmholtz-Gesellschaft. We are indebted to all children and their parents who participated in the study.

Abbreviations

AKI	acute kidney injury
AUC	area under the curve
BMI	body mass index
eCCl	estimated creatinine clearance
KDIGO	Kidney Disease: Improving Global Outcomes
NICU	neonatal intensive care unit
NMR	nuclear magnetic resonance
PCA	principle component analysis
PICU	pediatric intensive care unit
PLS-DA	partial least squares discriminant analysis
QC	quality control
ROC	receiver operating characteristic
SDS	standard deviation score
VIP	variable importance in projection

References

1.   Mammen, C.; Al Abbas, A.; Skippen, P.; Nadel, H.; Levine, D.; Collet, J.P.; Matsell, D.G. Long-term risk of CKD in children surviving episodes of acute kidney injury in the intensive care unit: A prospective cohort study. *Am. J. Kidney Dis.* **2012**, *59*, 523–530. [CrossRef]

2.   Menon, S.; Kirkendall, E.S.; Nguyen, H.; Goldstein, S.L. Acute kidney injury associated with high nephrotoxic medication exposure leads to chronic kidney disease after 6 months. *J. Pediatr.* **2014**, *165*, 522–527 e2. [CrossRef] [PubMed]

3.   Askenazi, D.J.; Feig, D.I.; Graham, N.M.; Hui-Stickle, S.; Goldstein, S.L. 3–5 year longitudinal follow-up of pediatric patients after acute renal failure. *Kidney Int.* **2006**, *69*, 184–189. [CrossRef] [PubMed]

4.   Kaddourah, A.; Basu, R.K.; Bagshaw, S.M.; Goldstein, S.L. Investigators, A., Epidemiology of Acute Kidney Injury in Critically Ill Children and Young Adults. *N. Engl. J. Med.* **2017**, *376*, 11–20. [CrossRef] [PubMed]

5.   Jetton, J.G.; Boohaker, L.J.; Sethi, S.K.; Wazir, S.; Rohatgi, S.; Soranno, D.E.; Chishti, A.S.; Woroniecki, R.; Mammen, C.; Swanson, J.R.; et al. Incidence and outcomes of neonatal acute kidney injury (AWAKEN): A multicentre, multinational, observational cohort study. *Lancet Child. Adolesc. Health* **2017**, *1*, 184–194. [CrossRef]

6.   McGregor, T.L.; Jones, D.P.; Wang, L.; Danciu, I.; Bridges, B.C.; Fleming, G.M.; Shirey-Rice, J.; Chen, L.; Byrne, D.W.; Van Driest, S.L. Acute Kidney Injury Incidence in Noncritically Ill Hospitalized Children, Adolescents, and Young Adults: A Retrospective Observational Study. *Am. J. Kidney Dis.* **2016**, *67*, 384–390. [CrossRef]

7.   Schrezenmeier, E.V.; Barasch, J.; Budde, K.; Westhoff, T.; Schmidt-Ott, K.M. Biomarkers in acute kidney injury - pathophysiological basis and clinical performance. *Acta Physiol. (Oxf)* **2017**, *219*, 554–572. [CrossRef]

8.   Malhotra, R.; Siew, E.D. Biomarkers for the Early Detection and Prognosis of Acute Kidney Injury. *Clin. J. Am. Soc. Nephrol.* **2017**, *12*, 149–173. [CrossRef]

9.   Waldherr, S.; Fichtner, A.; Beedgen, B.; Bruckner, T.; Schaefer, F.; Tonshoff, B.; Poschl, J.; Westhoff, T.H.; Westhoff, J.H. Urinary acute kidney injury biomarkers in very low-birth-weight infants on indomethacin for patent ductus arteriosus. *Pediatr. Res.* **2019**, *85*, 678–686. [CrossRef]

10.   Greenberg, J.H.; Parikh, C.R. Biomarkers for Diagnosis and Prognosis of AKI in Children: One Size Does Not Fit All. *Clin. J. Am. Soc Nephrol.* **2017**, *12*, 1551–1557. [CrossRef]

11. van Duijl, T.T.; Ruhaak, L.R.; de Fijter, J.W.; Cobbaert, C.M. Kidney Injury Biomarkers in an Academic Hospital Setting: Where Are We Now? *Clin. Biochem. Rev.* **2019**, *40*, 79–97. [PubMed]

12. Cerda, J. A biomarker able to predict acute kidney injury before it occurs? *Lancet* **2019**, *394*, 448–450. [CrossRef]

13. Weiss, R.H.; Kim, K. Metabolomics in the study of kidney diseases. *Nat. Rev. Nephrol.* **2011**, *8*, 22–33. [CrossRef] [PubMed]

14. Abbiss, H.; Maker, G.L.; Trengove, R.D. Metabolomics Approaches for the Diagnosis and Understanding of Kidney Diseases. *Metabolites* **2019**, *9*, 34. [CrossRef]

15. Kalim, S.; Rhee, E.P. An overview of renal metabolomics. *Kidney Int.* **2017**, *91*, 61–69. [CrossRef]

16. Izquierdo-Garcia, J.L.; Nin, N.; Cardinal-Fernandez, P.; Rojas, Y.; de Paula, M.; Granados, R.; Martinez-Caro, L.; Ruiz-Cabello, J.; Lorente, J.A. Identification of novel metabolomic biomarkers in an experimental model of septic acute kidney injury. *Am. J. Physiol. Renal. Physiol.* **2019**, *316*, F54–F62. [CrossRef] [PubMed]

17. Chihanga, T.; Ma, Q.; Nicholson, J.D.; Ruby, H.N.; Edelmann, R.E.; Devarajan, P.; Kennedy, M.A. NMR spectroscopy and electron microscopy identification of metabolic and ultrastructural changes to the kidney following ischemia-reperfusion injury. *Am. J. Physiol. Renal. Physiol.* **2018**, *314*, F154–F166. [CrossRef]

18. Jouret, F.; Leenders, J.; Poma, L.; Defraigne, J.O.; Krzesinski, J.M.; de Tullio, P. Nuclear Magnetic Resonance Metabolomic Profiling of Mouse Kidney, Urine and Serum Following Renal Ischemia/Reperfusion Injury. *PLoS ONE* **2016**, *11*, e0163021. [CrossRef]

19. Archdekin, B.; Sharma, A.; Gibson, I.W.; Rush, D.; Wishart, D.S.; Blydt-Hansen, T.D. Non-invasive differentiation of non-rejection kidney injury from acute rejection in pediatric renal transplant recipients. *Pediatr. Transplant.* **2019**, *23*, e13364. [CrossRef]

20. Mussap, M.; Antonucci, R.; Noto, A.; Fanos, V. The role of metabolomics in neonatal and pediatric laboratory medicine. *Clin. Chim. Acta* **2013**, *426*, 127–138. [CrossRef]

21. Beger, R.D.; Holland, R.D.; Sun, J.; Schnackenberg, L.K.; Moore, P.C.; Dent, C.L.; Devarajan, P.; Portilla, D. Metabonomics of acute kidney injury in children after cardiac surgery. *Pediatr. Nephrol.* **2008**, *23*, 977–984. [CrossRef] [PubMed]

22. Bouatra, S.; Aziat, F.; Mandal, R.; Guo, A.C.; Wilson, M.R.; Knox, C.; Bjorndahl, T.C.; Krishnamurthy, R.; Saleem, F.; Liu, P.; et al. The human urine metabolome. *PLoS ONE* **2013**, *8*, e73076. [CrossRef] [PubMed]

23. Westhoff, J.H.; Fichtner, A.; Waldherr, S.; Pagonas, N.; Seibert, F.S.; Babel, N.; Tonshoff, B.; Bauer, F.; Westhoff, T.H. Urinary biomarkers for the differentiation of prerenal and intrinsic pediatric acute kidney injury. *Pediatr. Nephrol.* **2016**, *31*, 2353–2363. [CrossRef] [PubMed]

24. Fanos, V.; Fanni, C.; Ottonello, G.; Noto, A.; Dessi, A.; Mussap, M. Metabolomics in adult and pediatric nephrology. *Molecules* **2013**, *18*, 4844–4857. [CrossRef]

25. Boudonck, K.J.; Mitchell, M.W.; Nemet, L.; Keresztes, L.; Nyska, A.; Shinar, D.; Rosenstock, M. Discovery of metabolomics biomarkers for early detection of nephrotoxicity. *Toxicol. Pathol.* **2009**, *37*, 280–292. [CrossRef]

26. Won, A.J.; Kim, S.; Kim, Y.G.; Kim, K.B.; Choi, W.S.; Kacew, S.; Kim, K.S.; Jung, J.H.; Lee, B.M.; Kim, S.; et al. Discovery of urinary metabolomic biomarkers for early detection of acute kidney injury. *Mol. Biosyst.* **2016**, *12*, 133–144. [CrossRef]

27. Sieber, M.; Hoffmann, D.; Adler, M.; Vaidya, V.S.; Clement, M.; Bonventre, J.V.; Zidek, N.; Rached, E.; Amberg, A.; Callanan, J.J.; et al. Comparative analysis of novel noninvasive renal biomarkers and metabonomic changes in a rat model of gentamicin nephrotoxicity. *Toxicol. Sci.* **2009**, *109*, 336–349. [CrossRef]

28. Martin-Lorenzo, M.; Gonzalez-Calero, L.; Ramos-Barron, A.; Sanchez-Nino, M.D.; Gomez-Alamillo, C.; Garcia-Segura, J.M.; Ortiz, A.; Arias, M.; Vivanco, F.; Alvarez-Llamas, G. Urine metabolomics insight into acute kidney injury point to oxidative stress disruptions in energy generation and H2S availability. *J. Mol. Med. (Berl)* **2017**, *95*, 1399–1409. [CrossRef]

29. Mercier, K.; McRitchie, S.; Pathmasiri, W.; Novokhatny, A.; Koralkar, R.; Askenazi, D.; Brophy, P.D.; Sumner, S. Preterm neonatal urinary renal developmental and acute kidney injury metabolomic profiling: An exploratory study. *Pediatr. Nephrol.* **2017**, *32*, 151–161. [CrossRef]

30. Elmariah, S.; Farrell, L.A.; Daher, M.; Shi, X.; Keyes, M.J.; Cain, C.H.; Pomerantsev, E.; Vlahakes, G.J.; Inglessis, I.; Passeri, J.J.; et al. Metabolite Profiles Predict Acute Kidney Injury and Mortality in Patients Undergoing Transcatheter Aortic Valve Replacement. *J. Am. Heart Assoc.* **2016**, *5*, e002712. [CrossRef]

31. Doskocz, M.; Marchewka, Z.; Jez, M.; Passowicz-Muszynska, E.; Dlugosz, A. Preliminary Study on J-Resolved NMR Method Usability for Toxic Kidney's Injury Assessment. *Adv. Clin. Exp. Med.* **2015**, *24*, 629–635. [CrossRef] [PubMed]

32. Zacharias, H.U.; Hochrein, J.; Vogl, F.C.; Schley, G.; Mayer, F.; Jeleazcov, C.; Eckardt, K.U.; Willam, C.; Oefner, P.J.; Gronwald, W. Identification of Plasma Metabolites Prognostic of Acute Kidney Injury after Cardiac Surgery with Cardiopulmonary Bypass. *J. Proteome Res.* **2015**, *14*, 2897–2905. [CrossRef] [PubMed]

33. Sun, J.; Shannon, M.; Ando, Y.; Schnackenberg, L.K.; Khan, N.A.; Portilla, D.; Beger, R.D. Serum metabolomic profiles from patients with acute kidney injury: A pilot study. *J. Chromatogr B Analyt Technol. Biomed. Life Sci.* **2012**, *893*, 107–113. [CrossRef] [PubMed]

34. Portilla, D.; Schnackenberg, L.; Beger, R.D. Metabolomics as an extension of proteomic analysis: Study of acute kidney injury. *Semin. Nephrol.* **2007**, *27*, 609–620. [CrossRef]

35. Zgoda-Pols, J.R.; Chowdhury, S.; Wirth, M.; Milburn, M.V.; Alexander, D.C.; Alton, K.B. Metabolomics analysis reveals elevation of 3-indoxyl sulfate in plasma and brain during chemically-induced acute kidney injury in mice: Investigation of nicotinic acid receptor agonists. *Toxicol. Appl. Pharmacol.* **2011**, *255*, 48–56. [CrossRef]

36. Hauet, T.; Baumert, H.; Gibelin, H.; Hameury, F.; Goujon, J.M.; Carretier, M.; Eugene, M. Noninvasive monitoring of citrate, acetate, lactate, and renal medullary osmolyte excretion in urine as biomarkers of exposure to ischemic reperfusion injury. *Cryobiology* **2000**, *41*, 280–291. [CrossRef]

37. Xu, E.Y.; Perlina, A.; Vu, H.; Troth, S.P.; Brennan, R.J.; Aslamkhan, A.G.; Xu, Q. Integrated pathway analysis of rat urine metabolic profiles and kidney transcriptomic profiles to elucidate the systems toxicology of model nephrotoxicants. *Chem. Res. Toxicol.* **2008**, *21*, 1548–1561. [CrossRef]

38. Portilla, D.; Li, S.; Nagothu, K.K.; Megyesi, J.; Kaissling, B.; Schnackenberg, L.; Safirstein, R.L.; Beger, R.D. Metabolomic study of cisplatin-induced nephrotoxicity. *Kidney Int.* **2006**, *69*, 2194–2204. [CrossRef]

39. Shah, V.O.; Townsend, R.R.; Feldman, H.I.; Pappan, K.L.; Kensicki, E.; Vander Jagt, D.L. Plasma metabolomic profiles in different stages of CKD. *Clin. J. Am. Soc. Nephrol.* **2013**, *8*, 363–370. [CrossRef]

40. Luck, M.; Bertho, G.; Bateson, M.; Karras, A.; Yartseva, A.; Thervet, E.; Damon, C.; Pallet, N. Rule-Mining for the Early Prediction of Chronic Kidney Disease Based on Metabolomics and Multi-Source Data. *PLoS ONE* **2016**, *11*, e0166905. [CrossRef]

41. Sharma, K.; Karl, B.; Mathew, A.V.; Gangoiti, J.A.; Wassel, C.L.; Saito, R.; Pu, M.; Sharma, S.; You, Y.H.; Wang, L.; et al. Metabolomics reveals signature of mitochondrial dysfunction in diabetic kidney disease. *J. Am. Soc. Nephrol.* **2013**, *24*, 1901–1912. [CrossRef]

42. Gronwald, W.; Klein, M.S.; Zeltner, R.; Schulze, B.D.; Reinhold, S.W.; Deutschmann, M.; Immervoll, A.K.; Boger, C.A.; Banas, B.; Eckardt, K.U.; et al. Detection of autosomal dominant polycystic kidney disease by NMR spectroscopic fingerprinting of urine. *Kidney Int.* **2011**, *79*, 1244–1253. [CrossRef]

43. Dantzler, W.H. Renal organic anion transport: A comparative and cellular perspective. *Biochim Biophys Acta* **2002**, *1566*, 169–181. [CrossRef]

44. Karniski, L.P.; Aronson, P.S. Chloride/formate exchange with formic acid recycling: A mechanism of active chl oride transport across epithelial membranes. *Proc. Natl. Acad Sci. USA* **1985**, *82*, 6362–6365. [CrossRef]

45. Scalabre, A.; Jobard, E.; Demede, D.; Gaillard, S.; Pontoizeau, C.; Mouriquand, P.; Elena-Herrmann, B.; Mure, P.Y. Evolution of Newborns' Urinary Metabolomic Profiles According to Age and Growth. *J. Proteome Res.* **2017**, *16*, 3732–3740. [CrossRef]

46. Gu, H.; Pan, Z.; Xi, B.; Hainline, B.E.; Shanaiah, N.; Asiago, V.; Gowda, G.A.; Raftery, D. 1H NMR metabolomics study of age profiling in children. *NMR Biomed.* **2009**, *22*, 826–833. [CrossRef]

47. Chiu, C.Y.; Yeh, K.W.; Lin, G.; Chiang, M.H.; Yang, S.C.; Chao, W.J.; Yao, T.C.; Tsai, M.H.; Hua, M.C.; Liao, S.L.; et al. Metabolomics Reveals Dynamic Metabolic Changes Associated with Age in Early Childhood. *PLoS ONE* **2016**, *11*, e0149823. [CrossRef]

48. Westhoff, J.H.; Seibert, F.S.; Waldherr, S.; Bauer, F.; Tonshoff, B.; Fichtner, A.; Westhoff, T.H. Urinary calprotectin, kidney injury molecule-1, and neutrophil gelatinase-associated lipocalin for the prediction of adverse outcome in pediatric acute kidney injury. *Eur. J. Pediatr.* **2017**, *176*, 745–755. [CrossRef]

49. Westhoff, J.H.; Tonshoff, B.; Waldherr, S.; Poschl, J.; Teufel, U.; Westhoff, T.H.; Fichtner, A. Urinary Tissue Inhibitor of Metalloproteinase-2 (TIMP-2) * Insulin-Like Growth Factor-Binding Protein 7 (IGFBP7) Predicts Adverse Outcome in Pediatric Acute Kidney Injury. *PLoS ONE* **2015**, *10*, e0143628. [CrossRef]

50. Kellum, J.A.; Lameire, N.; Group, K.A.G.W. Diagnosis, evaluation, and management of acute kidney injury: A KDIGO summary (Part 1). *Crit. Care.* **2013**, *17*, 204. [CrossRef]

51. Selewski, D.T.; Charlton, J.R.; Jetton, J.G.; Guillet, R.; Mhanna, M.J.; Askenazi, D.J.; Kent, A.L. Neonatal Acute Kidney Injury. *Pediatrics* **2015**, *136*, e463–e473. [CrossRef]

52. Schwartz, G.J.; Munoz, A.; Schneider, M.F.; Mak, R.H.; Kaskel, F.; Warady, B.A.; Furth, S.L. New equations to estimate GFR in children with CKD. *J. Am. Soc. Nephrol.* **2009**, *20*, 629–637. [CrossRef]

53. Chong, J.; Xia, J. MetaboAnalystR: An R package for flexible and reproducible analysis of metabolomics data. *Bioinformatics* **2018**, *34*, 4313–4314. [CrossRef]

54. Dieterle, F.; Ross, A.; Schlotterbeck, G.; Senn, H. Probabilistic quotient normalization as robust method to account for dilution of complex biological mixtures. Application in 1H NMR metabonomics. *Anal. Chem.* **2006**, *78*, 4281–4290. [CrossRef]

7

Factors Associated with Early Mortality in Critically Ill Patients Following the Initiation of Continuous Renal Replacement Therapy

Youn Kyung Kee [1], Dahye Kim [2], Seung-Jung Kim [3], Duk-Hee Kang [3], Kyu Bok Choi [3], Hyung Jung Oh [4,5,*] and Dong-Ryeol Ryu [3,4,6,*]

[1] Department of Internal Medicine, Hangang Sacred Heart Hospital, Hallym University College of Medicine, Seoul 07247, Korea; no7766@yuhs.ac

[2] Department of Nursing, Ewha Womans University Mokdong Hospital, Seoul 07985, Korea; dahye7738@gmail.com

[3] Department of Internal Medicine, School of Medicine, Ewha Womans University, Seoul 03761, Korea; sjkimwon@ewha.ac.kr (S.-J.K.); dhkang@ewha.ac.kr (D.-H.K.); kbchoi@ewha.ac.kr (K.B.C.)

[4] Research Institute for Human Health Information, Ewha Womans University Mokdong Hospital, Seoul 07985, Korea

[5] Ewha Institute of Convergence Medicine, Ewha Womans University Mokdong Hospital, Seoul 07985, Korea

[6] Tissue Injury Defense Research Center, College of Medicine, Ewha Womans University, Seoul 07985, Korea

* Correspondence: ohjmd@naver.com (H.J.O.); drryu@ewha.ac.kr (D.-R.R.)

Abstract: Continuous renal replacement therapy (CRRT) is an important modality to support critically ill patients, and the need for CRRT treatment has been increasing. However, CRRT management is costly, and the associated resources are limited. Thus, it remains challenging to identify patients that are likely to have a poor outcome, despite active treatment with CRRT. We sought to elucidate the factors associated with early mortality after CRRT initiation. We analyzed 240 patients who initiated CRRT at an academic medical center between September 2016 and January 2018. We compared baseline characteristics between patients who died within seven days of initiating CRRT (early mortality), and those that survived more than seven days beyond the initiation of CRRT. Of the patients assessed, 130 (54.2%) died within seven days of CRRT initiation. Multivariate logistic regression models revealed that low mean arterial pressure, low arterial pH, and high Sequential Organ Failure Assessment score before CRRT initiation were significantly associated with increased early mortality in patients requiring CRRT. In conclusion, the mortality within seven days following CRRT initiation was very high in this study. We identified several factors that are associated with early mortality in patients undergoing CRRT, which may be useful in predicting early outcomes, despite active treatment with CRRT.

Keywords: continuous renal replacement therapy; early mortality; clinical illness

1. Introduction

Acute kidney injury (AKI) is a major complication in critically ill patients, and it is associated with high mortality [1–3]. Continuous renal replacement therapy (CRRT) is a widely chosen treatment option in AKI patients requiring renal replacement therapy (RRT), particularly for hemodynamically unstable patients with considerable fluid accumulation [4–6]. Although CRRT is commonly considered as an initial option for critically ill patients who need RRT, the cost of CRRT treatment is higher than that of intermittent RRT, and CRRT-associated resources are limited [7,8].

Despite advances in CRRT techniques over the last several years, the mortality rate of patients undergoing CRRT remains high [9–12]. Many studies have investigated the benefit of CRRT treatment with regard to clinical outcomes and assessed potential prognostic factors for mortality [13–15]. Several factors, including sepsis, high acute physiology, and chronic health evaluation (APACHE) II score and/or sequential organ failure assessment (SOFA) score, poor urine output before CRRT initiation, comatose state, need for mechanical ventilation, fluid overload status, and type of CRRT solution are associated with increased mortality rate [16–22]. However, some patients die within one week of CRRT initiation, causing physicians to often doubt the benefits of such an invasive procedure on patient survival and/or renal preservation. Unfortunately, there are few studies to determine which factors are associated with increased early mortality in critically ill patients undergoing CRRT.

Considering the high cost and the limited resources available, identification of patients who would be more likely to have a poor outcome despite active treatment with CRRT is necessary to make an informed decision for patients requiring RRT. Thus, the aim of this study was to investigate the factors that are associated with increased early mortality, which we defined as death in the 7 days following CRRT initiation.

2. Methods

2.1. Study Population

This was a retrospective observational study of patients aged 18 years or older who initiated CRRT at a tertiary academic medical center between September 2016 and January 2018. Patients who were younger than 18 years, who were undergoing chronic dialysis due to end-stage renal disease, or who had a less than 3 month life expectancy due to malignancy were excluded. Ultimately, 240 patients were enrolled and assessed to determine the factors that were associated with early mortality in critically ill patients undergoing CRRT. We defined 'early mortality' as mortality within seven days of CRRT initiation. In addition, we defined 'very early mortality' as mortality within 24 h of CRRT initiation. This study was approved by the Institutional Review Board of Ewha Womans University, College of Medicine, and informed consent was waived because it was a retrospective cohort study.

2.2. Data Collection

Baseline characteristics were age, sex, body mass index (BMI), systolic blood pressure (SBP), diastolic blood pressure (DBP), mean arterial pressure (MAP), heart rate, comorbidities, Charlson Comorbidity Index (CCI) [23], SOFA score, and laboratory diagnostic data collected at the start of CRRT. Moreover, estimated glomerular filtration rate (eGFR) was calculated using the IDMS-traceable Modification of Diet in Renal Disease equation [24]. The presence of systemic inflammatory response syndrome (SIRS) [25]. APACHE II score and one-hour urine output immediately before CRRT initiation was also investigated. As a parameter for acute lung injury (ALI), patients with $PaO_2/FiO_2 \leq 300$ mmHg were evaluated. Data from patients collected until 28 days after CRRT initiation was used, and their survival or all-cause mortality was examined during this period.

2.3. CRRT Protocol

The decision to initiate the CRRT and the CRRT settings of target clearance, blood flow, dialysate, and replacement fluid rates, and anticoagulation administration were determined through discussion and consultation with nephrologists. The criteria for CRRT initiation were medically intractable or persistent electrolyte imbalance and/or metabolic acidosis, and decreased urine output with volume overload and/or progressive azotemia. Hemodynamic instability was also an important indication. Generally, vascular access for CRRT was via a femoral venous catheter, and the predilution method of continuous venovenous hemodiafiltration was usually performed. Blood flow was gradually increased from an initial rate of 100 to 150 mL/min according to the hemodynamic status of the patient. Although the target clearance was 35–40 mL/kg/h in most patients, this target was increased to 60 mL/kg/h or higher in patients with severe sepsis or septic shock if possible [26]. Additionally, the anticoagulant administered was selected by nephrologists, and they were dependent on bleeding tendency or contraindications to conventional heparin. After CRRT initiation, attending physicians and experienced nurses monitored the body weight, urine output, laboratory results, actual delivered dose, and the hemodynamic status of the patients, and discussed the results with nephrologists to maintain the adequacy of CRRT.

2.4. Statistical Analysis

Continuous variables are expressed as the mean and standard deviation (SD), and categorical variables as number and percentage. Chi-square tests for categorical variables and Student's t-test for continuous variables were used to compare baseline data between the two groups. We also performed univariate and multivariate logistic regression analyses to determine the factors associated with early or very early mortality. All statistical analyses were performed using SPSS version 23 software (SPSS, Chicago, IL, USA), and all p-values were two-tailed, with a predetermined alpha level <0.05 being considered statistically significant.

3. Results

3.1. Baseline Characteristics

Baseline demographic and clinical characteristics of these study patients are described in Table 1. For the 240 patients assessed, the mean age was 65.8 ± 14.7 years, and 150 patients (62.5%) were male. Mean SBP, DBP, and MAP were 112.5, 64.1, and 80.2 mmHg, respectively. In addition, there were 45 patients (18.8%) who had MAPs of less than 65 mmHg. Of the patients, 128 (53.3%) had hypertension, 89 (37.1%) were diagnosed with diabetes mellitus (DM), and the mean CCI was 6.6 ± 2.3. The mean volume of 1-hour urine outputs before CRRT was 27.2 ± 56.8 mL, and the mean APACHE II and SOFA scores were 26.1 ± 6.8 and 11.6 ± 3.9, respectively.

Table 1. Baseline characteristics of study patients.

Variables	Total	7-Day Mortality	7-Day Survivors	p Value
	(n = 240, 100%)	(n = 130, 54.2%)	(n = 110, 45.8%)	
Age (year)	65.8 ± 14.7	65.9 ± 14.2	65.7 ± 15.3	0.928
Male sex, n (%)	150 (62.5)	78 (60.0)	72 (65.5)	0.231
BMI (kg/m^2)	23.1 ± 4.3	23.0 ± 4.7	23.1 ± 3.7	0.850
SBP (mmHg)	112.5 ± 23.9	107.3 ± 22.6	118.6 ± 24.2	<0.001
DBP (mmHg)	64.1 ± 15.2	61.9 ± 14.1	66.8 ± 16.1	0.013
MAP (mmHg)	80.2 ± 16.0	77.0 ± 15.1	84.0 ± 16.3	0.001
MAP < 65 mmHg, n (%)	45 (18.8)	32 (24.6)	13 (11.8)	0.008
Heart rate (per min)	107.2 ± 24.0	110.7 ± 22.5	103.1 ± 25.2	0.015
Comorbidity disease				
Hypertension, n (%)	128 (53.3)	65 (50.0)	47 (42.7)	0.160
Diabetes mellitus, n (%)	89 (37.1)	43 (33.1)	46 (41.8)	0.103
CHF, n (%)	15 (6.3)	9 (6.9)	6 (5.5)	0.423
COPD, n (%)	4 (1.7)	2 (1.8)	2 (1.5)	0.624
Age CCI	6.60 ± 2.31	6.50 ± 2.42	6.72 ± 2.18	0.468
SIRS, n (%)	199 (82.9)	114 (87.7)	85 (77.3)	0.025
Sepsis, n (%)	75 (31.3)	42 (32.3)	33 (30.0)	0.404
Amount of 1-h UO (mL)	27.2 ± 56.8	26.6 ± 60.1	27.8 ± 52.9	0.879
APACHE II score	26.1 ± 6.8	28.9 ± 6.2	22.9 ± 6.0	<0.001
SOFA score	11.58 ± 3.87	12.70 ± 3.53	10.27 ± 3.86	<0.001

Data are presented as mean ± standard deviation or number (%). Abbreviations: BMI, body mass index; SBP, systolic blood pressure; DBP, diastolic blood pressure; MAP, mean arterial blood pressure; CHF, congestive heart failure; COPD, chronic obstructive heart failure; CCI, Charlson comorbidity index; SIRS, systemic inflammatory response syndrome; UO, urine output.

When we divided these patients into two groups (early mortality vs. 7-day survival past CRRT initiation), 138 (54.2%) died within seven days following the start of CRRT, and 110 (45.8%) survived more than seven days following CRRT initiation. There were no significant differences in age, sex distribution, BMI, the prevalence of underlying diseases, CCI, or 1-h urine volume output at baseline between the two groups. The proportion of patients diagnosed with sepsis was also not significantly different between the two groups.

However, SBP, DBP, and MAP were significantly lower in the patients that exhibited early mortality following CRRT initiation compared to 7-day survivors. Additionally, heart rate and APACHE II and SOFA scores were significantly higher in the early mortality group compared to those of 7-day survivors. Finally, we observed that a higher proportion of patients suffered from SIRS in the early mortality group compared to the 7-day survivor group.

Table 2 shows laboratory data of the patients at baseline. The mean white blood cell count was 13,100/μL; the mean hemoglobin was 9.4 ± 2.1 g/dL; and serum sodium, potassium, and bilirubin levels were 138.9 ± 7.3, 4.5 ± 1.0, and 2.8 ± 4.9 mEq/L, respectively. Additionally, the mean aspartate transaminase (AST) and alanine transaminase (ALT) levels were 401.8 ± 1157.2 and 158.8 ± 575.5 IU/L, respectively, and the mean eGFR was 22.7 ± 17.1 ml/min/1.73 m^2. The mean arterial pH was 7.29 ± 0.13, and the base excess was -7.74 ± 7.10 mmol/L. When these data were compared between the early mortality and the 7-day survivor groups, serum phosphate level was significantly higher, while arterial pH was significantly lower in the early mortality group compared to the survivor group. Moreover, there was a higher proportion of patients with pH < 7.35 in the early mortality group than in the survivor group, and base excess was lower (base excess = -8.88) in the early mortality group compared to the survivor group (base excess = -6.43). Meanwhile, there was no difference in the proportion of patients with $PaO_2/FiO_2 \leq 300$ mmHg between groups. The baseline characteristics and laboratory findings of patients with very early mortality were additionally described in Supplementary Materials (Tables S1 and S2).

Table 2. Baseline laboratory data of study patients.

Variables	Total	7-Day Mortality	7-Day Survivors	p Value
	(n = 240, 100%)	(n = 130, 54.2%)	(n = 110, 45.8%)	
WBC (10^3/μL)	13.1 ± 12.3	14.1 ± 15.5	11.9 ± 7.1	0.147
Hemoglobin (g/dL)	9.4 ± 2.1	9.5 ± 2.3	9.4 ± 1.9	0.892
Platelet (10^3/μL)	127.8 ± 86.5	127.9 ± 89.1	127.6 ± 83.8	0.980
Sodium (mEq/L)	138.9 ± 7.3	139.6 ± 7.9	138.1 ± 6.4	0.119
Potassium (mEq/L)	4.5 ± 1.0	4.6 ± 1.0	4.5 ± 0.9	0.289
Calcium (mg/dL)	7.8 ± 1.3	7.7 ± 1.2	7.8 ± 1.4	0.669
Phosphate (mg/dL)	5.5 ± 2.9	5.9 ± 3.2	5.0 ± 2.5	0.021
Bilirubin, total (mg/dL)	2.8 ± 4.9	2.9 ± 4.9	2.6 ± 4.8	0.568
AST (IU/L)	401.8 ± 1157.2	416.8 ± 1012.7	384.5 ± 1308.8	0.831
ALT (IU/L)	185.8 ± 575.5	199.1 ± 473.4	170.6 ± 675.7	0.706
eGFR (ml/min/1.73 m^2)	22.7 ± 17.1	23.7 ± 16.2	21.4 ± 18.1	0.300
pH	7.29 ± 0.13	7.25 ± 0.12	7.33 ± 0.12	<0.001
pH < 0.35, n (%)	164 (68.3)	107 (82.3)	57 (51.8)	<0.001
BE (mmol/L)	-7.75 ± 7.10	-8.88 ± 6.64	-6.43 ± 7.43	0.008
$PaO_2/FiO_2 < 300$	188 (78.3)	106 (81.5)	82 (74.5)	0.125

Data are presented as mean $\pm$ standard deviation or number (%). Abbreviations: WBC, whole blood cell; AST, aspartate aminotransferase; ALT, alanine aminotransferase; eGFR, estimated glomerular filtration rate; BE, base excess.

3.2. Factors Associated with Early Mortality

In this study, 162 patients (67.5%) died in the 28 days following CRRT initiation, and most of those deaths occurred in the early period following CRRT initiation (Figure 1). Specifically, 130 patients (80.2%) died within seven days following CRRT initiation, with 54 of those patients dying within 24 h following CRRT initiation.

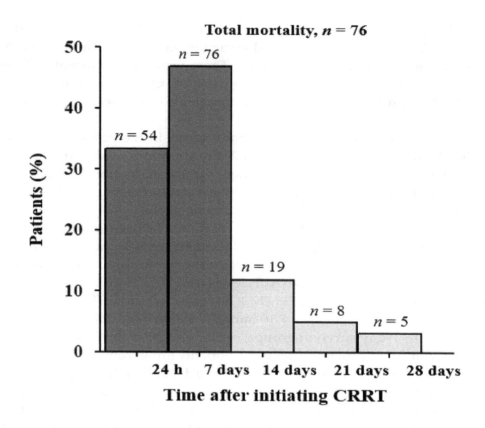

Figure 1. Mortality rate according to time after continuous renal replacement therapy (CRRT) initiation.

By univariate logistic regression analysis, patients with MAP < 65 mmHg and SIRS had an odds ratio (OR) of 2.436 (95% CI; 1.206–4.922, p = 0.013) and OR of 2.096 (95% CI; 1.054–4.168, p = 0.035) for an increased risk of early mortality, compared to patients with MAP > 65 mmHg, and an absence of SIRS. Moreover, a 1-SD increase of serum phosphate was significantly associated with an increased risk of early mortality (OR = 1.393, 95% CI (1.044–1.858), p = 0.024), and a 1-SD increase in SOFA score was also significantly associated with an increased incidence of early mortality (OR = 1.992, 95% CI (1.488–2.668), p < 0.001). Finally, the patients with pH < 7.35 also had a higher risk of early mortality compared to those with pH > 7.35 (OR = 4.326, 95% CI (2.409–7.768), p < 0.001). Importantly, after adjustment for demographic factors and other factors found to associate by univariate analysis with early mortality, increased SOFA score, low MAP (<65 mmHg), and low arterial pH (<7.35) all remained significantly associated with an increased risk of early mortality (SOFA score; OR = 1.758, 95% CI (1.282–2.412), p < 0.001, low MAP; OR = 2.771, 95% CI (1.213–6.327), p = 0.016, and low pH; OR = 3.067, 95% CI (1.593–5.903), p = 0.001) (Table 3). With consideration for overlapping parts between MAP, SIRS, and SOFA scores, additional multivariate regression analyses were performed by adjusting one of these three parameters to add to the other variables. As a result, SIRS showed a loss of significance, even in the analysis, without adjustment with MAP and SOFA scores.

We also performed multivariate logistic regression analyses to assess factors associated with very early mortality, to determine the similarities and differences between those factors related to the increased early mortality. We found that an increased serum sodium level, phosphate level, SOFA score, and low MAP (<65 mmHg) were all significantly associated with increased very early mortality, even after multivariate adjustment, as described previously (Table 4). Therefore, low MAP and increased SOFA scores are associated with an increased risk of both early and very early mortality.

Table 3. Logistic regression analysis for early mortality *.

Factors	Univariate		Multivariate	
	OR (95% CI)	p Value	OR (95% CI)	p Value
Age (per 1-SD increase)	1.012 (0.785−1.305)	0.928	1.079 (0.803−1.450)	0.614
Male (versus Female)	0.792 (0.467−1.341)	0.385	0.877 (0.477−1.610)	0.671
BMI (per 1-SD increase)	0.976 (0.757−1.259)	0.976	0.929 (0.695−1.240)	0.616
MAP < 65 mmHg (versus MAP ≥ 65 mmHg)	2.436 (1.206−4.922)	0.013	2.771 (1.213−6.327)	0.016
SIRS (versus no SIRS)	2.096 (1.054−4.168)	0.035	1.602 (0.717−3.583)	0.251
Sepsis (versus no sepsis)	0.898 (0.519−1.555)	0.898	-	
Phosphate (per 1-SD increase)	1.393 (1.044−1.858)	0.024	1.197 (0.869−1.649)	0.270
pH < 7.35 (versus pH ≥ 7.35)	4.326 (2.409−7.768)	<0.001	3.067 (1.593−5.903)	0.001
SOFA score (per 1-SD increase)	1.992 (1.488−2.668)	<0.001	1.758 (1.282−2.412)	<0.001

* The early mortality was defined by the death within seven days after CRRT initiation. Abbreviations: OR, odds ratio; CI, confidential interval; SD, standard deviation; BMI, body mass index; MAP, mean arterial blood pressure; SIRS, systemic inflammatory response syndrome

Table 4. Logistic regression analysis for very early mortality *.

Factors	Univariate		Multivariate	
	OR (95% CI)	p Value	OR (95% CI)	p Value
Age (per 1-SD increase)	1.069 (0.785−1.456)	0.672	1.363 (0.909−2.043)	0.134
Male (versus female)	0.632 (0.337−1.151)	0.131	0.707 (0.327−1.532)	0.380
BMI (per 1-SD increase)	1.038 (0.768−1.402)	0.810	0.956 (0.657−1.391)	0.816
Diabetes mellitus (versus non-diabetes)	0.354 (0.172−0.730)	0.005	0.456 (0.189−1.101)	0.081
MAP < 65 mmHg (versus MAP ≥ 65 mmHg)	4.295 (2.144−8.607)	<0.001	8.498 (3.379−21.375)	<0.001
SIRS (versus no SIRS)	2.352 (0.874−6.326)	0.090	-	-
Sepsis (versus no sepsis)	1.103 (0.570−2.136)	0.770	-	-
Sodium (per 1-SD increase)	1.458 (1.202−1.769)	<0.001	1.588 (1.241−2.031)	<0.001
Phosphate (per 1-SD increase)	1.632 (1.207−2.207)	0.001	1.669 (1.149−2.424)	0.007
pH < 7.35 (versus pH ≥ 7.35)	4.828 (1.965−11.863)	0.001	2.395 (0.860−6.675)	0.095
SOFA score (per 1-SD increase)	1.895 (1.329−2.702)	<0.001	1.691 (1.049−2.725)	0.031

* Very early mortality was defined by death within 24 h after CRRT initiation. Abbreviations: OR, odds ratio; CI, confidential interval; SD, standard deviation; BMI, body mass index; MAP, mean arterial blood pressure; SIRS, systemic inflammatory response syndrome

4. Discussion

This study demonstrated that early mortality within seven days following CRRT initiation was high in critically ill patients undergoing CRRT (54.2%). Moreover, MAP < 65 mmHg, arterial pH < 7.35, and high SOFA score at CRRT initiation significantly associated with increased risk of early mortality in these patients.

When we stratified the mortality rate of critically ill patients undergoing CRRT initiation, 80.2% of the total 162 patients that died during the 28-day follow-up period died within seven days following CRRT initiation, and 33.3% (54/162 patients) died within 24 h following CRRT initiation. A smaller percentage of patients, 19.8% (32/162 patients), died between eight and 28 days following CRRT initiation. Thus, we assessed which factors were associated with early or very early mortality in this group.

There are many studies assessing prognostic factors for the mortality risk of CRRT to predict and prevent poor clinical outcomes [13–22]. However, most of these studies assessed mortality beyond 28 days post-initiation of CRRT. Only a few studies have been conducted to investigate early mortality among critically ill patients undergoing CRRT [27,28]. In contrast, clinicians are often challenged to determine the benefit of CRRT, and it is difficult to identify patients that are more likely to demonstrate poor clinical outcomes, despite active treatment with CRRT to make the best decision for patients requiring RRT.

In this study, MAP < 65 mmHg, arterial pH < 7.35, and high SOFA score at CRRT initiation were risk factors for early mortality. Additionally, MAP < 65 mmHg, increased serum sodium, and phosphate levels, and high SOFA score at CRRT initiation, were significantly associated with an increased rate of very early mortality. Above these factors can be found in the other studies which were performed for the 28-, 60-, or 90-day mortality, which means that such factors may be more likely to be issued for early mortality.

CRRT treatment is primarily considered for patients in critical condition, who are hemodynamically unstable, and/or who suffer from increased intracranial pressure due to acute brain injury [29,30]; thus, the mortality rate of patients requiring CRRT is generally high. The mortality rate within hours or days following CRRT initiation is particularly high, mainly due to the poor condition of the patients at the initiation of CRRT. Specifically, Passos et al. [31] demonstrated a 7-day mortality of 45.0% (84/186 patients), and Prasad et al. [27] reported that 16.0% (17/106 patients) died within 24 h after the start of CRRT. In this study, 22.5% (54/240 patients) died within 24 h, and 54.2% (130/240 patients) died within seven days following CRRT initiation. Moreover, 80.2% of the total number of patients that died within the 28-day period (130/162 patients) died within 7 days following CRRT initiation. To our knowledge, this is the first study comparing the mortality rate at different time periods following CRRT initiation, and these results suggest that a majority of patients undergoing CRRT die within seven days following initiation. However, a prospective cohort study with a larger population should be performed to confirm these results.

AKI, combined with cardiovascular instability, fluid overload, cerebral edema, and high fluid requirement, generally indicates a need for CRRT [32,33]. In addition, the need to eliminate inflammatory mediators, remove fluid, or eliminate other endogenous toxic solutes have been presented as non-renal reasons to initiate CRRT [34]. In our study, several factors were found to be associated with early or very early mortality in patients undergoing CRRT. MAP is a hemodynamic parameter, and maintaining MAP $\geq$ 65 mmHg is recommended in the management of patients with septic shock, a condition for which CRRT is a common treatment [35]. In addition, a SOFA score represents a severity parameter and it is a widely accepted prognostic factor for critically ill patients [36,37]. Several studies report a significant association between a high SOFA score at CRRT initiation, and increased mortality [38–40]. Arterial pH is one of the variables that is considered in the APACHE II score, which was designed to measure the disease severity and the risk of death in critically ill patients, and several studies have demonstrated that arterial pH is associated with increased mortality in patients undergoing CRRT [41–43]. In addition, previous studies have reported that hypernatremia and hyperphosphatemia are common in critically ill patients, and they were associated with increased morbidity and mortality [44–47]. The factors identified in this study could be predictable through previous studies; however, this study has significance because it reaffirms the clinical importance of these factors by assessing the association with early death showing high mortality rate. The results presented here do not indicate the futility of CRRT treatment for patients with lower MAP, lower pH, higher serum sodium or phosphate, or high SOFA score. However, these results could be useful in predicting the prognosis of critically ill patients after CRRT initiation.

There are some limitations to our study. First, this was a single center study with a relatively small sample size, so we cannot rule out selection bias, and these results may not be generalizable to other populations. Therefore, a future multiple-center study with a larger sample size is warranted to verify factors that are associated with early mortality in critically ill patients undergoing CRRT. Second, because of the inherent limitations of a retrospective study, other potential factors associated with early death in critically ill patients, such as causes of CRRT initiation or primary diagnosis at admission may not have been assessed. Third, we investigated mortality events based on arbitrarily stratified time periods, such as within 24 h, 7 days, or 28 days following CRRT initiation, and defined 'early mortality' or 'very early mortality' discretionally. However, several studies for mortality of the patients undergoing CRRT have used 28-days mortality as the end-point and there have been also some studies for 24-hour and 7-day mortality, so that these timeframes are not without precedent. Moreover, in this study, we found that the highest mortality following CRRT occurred in the early timeframe following CRRT initiation. Lastly, this observational study does not allow us to conclude a causal relationship, and it only demonstrates the associations between clinical factors and early or very early mortality in patients undergoing CRRT treatment.

5. Conclusions

In conclusion, we found that the early mortality rate within seven days following CRRT initiation was very high in this cohort of critically ill patients undergoing CRRT. Moreover, low MAP, low arterial pH, and high SOFA score at CRRT initiation were associated with early mortality in these patients. Although these factors may not be used as determinants in deciding whether or not CRRT should be initiated in critically ill patients, they may be useful in predicting early or very early mortality despite active treatment with CRRT.

Author Contributions: D.-R.R. originated the concept for this study. K.B.C. and D.-H.K. contributed to the study design and coordination of the study. Y.K.K. and H.J.O. drafted the manuscript and conducted the analyses. D.K. and S.-J.K. maintained the patient database and assisted in data analysis. All authors read and approved final manuscript.

References

1.   Liangos, O.; Wald, R.; O'Bell, J.W.; Price, L.; Pereira, B.J.; Jaber, B.L. Epidemiology and outcomes of acute renal failure in hospitalized patients: A national survey. *Clin. J. Am. Soc. Nephrol.* **2006**, *1*, 43–51. [CrossRef] [PubMed]

2.   Uchino, S.; Kellum, J.A.; Bellomo, R.; Doig, G.S.; Morimatsu, H.; Morgera, S.; Schetz, M.; Tan, I.; Bouman, C.; Macedo, E.; et al. Acute renal failure in critically ill patients: A multinational, multicenter study. *JAMA* **2005**, *294*, 813–818. [CrossRef] [PubMed]

3.   Bagshaw, S.M.; Laupland, K.B.; Doig, C.J.; Mortis, G.; Fick, G.H.; Mucenski, M.; Godinez-Luna, T.; Svenson, L.W.; Rosenal, T. Prognosis for long-term survival and renal recovery in critically ill patients with severe acute renal failure: A population-based study. *Crit. Care* **2005**, *9*, R700. [CrossRef] [PubMed]

4.   Truche, A.S.; Darmon, M.; Bailly, S.; Clec'h, C.; Dupuis, C.; Misset, B.; Azoulay, E.; Schwebel, C.; Bouadma, L.; Kallel, H.; et al. Continuous renal replacement therapy versus intermittent hemodialysis in intensive care patients: Impact on mortality and renal recovery. *Intensiv. Care Med.* **2016**, *42*, 1408–1417. [CrossRef] [PubMed]

5.   Davenport, A.; Will, E.J.; Davidson, A.M. Improved cardiovascular stability during continuous modes of renal replacement therapy in critically ill patients with acute hepatic and renal failure. *Crit. Care Med.* **1993**, *21*, 328–338. [CrossRef] [PubMed]

6.   Kruczynski, K.; Irvine-Bird, K.; Toffelmire, E.B.; Morton, A.R. A comparison of continuous arteriovenous hemofiltration and intermittent hemodialysis in acute renal failure patients in the intensive care unit. *ASAIO* **1993**, *39*, M778–M781.

7.   Srisawat, N.; Lawsin, L.; Uchino, S.; Bellomo, R.; Kellum, J.A. Cost of acute renal replacement therapy in the intensive care unit: Results from The Beginning and Ending Supportive Therapy for the Kidney (BEST Kidney) study. *Crit. Care* **2010**, *14*, R46. [CrossRef] [PubMed]

8.   Farese, S.; Jakob, S.M.; Kalicki, R.; Frey, F.J.; Uehlinger, D.E. Treatment of acute renal failure in the intensive care unit: Lower costs by intermittent dialysis than continuous venovenous hemodiafiltration. *Artif. Organs* **2009**, *33*, 634–640. [CrossRef] [PubMed]

9.   Brivet, F.G.; Kleinknecht, D.J.; Loirat, P.; Landais, P.J. Acute renal failure in intensive care units—Causes, outcome, and prognostic factors of hospital mortality: A prospective, multicenter study. *Crit. Care Med.* **1996**, *24*, 192–198. [CrossRef] [PubMed]

10.   Metnitz, P.G.; Krenn, C.G.; Steltzer, H.; Lang, T.; Ploder, J.; Lenz, K.; Le Gall, J.R.; Druml, W. Effect of acute renal failure requiring renal replacement therapy on outcome in critically ill patients. *Crit. Care Med.* **2002**, *30*, 2051–2058. [CrossRef] [PubMed]

11.   Cho, K.C.; Himmelfarb, J.; Paganini, E.; Ikizler, T.A.; Soroko, S.H.; Mehta, R.L.; Chertow, G.M. Survival by dialysis modality in critically ill patients with acute kidney injury. *J. Am. Soc. Nephrol.* **2006**, *17*, 3132–3138. [CrossRef] [PubMed]

12.   Uchino, S.; Bellomo, R.; Morimatsu, H.; Morgera, S.; Schetz, M.; Tan, I.; Bouman, C.; Macedo, E.; Gibney, N.; Tolwani, A.; et al. Continuous renal replacement therapy: A worldwide practice survey. *Intensiv. Care Med.*

2007, *33*, 1563–1570. [CrossRef] [PubMed]

13. Sasaki, S.; Gando, S.; Kobayashi, S.; Nanzaki, S.; Ushitani, T.; Morimoto, Y.; Demmotsu, O. Predictors of mortality in patients treated with continuous hemodiafiltration for acute renal failure in an intensive care setting. *ASAIO* **2001**, *47*, 86–91. [CrossRef]

14. Wald, R.; Deshpande, R.; Bell, C.M.; Bargman, J.M. Survival to discharge among patients treated with continuous renal replacement therapy. *Hemod. Int.* **2006**, *10*, 82–87. [CrossRef] [PubMed]

15. Oh, H.J.; Park, J.T.; Kim, J.K.; Yoo, D.E.; Kim, S.J.; Han, S.H.; Kang, S.W.; Choi, K.H.; Yoo, T.H. Red blood cell distribution width is an independent predictor of mortality in acute kidney injury patients treated with continuous renal replacement therapy. *Nephrol. Dial. Transplant.* **2011**, *27*, 589–594. [CrossRef] [PubMed]

16. Kellum, J.A.; Angus, D.C.; Johnson, J.P.; Leblanc, M.; Griffin, M.; Ramakrishnan, N.; Linde-Zwirble, W.T. Continuous versus intermittent renal replacement therapy: A meta-analysis. *Intensiv. Care Med.* **2002**, *28*, 29–37. [CrossRef] [PubMed]

17. Soubrier, S.; Leroy, O.; Devos, P.; Nseir, S.; Georges, H.; d'Escrivan, T.; Guery, B. Epidemiology and prognostic factors of critically ill patients treated with hemodiafiltration. *J. Crit. Care* **2006**, *21*, 66–72. [CrossRef] [PubMed]

18. Kim, E.S.; Ham, Y.R.; Jang, W.I.; Jung, J.Y.; Kwon, O.K.; Chung, S.; Choi, D.E.; Na, K.R.; Lee, K.W.; Shin, Y.T. Prognostic factors of acute renal failure patients treated with continuous renal replacement therapy. *Korean J. Nephrol.* **2010**, *29*, 54–63.

19. Gjyzaria, A.; Muzi, L.; Morabito, S. Continuous renal replacement therapy for acute renal failure in critically ill patients and early predictive factors. *BANTAO* **2007**, *5*, 58–60.

20. Lee, S.H.; Kwon, S.K.; Kim, H.Y. Outcome and prognosis in patients receiving continuous renal replacement therapy. *Korean J. Nephrol.* **2010**, *29*, 434–440.

21. Vaara, S.T.; Korhonen, A.M.; Kaukonen, K.M.; Nisula, S.; Inkinen, O.; Hoppu, S.; Laurila, J.J.; Mildh, L.; Reinikainen, M.; Lund, V.; et al. Fluid overload is associated with an increased risk for 90-day mortality in critically ill patients with renal replacement therapy: Data from the prospective FINNAKI study. *Crit. Care* **2012**, *16*, R197. [CrossRef] [PubMed]

22. Kashani, K.; Thongprayoon, C.; Cheungpasitporn, W.; Iacovella, G.M.; Akhoundi, A.; Albright, R.C. Association between mortality and replacement solution bicarbonate concentration in continuous renal replacement therapy: A propensity-matched cohort study. *PLoS ONE* **2017**, *12*, e0185064. [CrossRef] [PubMed]

23. Charlson, M.E.; Pompei, P.; Ales, K.L.; MacKenzie, C.R. A new method of classifying prognostic comorbidity in longitudinal studies: Development and validation. *J. Chronic Dis.* **1987**, *40*, 373–383. [CrossRef]

24. Levey, A.S.; Bosch, J.P.; Lewis, J.B.; Greene, T.; Rogers, N.; Roth, D. A more accurate method to estimate glomerular filtration rate from serum creatinine: A new prediction equation. *Ann. Intern. Med.* **1999**, *130*, 461–470. [CrossRef] [PubMed]

25. Bone, R.C.; Balk, R.A.; Cerra, F.B.; Dellinger, R.P.; Fein, A.M.; Knaus, W.A.; Schein, R.M.; Sibbald, W.J. Definitions for sepsis and organ failure and guidelines for the use of innovative therapies in sepsis. *Chest* **1992**, *101*, 1644–1655. [CrossRef] [PubMed]

26. Zahar, J.R.; Timsit, J.F.; Garrouste-Orgeas, M.; Français, A.; Vesin, A.; Descorps-Declere, A.; Dubois, Y.; Souweine, B.; Haouache, H.; Goldgran-Toledano, D.; et al. Outcomes in severe sepsis and patients with septic shock: Pathogen species and infection sites are not associated with mortality. *Crit. Care Med.* **2011**, *39*, 1886–1895. [CrossRef] [PubMed]

27. Prasad, B.; Urbanski, M.; Ferguson, T.W.; Karreman, E.; Tangri, N. Early mortality on continuous renal replacement therapy (CRRT): The prairie CRRT study. *Can. J. Kidney Health Dis.* **2016**, *3*, 36. [CrossRef] [PubMed]

28. Gonzalez, C.A.; Pinto, J.L.; Orozco, V.; Contreras, K.; Garcia, P.; Rodriguez, P.; Patiño, J.; Echeverri, J. Early mortality risk factors at the beginning of continuous renal replacement therapy for acute kidney injury. *Cogent Med.* **2018**, *5*, 1407485. [CrossRef]

29. Macedo, E.; Mehta, R.L. Continuous dialysis therapies: Core curriculum 2016. *Am. J. Kidney Dis.* **2016**, *68*, 645–657. [CrossRef] [PubMed]

30. Ronco, C. Continuous renal replacement therapies for the treatment of acute renal failure in intensive care patients. *Clin. Nephrol.* **1993**, *40*, 187–198. [PubMed]

31. Da Hora Passos, R.; Ramos, J.G.; Mendonça, E.J.; Miranda, E.A.; Dutra, F.R.; Coelho, M.F.; Pedroza, A.C.; Correia, L.C.; Batista, P.B.; Macedo, E.; et al. A clinical score to predict mortality in septic acute kidney injury

patients requiring continuous renal replacement therapy: The HELENICC score. *BMC Anesthesiol.* **2017**, *17*, 21. [CrossRef] [PubMed]

32. Schetz, M. Classical and alternative indications for continuous renal replacement therapy. *Kidney Int.* **1998**, *S66*, S129.

33. Davenport, A. *Renal Replacement Therapy for the Patient with Acute Traumatic Brain Injury and Severe Acute Kidney Injury, in Acute Kidney Injury*; Karger Publishers: Basel, Switzerland, 2007; pp. 333–339.

34. Schetz, M. Non-renal indications for continuous renal replacement therapy. *Kidney Int.* **1999**, *56*, S88–S94. [CrossRef]

35. Rhodes, A.; Evans, L.E.; Alhazzani, W.; Levy, M.M.; Antonelli, M.; Ferrer, R.; Kumar, A.; Sevransky, J.E.; Sprung, C.L.; Nunnally, M.E.; et al. Surviving sepsis campaign: International guidelines for management of sepsis and septic shock: 2016. *Intensiv. Care Med.* **2017**, *43*, 304–377. [CrossRef] [PubMed]

36. Oppert, M.; Engel, C.; Brunkhorst, F.M.; Bogatsch, H.; Reinhart, K.; Frei, U.; Eckardt, K.U.; Loeffler, M.; John, S. Acute renal failure in patients with severe sepsis and septic shock—A significant independent risk factor for mortality: Results from the German Prevalence Study. *Nephrol. Dial. Transplant.* **2007**, *23*, 904–909. [CrossRef] [PubMed]

37. Ferreira, F.L.; Bota, D.P.; Bross, A.; Mélot, C.; Vincent, J.L. Serial evaluation of the SOFA score to predict outcome in critically ill patients. *JAMA* **2001**, *286*, 1754–1758. [CrossRef] [PubMed]

38. Kawarazaki, H.; Uchino, S.; Tokuhira, N.; Ohnuma, T.; Namba, Y.; Katayama, S.; Toki, N.; Takeda, K.; Yasuda, H.; Izawa, J.; et al. Who may not benefit from continuous renal replacement therapy in acute kidney injury? *Hemodial. Int.* **2013**, *17*, 624–632. [CrossRef] [PubMed]

39. Rhee, H.; Jang, K.S.; Park, J.M.; Kang, J.S.; Hwang, N.K.; Kim, I.Y.; Song, S.H.; Seong, E.Y.; Lee, D.W.; Lee, S.B.; et al. Short-and long-term mortality rates of elderly acute kidney injury patients who underwent continuous renal replacement therapy. *PLoS ONE* **2016**, *11*, e0167067. [CrossRef] [PubMed]

40. Pistolesi, V.; Di Napoli, A.; Fiaccadori, E.; Zeppilli, L.; Polistena, F.; Sacco, M.I.; Regolisti, G.; Tritapepe, L.; Pierucci, A.; Morabito, S. Severe acute kidney injury following cardiac surgery: Short-term outcomes in patients undergoing continuous renal replacement therapy (CRRT). *J. Nephrol.* **2016**, *29*, 229–239. [CrossRef] [PubMed]

41. Soni, S.S.; Nagarik, A.P.; Adikey, G.K.; Raman, A. Using continuous renal replacement therapy to manage patients of shock and acute renal failure. *J. Emerg. Trauma Shock* **2009**, *2*, 19. [PubMed]

42. Yoon, J.; Kim, Y.; Yim, H.; Cho, Y.S.; Kym, D.; Hur, J.; Chun, W.; Yang, H.T. Analysis of prognostic factors for acute kidney injury with continuous renal replacement therapy in severely burned patients. *Burns* **2017**, *43*, 1418–1426. [CrossRef] [PubMed]

43. Bae, W.K.; Lim, D.H.; Jeong, J.M.; Jung, H.Y.; Kim, S.K.; Park, J.W.; Bae, E.H.; Ma, S.K.; Kim, S.W.; Kim, N.H.; et al. Continuous renal replacement therapy for the treatment of acute kidney injury. *Korean J. Intern. Med.* **2008**, *23*, 58. [CrossRef] [PubMed]

44. Han, S.S.; Bae, E.; Kim, D.K.; Kim, Y.S.; Han, J.S.; Joo, K.W. Dysnatremia, its correction, and mortality in patients undergoing continuous renal replacement therapy: A prospective observational study. *BMC Nephrol.* **2016**, *17*, 2. [CrossRef] [PubMed]

45. Lindner, G.; Funk, G.C.; Schwarz, C.; Kneidinger, N.; Kaider, A.; Schneeweiss, B.; Kramer, L.; Druml, W. Hypernatremia in the critically ill is an independent risk factor for mortality. *Am. J. Kidney Dis.* **2007**, *50*, 952–957. [CrossRef] [PubMed]

46. Jung, S.Y.; Kwon, J.; Park, S.; Jhee, J.H.; Yun, H.R.; Kim, H.; Kee, Y.K.; Yoon, C.Y.; Chang, T.I.; Kang, E.W.; et al. Phosphate is a potential biomarker of disease severity and predicts adverse outcomes in acute kidney injury patients undergoing continuous renal replacement therapy. *PLoS ONE* **2018**, *13*, e0191290. [CrossRef] [PubMed]

47. Kraft, M.D.; Btaiche, I.F.; Sacks, G.S.; Kudsk, K.A. Treatment of electrolyte disorders in adult patients in the intensive care unit. *Am. J. Health-Syst. Pharm.* **2005**, *62*, 1663–1682. [CrossRef] [PubMed]

8

Acute Kidney Injury after Lung Transplantation

**Ploypin Lertjitbanjong [1], Charat Thongprayoon [2], Wisit Cheungpasitporn [3,*],
Oisín A. O'Corragain [4], Narat Srivali [5], Tarun Bathini [6], Kanramon Watthanasuntorn [1],
Narothama Reddy Aeddula [7], Sohail Abdul Salim [3], Patompong Ungprasert [8], Erin A. Gillaspie [9],
Karn Wijarnpreecha [10], Michael A. Mao [10] and Wisit Kaewput [11,*]**

[1]   Department of Internal Medicine, Bassett Medical Center, Cooperstown, NY 13326, USA;
       ploypinlert@gmail.com (P.L.); kanramon@gmail.com (K.W.)
[2]   Division of Nephrology and Hypertension, Mayo Clinic, Rochester, MN 55905, USA;
       charat.thongprayoon@gmail.com
[3]   Division of Nephrology, Department of Medicine, University of Mississippi Medical Center, Jackson,
       MS 39216, USA; sohail3553@gmail.com
[4]   Department of Thoracic Medicine and Surgery, Temple University Hospital, Philadelphia, PA 19140, USA;
       109426469@umail.ucc.ie
[5]   Department of Internal Medicine, St. Agnes Hospital, Baltimore, MD 21229, USA; nsrivali@gmail.com
[6]   Department of Internal Medicine, University of Arizona, Tucson, AZ 85721, USA; tarunjacobb@gmail.com
[7]   Department of Medicine, Deaconess Health System, Evansville, IN 47747, USA; dr.anreddy@gmail.com
[8]   Cleveland Clinic Lerner College of Medicine of Case Western Reserve University, Cleveland Clinic,
       Cleveland, OH 44195, USA; p.ungprasert@gmail.com
[9]   Department of Thoracic Surgery, Vanderbilt University Medical Center, Nashville, TN 37212, USA;
       erin.a.gillaspie@vumc.org
[10]   Department of Medicine, Mayo Clinic, Jacksonville, FL 32224, USA; dr.karn.wi@gmail.com (K.W.);
       mao.michael@mayo.edu (M.A.M.)
[11]   Department of Military and Community Medicine, Phramongkutklao College of Medicine, Bangkok 10400,
       Thailand
*   Correspondence: wcheungpasitporn@gmail.com (W.C.); wisitnephro@gmail.com (W.K.);

Abstract: Background: Lung transplantation has been increasingly performed worldwide and is considered an effective therapy for patients with various causes of end-stage lung diseases. We performed a systematic review to assess the incidence and impact of acute kidney injury (AKI) and severe AKI requiring renal replacement therapy (RRT) in patients after lung transplantation. Methods: A literature search was conducted utilizing Ovid MEDLINE, EMBASE, and Cochrane Database from inception through June 2019. We included studies that evaluated the incidence of AKI, severe AKI requiring RRT, and mortality risk of AKI among patients after lung transplantation. Pooled incidence and odds ratios (ORs) with 95% confidence interval (CI) were obtained using random-effects meta-analysis. The protocol for this meta-analysis is registered with PROSPERO (International Prospective Register of Systematic Reviews; no. CRD42019134095). Results: A total of 26 cohort studies with a total of 40,592 patients after lung transplantation were enrolled. Overall, the pooled estimated incidence rates of AKI (by standard AKI definitions) and severe AKI requiring RRT following lung transplantation were 52.5% (95% CI: 45.8–59.1%) and 9.3% (95% CI: 7.6–11.4%). Meta-regression analysis demonstrated that the year of study did not significantly affect the incidence of AKI ($p = 0.22$) and severe AKI requiring RRT ($p = 0.68$). The pooled ORs of in-hospital mortality in patients after lung transplantation with AKI and severe AKI requiring RRT were 2.75 (95% CI, 1.18–6.41) and 10.89 (95% CI, 5.03–23.58). At five years, the pooled ORs of mortality among patients after lung transplantation with AKI and severe AKI requiring RRT were 1.47 (95% CI, 1.11–1.94) and 4.79 (95% CI, 3.58–6.40), respectively. Conclusion: The overall estimated incidence rates of AKI and severe AKI requiring RRT in patients after lung transplantation are 52.5% and 9.3%, respectively. Despite advances in therapy, the incidence of AKI in patients after lung transplantation does not seem to have decreased. In addition, AKI after lung transplantation is significantly associated with reduced short-term and long-term survival.

Keywords: acute kidney injury; incidence; lung transplantation; transplantation; epidemiology; meta-analysis

1. Introduction

Acute kidney injury (AKI) is a complex clinical syndrome characterized by a sharp reduction in the glomerular filtration rate (GFR) followed by elevated serum creatinine or oliguria, and is associated with various etiologies and pathophysiological pathways. AKI is a major global health problem with a steadily increasing incidence in recent years [1–3]. The global burden of AKI is 13.3 million cases per year and is associated with significant mortality, resulting in 1.4 million deaths per year [4–6]. Mortality rates from AKI range from 16% to 50% according to the stage and vary widely according to etiology and patient comorbidities [7,8]. Those who survive the AKI are at increased risk for hypertension and progressive chronic kidney disease (CKD), including end-stage kidney disease (ESKD) [9].

Since the first human lung transplant was performed in 1963, almost 55,000 lung transplantations have been performed worldwide, now with nearly 4600 lung transplantations performed annually [10]. Up to 68% of lung transplant recipients develop AKI, which has been associated with increased one-year mortality, length of hospital stay, higher resource utilization, and related health care burden [10–22]. Though survival following lung transplantation has improved over the past few decades, morbidity and mortality related to AKI after lung transplantation and resultant progressive CKD remain relatively high and is a cause for increasing concern [16,23–25]. The incidence of AKI following lung transplantation varies widely, estimated to be as high as two-thirds of recipients, with up to 5% to 8% requiring dialysis in the initial few months post lung transplantation [11,13–15,21,24,26–29]. Differences in the definition of AKI may account for the variance of incidence of post-lung-transplant AKI [28].

Despite significant advances in lung transplantation surgical and medical practices, the epidemiology, risk factors, and mortality associated with AKI among post-lung-transplant recipients and their trends remain unclear. Therefore, we conducted a systematic review to summarize and trend the incidence of AKI (utilizing standard AKI definitions including AKIN (acute kidney injury network) [30], RIFLE (risk, injury, failure, loss of kidney function, and end-stage kidney disease) [31], and KDIGO (kidney disease: Improving global outcomes) [32] classifications) and mortality risk of AKI in lung transplant recipients.

2. Methods

2.1. Information Sources and Search Strategy

The protocol for this meta-analysis is registered with PROSPERO (International Prospective Register of Systematic Reviews (CRD42019134095)). A systematic literature search of Ovid MEDLINE, EMBASE, and the Cochrane Database from database inceptions through June 2019 was performed to summarize the incidence and impact of AKI on mortality risk among adult patients following lung transplantation. Two investigators (P.L. and C.T.) individually performed a systematic literature search utilizing the search approach that consolidated the search terms of "lung" OR "pulmonary" AND "transplant" OR "transplantation" AND "acute kidney injury" OR "acute renal failure" OR "renal replacement therapy". Detailed information on the search strategy from each database is provided in Online Supplementary Data 1. No language limitation was implemented. A manual review for conceivably-related studies employing references of the included studies was additionally performed. Grey literature was also searched for further relevant information. This systematic review was conducted following the PRISMA (Preferred Reporting Items for Systematic Reviews and Meta-Analysis) statement [33].

2.2. Study Selection

Studies were included in this meta-analysis if they were observational studies or clinical trials that provided data on incidence of AKI (utilizing standard AKI definitions including AKIN [30], RIFLE [31], and KDIGO [32] classifications), AKI requiring renal replacement therapy (RRT), and mortality risk of AKI in adult patients after lung transplantation (age ≥ 18 years old). Eligible studies needed to provide data to assess the incidence or mortality rate of AKI with 95% confidence intervals (CIs). Retrieved articles were individually examined for eligibility by the two investigators (P.L. and C.T.). Inconsistencies were discussed with the third reviewer (W.C.) and solved by common agreement. The size of the study did not limit inclusion.

2.3. Data Collection Process

A structured data collecting form was used to collect the following data from individual studies including title, name of authors, year of the study, publication year, country where the study was conducted, patient characteristics, AKI definition, incidence of AKI, incidence of severe AKI requiring RRT, and mortality risk of AKI among patients after lung transplantation.

2.4. Statistical Analysis

Comprehensive Meta-Analysis software version 3.3.070 (Biostat Inc., Englewood, NJ, USA) was used to perform meta-analysis. Adjusted point estimates of included studies were incorporated by the generic inverse variance method of DerSimonian–Laird, which assigned the weight of an individual study based on its variance [34]. Due to the probability of between-study variance, we applied a random-effects model to pool outcomes of interest, including incidence of AKI and mortality risk. Statistical heterogeneity of studies was assessed by the Cochran's Q test ($p < 0.05$ for a statistical significance) and the I^2 statistic (≤25% represents insignificant heterogeneity, 26% to 50% represents low heterogeneity, 51% to 75% represents moderate heterogeneity, and ≥75% represents high heterogeneity) [35]. The presence of publication bias was assessed by both funnel ploy and the Egger test [36].

3. Results

The search yielded a total of 1809 articles for initial screening. After removal of 714 duplicates, the titles and abstracts of 1095 articles were screened for eligibility. A total of 922 articles were excluded (due to in vitro studies, pediatric patient population, animal studies, case reports, correspondences, or review articles). A total of 173 potentially relevant studies were included for full-length article review;

147 of them were additionally excluded from the full-text review as they did not provide the outcome of interest ($n = 77$) or were not observational studies ($n = 48$), or did not use a standard AKI definition ($n = 22$).

Thus, 26 cohort studies [10,11,13,14,19,21,24,28,29,37–53] with 40,592 patients undergoing lung transplantation were identified. Figure 1 shows a flowchart outlining identification of papers for inclusion. Table 1 presents the characteristics of the included studies. The kappa for systematic searches, selection of studies and data extraction were 0.98, 0.87, and 0.98, respectively.

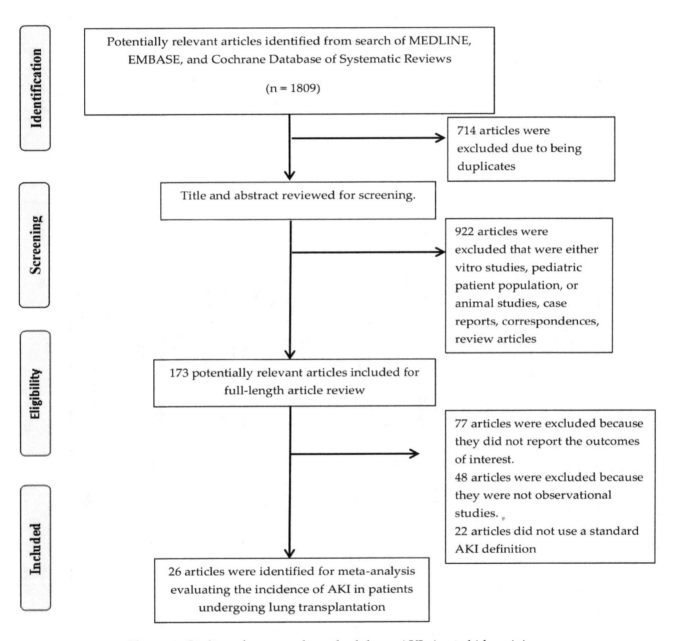

Figure 1. Outline of our search methodology. AKI, Acute kidney injury.

Table 1. Main characteristic of studies included in analysis assessing the incidence of acute kidney injury in patients after lung transplantation.

Study	Year	Country	Patients	Number	AKI Definition	AKI Incidence
Rocha et al. [13]	2005	USA	Patents underwent lung transplantation -Double 146/296 (49.3%) -COPD 134/296 (45.3%) -Cystic fibrosis 61/296 (20.6%) -Idiopathic pulmonary fibrosis 31/296 (10.5%)	296	RIFLE criteria	AKI 166/296 (56.1%) RRT 23/296 (7.8%)
Arnaoutakis et al. [11]	2011	USA	Patients underwent lung transplantation -Double 93/106 (87.7%) -COPD 33/106 (31.1%) -Idiopathic pulmonary fibrosis 22/106 (20.8%) -Cystic fibrosis 21/106 (19.8%)	106	RIFLE criteria	AKI 67/106 (63.2%) RRT 14/106 (13.2%)
Machuca et al. [37]	2011	Brazil	Patients underwent lung transplantation - Idiopathic pulmonary fibrosis 53/130 (40.8%) -COPD 52/130 (40%) -Lymphangioleiomyomatosis 8/130 (6.2%) -Cystic fibrosis 4/130 (3%)	130	Doubling of baseline serum creatinine levels	AKI 41/130 (31.5%) RRT 19/130 (14.6%)
George et al. [19]	2012	USA	Patients underwent lung transplantation from UNOS database -Double 6876/12,108 (56.8%) -COPD 4227/12,108 (34.9%) -Idiopathic pulmonary fibrosis 3369/12,108 (27.8%)	12,108	RRT	RRT 655/12,108 (5.41%)
Jacques et al. [21]	2012	Canada	Patients underwent lung transplantation -Double 85/174 (58.9%) -Emphysema 64/174 (36.8%) -Cystic fibrosis 44 /174 (25.3%) -Idiopathic pulmonary fibrosis 24/174 (13.8%)	174	RIFLE criteria	AKI 67/174 (38.5%)
Wehbe et al. [38]	2012	USA	Patients underwent lung transplantation -Double 372/657 (56.6%) -COPD 233/657 (35.5%) -Idiopathic pulmonary fibrosis 212/657 (32.3%) -Cystic fibrosis 90/657 (13.7%)	657	AKIN classification	AKI 424/657 (64.5%) RRT 40/657 (6.1%)

Table 1. *Cont.*

Study	Year	Country	Patients	Number	AKI Definition	AKI Incidence
Hennessy et al. [39]	2013	USA	Patients underwent lung transplantation -Double 98/352 (27.8%) -COPD 170/352 (48.2%) -Cystic fibrosis28/352 (8%) -Pulmonary fibrosis 53/352 (15%)	352	SCr > 3 mg/dL within 5 days after surgery	AKI 33/325 (9.4%) RRT 16/325 (4.9%)
Shigemura et al. [40]	2013	USA	-Patients underwent lobar lung transplantation. -Double 13/25 (52%) -Idiopathic pulmonary fibrosis 9/25 (36%) -Sarcoidosis 4/25 (16%) -Cystic fibrosis 2/25 (8%)	25	RRT	RRT 4/25 (16%)
Xue et al. [28]	2014	China	Patients underwent lung transplantation -Double 38/88 (43.2%) -Idiopathic pulmonary fibrosis 46/88 (52.3%) -COPD 19/88 (21.6%) -Brochiectesis7/88 (8%)	88	AKIN classification	AKI 47/88 (53.4%) RRT 3/88 (3.4%)
Ishikawa et al. [29]	2014	Canada	Patients underwent lung transplantation -Double 15/50 (30%) -Interstitial lung disease 18/50 (36%) -COPD 14/50 (28%) -Cystic fibrosis 10/50 (20%) -Alpha 1 antitrypsin deficiency 5/50 (10%)	50	RIFLE criteria	AKI during first 72 hours after transplant 27/50 (54%) AKI during hospitalization 32/50 (64%) RRT 4/50 (8%)
Fidalgo et al. [14]	2014	Canada	Patient underwent lung transplant -Double 354/445 (79.6%) -Heart-lung transplant 20/445 (4.5%) -COPD 149/445 (33.5%) -Idiopathic pulmonary fibrosis 99/445 (22.2%) -Cystic fibrosis 71/445 (16%)	445	KDIGO criteria	Total AKI 306/445 (68.8%) AKI in lung transplant only 290/425 (68.2%) RRT 36/445 (8.1%)
Silhan et al. [41]	2014	USA	Pulmonary fibrosis patients with telomerase mutation carriers underwent lung transplant -Double 5/8 (62.5%)	8	RRT	RRT 4/8 (50%)
Tokman et al. [42]	2015	USA	Pulmonary fibrosis patients underwent lung transplantation -Double 12/14 (85.7%)	14	Increase in serum creatinine of ≥ 1.5 times from baseline within seven days after transplant	AKI 8/14 (57.1%) RRT 1/14 (7.1%)

Table 1. *Cont.*

Study	Year	Country	Patients	Number	AKI Definition	AKI Incidence
Sikma et al. [44]	2017	Netherlands	Patient underwent lung transplantation -Double 148/186 (79.6%) -COPD/alpha 1 antitrypsin deficiency 80/186 (43%) -Sarcoidosis/Interstitial lung disease/usual interstitial pneumonia 14/186 (7.5%)	186	KDIGO criteria	AKI 85/186 (45.7%)
Carillo et al. [43]	2017	Italy	Patients underwent lung transplantation -Double 6/22 (27.3%) -Pulmonary fibrosis 13/22 (59%) -Emphysema 7/22(31.8%)	22	RRT	RRT 5/22 (22.7%)
Balci et al. [24]	2017	Turkey	Patients underwent lung transplantation -Idiopathic pulmonary fibrosis 10/30 (33.3%) -COPD 6/30 (20%) -Cystic fibrosis/bronchiectasis 9/30 (30%)	30	AKIN classification	AKI 16/30 (53.3%) RRT 0/30 (0%)
Nguyen et al. [10]	2017	USA	Patients underwent lung transplantation -Double 55/97 (56.7%) -COPD 11/97 (11.3%) -Idiopathic pulmonary fibrosis 50/97 (51.5%) -Cystic fibrosis 20/97 (20.6%) -Pulmonary hypertension 11/97 (11.3%)	97	RIFLE criteria	AKI 57/97 (58.8%) RRT 35/97 (38.5%)
Banga et al. [46]	2017	USA	Patients underwent lung transplantation. Data was from UNOS database from 1994-2014	24,110	RRT	RRT 1369/24,110 (5.7%)
Newton et al. [45]	2017	USA	Pulmonary fibrosis patients underwent lung transplantation. -Double 70/82 (85.4%)	82	increase in serum creatinine to ≥ 1.5 times from baseline within 7 days after transplant	AKI 54/82 (65.9%) RRT 2/82 (2.4%)
Cosgun et al. [47]	2017	USA	Patient underwent lung transplantation -Double 285/291 (97.9%) -Requiring intraoperative ECMO 134/291 (46.0%) -Cystic fibrosis 89/291 (30.6%) -COPD 88/291 (30.2%) -Idiopathic pulmonary fibrosis 63/291 (21.6%)	291	RRT	RRT 27/291 (9.3%)

Table 1. *Cont.*

Study	Year	Country	Patients	AKI Definition	Number	AKI Incidence
Ahmad et al. [48]	2018	USA	Patients underwent lung transplantation from brain death donors -Double 20/32 (62.5%) -Interstitial lung disease 24/32 (75%) -COPD 8/32 (25%)	RIFLE criteria	32	AKI at 24 hours post-transplant = 6/32 (18.8%) AKI at 72 hours post-transplant = 4/32 (12.5%)
Iyengar et al. [49]	2018	USA	Patients underwent lung transplantation -Double 267/501 (53.3%)	RRT	501	RRT 19/501 (3.8%)
Ri et al. [50]	2018	Korea	Patient underwent lung transplantation -Idiopathic pulmonary fibrosis 12/33 (36.4%) -Interstitial lung disease 20/33 (60.6%) -Primary pulmonary hypertension 1/14 (7.1%)	AKIN criteria	33	AKI 14/33 (42.4%) RRT 0/33 (0%)
Calabrese et al. [51]	2018	USA	Patient underwent lung transplantation -Double 288/321 (89.7%) -Heart-lung 6/321 (1.9%) -Idiopathic pulmonary fibrosis 210/321 (65.4%) -COPD 66/321 (20.6%) -Cystic fibrosis 31/321 (9.7%)	KDIGO criteria	321	AKI KDIGO stage 2 and 3 61/321 (19.0%)
Bennett et al. [52]	2019	Italy	Patients underwent lung transplantation -Double 66/135 (48.9%) -Pulmonary fibrosis 72/135 (53.33%) -COPD 28/135 (20.74%) -Cystic fibrosis 25/135 (18.52%)	KDIGO criteria	135	AKI 45/135 (33.3%) RRT 18/135 (13.3%)
Shashaty et al. [53]	2019	USA	Patients underwent lung transplantation -Double 180/299 (60.2%) -COPD 119/299 (39.8%) -Interstitial lung disease 123/299 (41.1%) -Cystic fibrosis 26/299 (8.70%)	KDIGO criteria	299	AKI 188/299 (62.9%) RRT 19/299 (6.4%)

Abbreviations: AKI, Acute kidney injury; AKIN, acute kidney injury network; COPD, chronic obstructive pulmonary disease; KDIGO, kidney disease improving global outcomes; RIFLE, risk, injury, failure, loss of kidney function, and end-stage kidney disease; RRT, renal replacement therapy; UNOS, United Network for Organ Sharing; USA, United States of America; SCr, serum creatinine.

3.1. Incidence of Acute Kidney Injury among Patients after Lung Transplantation

The pooled estimated incidence rates of AKI and severe AKI requiring RRT after lung transplantation were 52.5% (95% CI: 45.8–59.1%, I^2 = 89%, Figure 2) and 9.3% (95% CI: 7.6–11.4%, I^2 = 90%, Figure 3). Subgroup analysis based on the AKI definition was performed and demonstrated a pooled estimated incidence of AKI after lung transplantation of 49% (95% CI: 38.3–59.8%, I^2 = 86%, Figure 2) by RIFLE criteria, 55.5% (95% CI: 45.2–65.4%, I^2 = 71%, Figure 2) by AKIN criteria, and 53.0% (95% CI: 38.2–67.3%, I^2 = 91%, Figure 2) by KDIGO criteria.

Group by Definition	Study name	Event rate	Lower limit	Upper limit	Z-Value	p-Value	Relative weight
AKIN	Wehbe et al	0.645	0.608	0.681	7.341	0.000	36.10
AKIN	Xue et al	0.534	0.430	0.635	0.639	0.523	27.48
AKIN	Balci et al	0.533	0.358	0.701	0.365	0.715	17.84
AKIN	Ri et al	0.424	0.270	0.595	-0.867	0.386	18.57
AKIN		0.555	0.452	0.654	1.042	0.297	
KDIGO	Fidalgo et al	0.682	0.637	0.725	7.339	0.000	25.61
KDIGO	Sikma et al	0.457	0.387	0.529	-1.172	0.241	24.88
KDIGO	Bennett et al	0.333	0.259	0.417	-3.797	0.000	24.13
KDIGO	Shashaty et al	0.629	0.573	0.682	4.402	0.000	25.37
KDIGO		0.530	0.382	0.673	0.390	0.697	
RIFLE	Rocha et al	0.561	0.504	0.616	2.087	0.037	19.91
RIFLE	Arnaoutakis et al	0.632	0.537	0.718	2.687	0.007	17.97
RIFLE	Jacques et al	0.385	0.316	0.459	-3.005	0.003	19.10
RIFLE	Ishikawa et al	0.540	0.402	0.672	0.565	0.572	15.69
RIFLE	Nguyen et al	0.588	0.487	0.681	1.717	0.086	17.84
RIFLE	Ahmad et al	0.125	0.048	0.289	-3.640	0.000	9.50
RIFLE		0.490	0.383	0.598	-0.180	0.857	
Overall		0.525	0.458	0.591	0.738	0.461	

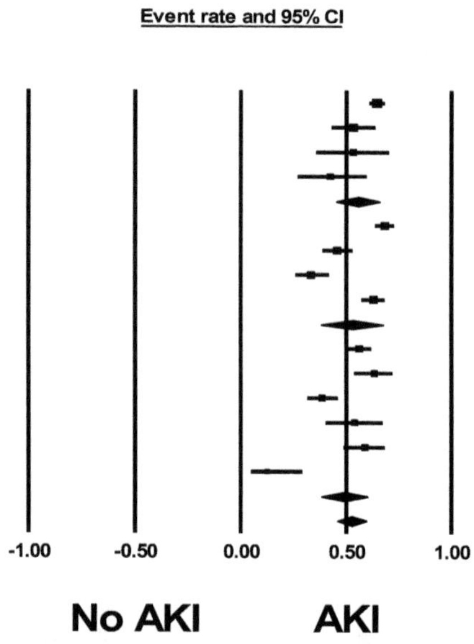

Figure 2. Forest plots of the included studies evaluating incidence rates of AKI after lung transplantation. AKI, Acute kidney injury.

Study name	Event rate	Lower limit	Upper limit	Z-Value	p-Value	Relative weight
Rocha et al	0.078	0.052	0.114	-11.394	0.000	5.84
Arnaoutakis et al	0.132	0.080	0.211	-6.563	0.000	5.06
Machuca et al	0.146	0.095	0.218	-7.109	0.000	5.49
George et al	0.054	0.050	0.058	-71.223	0.000	7.32
Wehbe et al	0.061	0.045	0.082	-16.769	0.000	6.43
Hennessy et al	0.049	0.030	0.079	-11.548	0.000	5.40
Shigemura et al	0.160	0.061	0.357	-3.040	0.002	2.77
Xue et al	0.034	0.011	0.100	-5.692	0.000	2.52
Ishikawa et al	0.080	0.030	0.195	-4.685	0.000	2.93
Fidalgo et al	0.081	0.059	0.110	-13.979	0.000	6.32
Silhan et al	0.500	0.200	0.800	0.000	1.000	1.95
Tokman et al	0.071	0.010	0.370	-2.472	0.013	1.05
Carillo et al	0.227	0.098	0.444	-2.405	0.016	3.02
Balci et al	0.016	0.001	0.211	-2.883	0.004	0.60
Nguyen et al	0.361	0.272	0.461	-2.704	0.007	5.91
Banga et al	0.057	0.054	0.060	-100.978	0.000	7.35
Newton et al	0.024	0.006	0.092	-5.153	0.000	1.91
Cosgun et al	0.093	0.064	0.132	-11.285	0.000	6.01
Iyengar et al	0.038	0.024	0.059	-13.825	0.000	5.65
Kim et al	0.300	0.190	0.440	-2.746	0.006	4.82
Ri et al	0.015	0.001	0.196	-2.951	0.003	0.60
Bennett et al	0.133	0.086	0.202	-7.393	0.000	5.44
Shashaty et al	0.064	0.041	0.097	-11.348	0.000	5.62
	0.093	0.076	0.114	-19.794	0.000	

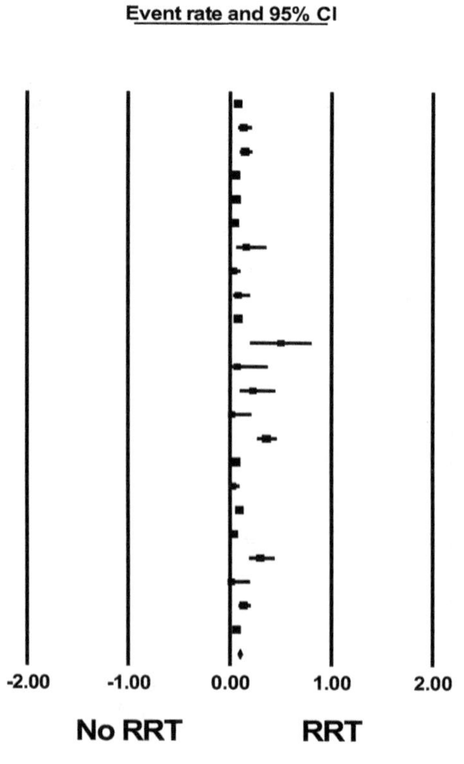

Figure 3. Forest plots of the included studies evaluating incidence rates of AKI requiring RRT after lung transplantation. AKI, Acute kidney injury; RRT, renal replacement therapy.

Meta-regression analysis demonstrated that year of study did not significantly affect the incidence of AKI ($p = 0.22$) and severe AKI requiring RRT ($p = 0.68$) among patients after lung transplantation, as shown in Figure 4.

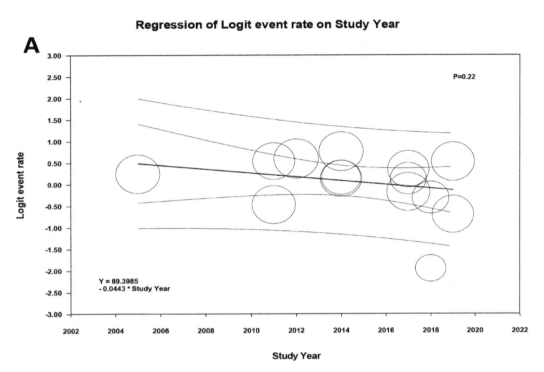

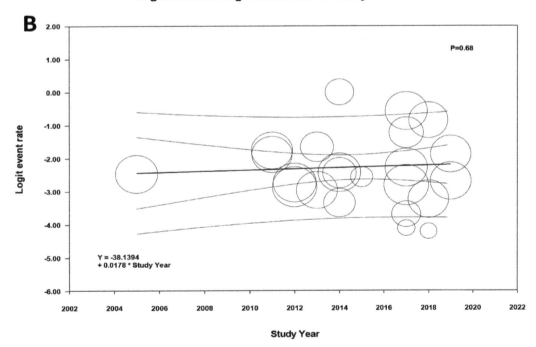

Figure 4. Meta-regression analyses showed that year of study did not significantly affect (**A**) the incidence of AKI ($p = 0.11$) and (**B**) severe AKI requiring RRT ($p = 0.54$) among patients after lung transplantation. AKI, acute kidney injury; RRT, renal replacement therapy.

3.2. Mortality Risk of Acute Kidney Injury in Patients after Lung Transplantation

Data on mortality risk from included studies are shown in Table 2. The pooled OR of hospital mortality among patients after lung transplantation with AKI and severe AKI requiring RRT were 2.75

(95% CI, 1.18–6.41, $I^2 = 69\%$, Figure 5A) and 10.89 (95% CI, 5.03–23.58, $I^2 = 82\%$, Figure 5B), respectively. At one year, the pooled OR of mortality among patients after lung transplantation with AKI and severe AKI requiring RRT were 2.99 (95% CI, 1.72–5.18, $I^2 = 74\%$, Figure S1) and 8.32 (95% CI, 5.95–11.63, $I^2 = 70\%$, Figure S2), respectively. At five years, the pooled OR of mortality among patients after lung transplantation with AKI and severe AKI requiring RRT were 1.47 (95% CI, 1.11–1.94, $I^2 = 0\%$, Figure S3) and 4.79 (95% CI, 3.58–6.40, $I^2 = 81\%$, Figure S4), respectively.

Table 2. Mortality risk of AKI in patients after lung transplantation.

Study	Year	Results	Confounder Adjustment
Rocha et al. [13]	2005	One-year mortality AKI: 4.33 (2.08–8.99) RRT: 23.70 (8.29–67.80) Five-year mortality AKI: 1.44 (0.90–2.30) RRT: 9.73 (2.82–33.53)	None
Arnaoutakis et al. [11]	2011	In-hospital mortality AKI: 0.48 (0.13–1.71) RRT: 28.2 (6.18–128.1) One-year mortality AKI: 0.47 (0.20–1.14) RRT: 4.97 (1.54–16.0)	Lung allocation score, pre-transplant GFR, recipient age, donor cigarette use, postoperative tracheostomy
Machuca et al. [37]	2011	Mortality AKI: 2.47 (1.13–5.39) RRT: 2.68 (1.36–5.27)	Mechanical ventilation duration, reintubation, acute rejection in the first month, coronary heart disease
George et al. [19]	2012	30-day mortality RRT: 7.87 (6.07–10.20) One-year mortality RRT: 7.89 (6.80–9.15) Five-year mortality RRT: 5.35 (4.72–6.07)	Recipient age, GFR, BMI, diagnosis, mean pulmonary artery pressure, ICU status, ECMO support, donor age, bilateral lung transplant, ischemic time, annual center volume
Jacques et al. [21]	2012	30-day mortality AKI:1.36 (0.40–4.64) Long-term mortality AKI: 1.54 (0.79–2.99)	Age, sex, indication, ICU length of stay, coronary artery disease, aprotinin use, double lung transplantation
Wehbe et al. [38]	2012	Hospital mortality AKI: 6.05 (1.83–20.00) RRT: 13.66 (6.19–30.17) One-year mortality AKI: 2.92 (1.76–4.82)	Age, sex, race, type on lung transplantation, COPD, pre-transplantation diabetes, baseline creatinine
Hennessy et al. [39]	2013	30-day mortality AKI: 10.23 (4.05–25.86) RRT: 41.41 (13.06–131.31) One-year mortality AKI: 7.01 (3.29–14.92) RRT: 43.04 (9.48–195.50)	None
Xue et al. [28]	2014	Five-year mortality AKI: 1.48 (1.04–2.11)	Age, sex, type, and cause of lung transplant, hypertension, and diabetes
Ishikawa et al. [29]	2014	Mortality AKI: 3/27 (11%) vs. 0/23 (0%)	None
Fidalgo et al. [14]	2014	Hospital mortality AKI: 22/306 (7%) vs. 0/139 (0%) One-year mortality AKI: 2.81 (1.15–6.84)	Age, sex, COPD, eGFR, LAS score, diabetes mellitus, pulmonary artery pressure, previous sternotomy, type of lung transplant, ICU length of stay
Balci et al. [24]	2017	30-day mortality AKI: 0.82 (0.18–3.74)	None
Nguyen et al. [10]	2017	One-year mortality AKI: 1.73 (0.42–7.13) RRT: 1.20 (0.32–4.60)	None

Table 2. *Cont.*

Study	Year	Results	Confounder Adjustment
Banga et al. [46]	2017	One-year mortality RRT: 7.23 (6.2–8.43) Five-year mortality RRT: 3.96 (3.43–4.56)	Age, serum albumin, type of procedure, CMV mismatch, Length of hospital stay after transplantation, recipient hospitalized at the time of transplant, history of prior cardiac surgery, acute rejection
Bennett et al. [52]	2019	One-year mortality AKI: 6.20 (2.74–14.05) RRT: 21.60 (5.75–81.11)	None
Shashaty et al. [53]	2019	One-year mortality AKI: 3.64 (1.68–7.88)	Primary graft dysfunction, age, bilateral lung transplant

Abbreviations: AKI, acute kidney injury; RRT, renal replacement therapy; BMI, body mass index; CMV, cytomegalovirus; COPD, chronic obstructive pulmonary disease; DM, diabetes mellitus; ECMO, extracorporeal membrane oxygenation; eGFR, estimated glomerular filtration rate; HES, hydroxyethyl starch; ICU, intensive care unit; SCr, serum creatinine.

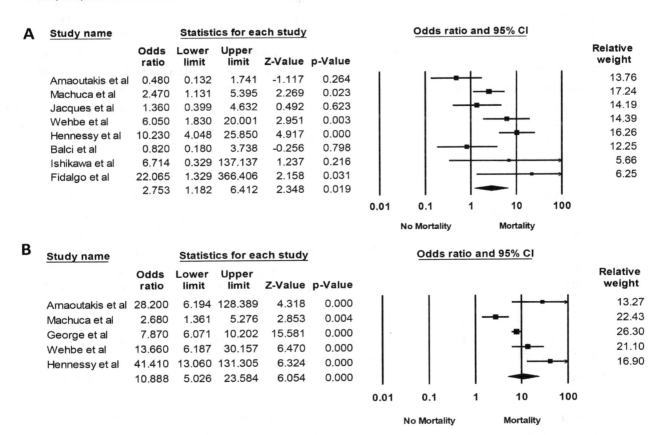

Figure 5. Forest plots of the included studies evaluating hospital mortality of (**A**) AKI and (**B**) AKI requiring RRT after lung transplantation. AKI, acute kidney injury; RRT, renal replacement therapy.

3.3. Evaluation for Publication Bias

Funnel plot (Figures S5 and S6) and Egger's regression asymmetry tests were performed to assess publication bias in analysis evaluating mortality risk of AKI in patients after lung transplant with AKI and severe AKI requiring RRT, respectively. We found no significant publication bias in meta-analysis evaluating mortality risk of patients after lung transplant with AKI ($p = 0.99$) and severe AKI requiring RRT ($p = 0.50$).

4. Discussion and Conclusions

In this systematic review, we demonstrated that AKI in patients after lung transplantation is common, with pooled incidence rates of AKI and severe AKI requiring RRT in patients after lung transplantation of 52.5% and 9.3%, respectively. We also showed that the incidence of AKI in patients after lung transplantation has not improved, despite advances in therapy. Compared to those without AKI, patients with post-lung-transplant AKI had increased short and long-term mortality.

Some specific factors related to AKI after lung transplant include hypercapnia/hypoxemia-mediated impaired renal blood flow (RBF), hemodynamics during lung transplant surgery, and the use of extracorporeal membrane oxygenation (ECMO) and cardio-pulmonary bypass (CPB) during lung transplant surgery [12,28,44,54]. Postoperative respiratory failure is common after lung transplantation; reported to be as high as 55% [55]. Hypoxemia is associated with reduced RBF in a dose-dependent relationship [56–58] thought to be related to stimulation of adrenergic neurons and alterations in nitric oxide metabolism [59]. In addition, studies have shown that hypercapnia can induce peripheral vasodilatation and decreased systemic vascular resistance, with a compensatory neurohormonal vasoconstriction response. This leads to activation of the renin-angiotensin-aldosterone system (RAAS) and direct renal vasoconstriction, resulting in a reduction in RBF and GFR [56,60–62]. Furthermore, poorly controlled hemodynamics during lung transplant surgery can result in intraoperative hypotension, one of the most significant risk factors for the development of AKI after lung transplantation [10,24]. Currently, CPB remains a standard method used in lung transplantation for intraoperative cardiorespiratory support, especially in cases of poor hemodynamic tolerance or severe pulmonary arterial hypertension [63]. However, CPB is commonly associated with inflammatory reactions and bleeding complications [64]. ECMO has more recently been used as an alternative option to CPB for intraoperative cardiopulmonary support during lung transplantation [63]. When compared to CPB, studies have demonstrated beneficial effects of intraoperative ECMO support, with lower rates of primary graft dysfunction, acute post-operative bleeding, AKI requiring RRT, and length of hospital stay [63]. However, the use of ECMO itself may also cause a renal insult related to the activation of proinflammatory mediators caused by the continuous exposure of blood to the non-biological and non-endothelialized ECMO interface [65]. Therefore, our study demonstrated that patients undergoing lung transplantation more frequently develop AKI and AKI requiring RRT than abdominal solid organ transplantation, such as liver transplantation (incidence of AKI and AKI requiring RRT of 41% and 7%, respectively) [66].

As there are currently no effective targeted pharmacotherapies available for AKI, treatment is limited to supportive strategies and RRT when indicated [4–6,8]. Patients who recover from AKI continue to have an increased risk of mortality on either short or long-term follow-up [9]. Following post-lung-transplant AKI, patients may develop CKD, with rates of progression to ESKD as high as 3.8%, 7.2%, and 7.9% at one, five, and ten years after lung transplant, respectively [17,46,67]. Therefore, prevention and early identification of AKI in patients at risk for post-lung-transplant AKI may potentially play an important role in improving patient outcomes. Important risk factors for AKI in patients after lung transplantation include bilateral lung transplantation [19,21,29,68], lower baseline estimated GFR [13,19,38,46,68], pulmonary hypertension [19,38,46], duration of mechanical ventilation requirement [13,14,24,28,46,53], the need for ECMO support [19,46,68], intraoperative hypotension, and vasopressor requirement [10,24] (Table 3).

Table 3. Reported risk factors for AKI after lung transplantation.

Reported Risk Factors for AKI after Lung Transplantation

- High baseline SCr, lower baseline eGFR [13,19,38,46,68]
- Male [52]
- Older age [19]
- Higher BMI [68]
- Carriers of the ABCB1 CGC-CGC diplotype [51]
- African American and Hispanic ethnicity [19,46,68]
- Higher mean pulmonary artery pressure, pulmonary hypertension [19,38,46]
- Intraoperative hypoxemia [29]
- Duration of mechanical ventilation requirement [13,14,24,28,46]
- Duration of ICU stay [68]
- The need of ECMO support [19,46,68]
- Bilateral lung transplantation [19,21,29,68]
- Non-COPD diagnosis [13]
- Cystic fibrosis [44,53]
- Idiopathic pulmonary fibrosis [19]
- Sarcoidosis [68]
- Intraoperative hypotension and vasopressors requirement [10,24]
- Higher HES volume [29]
- Longer cardiopulmonary bypass time [10,14,52]
- Ischemic time [19]
- Aprotinin use [21]
- Pretransplant diabetes mellitus [38,68]
- Pretransplant hypertension [28]
- Longer time on waiting list [68]
- Lower Karnofsky performance score [68]
- Supratherapeutic cyclosporine/tacrolimus trough [14,44]
- Amphotericin B use [13] and nephrotoxic medications [44]
- Infection [24,44]

Abbreviations: BMI, body mass index; COPD, chronic obstructive pulmonary disease; DM, diabetes mellitus; ECMO, extracorporeal membrane oxygenation; eGFR, estimated glomerular filtration rate; HES, hydroxyethyl starch; ICU, intensive care unit; SCr, serum creatinine.

There is experimental data that injurious ventilation strategies, such as a high tidal volume, low positive end-expiratory pressure approach can cause renal epithelial cell apoptosis and dysregulation of extracellular ligands that control renal vascular tone and endothelial integrity, resulting in AKI [69,70]. Among patients with acute respiratory distress syndrome, protective lung ventilation is associated with a reduced risk for AKI requiring dialysis and improves dialysis-free survival [71]. Therefore, future studies are needed to assess whether maintaining perioperative lung-protective ventilation helps to prevent AKI following lung transplantation [12]. Moreover, ECMO management may also play an important role in the prevention of post lung transplant AKI. High ECMO pump speed is associated with hemolysis and AKI development [65]. Future prospective studies are needed to assess the effects of ECMO pump speed on the risk of post-lung-transplantation AKI. Finally, immunosuppressive medications may also play an important role in AKI development following lung transplantation [12,72]. AKI related to calcineurin inhibitor (CNI)-induced thrombotic microangiopathy (TMA) has been reported in lung transplant recipients and is often missed or recognized late in the ICU setting [12,72]. Although TMA in lung transplant recipients is a rare condition, early recognition and management can potentially reduce post lung transplant-related morbidity and mortality [12,72,73].

Our study has some limitations. Firstly, there are statistical heterogeneities in our meta-analysis. Subgroup analyses were performed using differing AKI definitions, including RIFLE criteria AKIN criteria and KDIGO criteria. Meta-regression analysis assessing the effect of year of study on the incidence of AKI was also performed, and we found no significant correlation between year of study and incidence of AKI post lung transplantation. Secondly, AKI diagnosis from the included studies was based on changes in serum creatinine, and data on urine output and AKI biomarkers was limited. Lastly, this systematic review is primarily based on observational studies, as the data from clinical trials or population-based studies were limited. Thus, it can, at best, demonstrate an association between AKI and increased short-term and long-term mortality post lung transplant, but not a causal relationship.

In summary, AKI and severe AKI requiring RRT are common in patients after lung transplantation, with overall estimated incidence rates of 52.5% and 9.3%, respectively. Post-lung-transplant AKI is significantly associated with reduced short-term and long-term survival. Despite advances in transplantation therapy, the incidence of AKI in patients after lung transplantation does not appear to have improved.

Supplementary Materials
Search terms for systematic review; Figure S1. Forest plots of the included studies assessing the pooled OR of mortality at one year among patients after lung transplantation with AKI; Figure S2: Forest plots of the included studies assessing the pooled OR of mortality at one year among patients after lung transplantation with severe AKI requiring RRT; Figure S3: Forest plots of the included studies assessing the pooled OR of mortality at five years among patients after lung transplantation with AKI; Figure S4: Forest plots of the included studies assessing the pooled OR of mortality at five years among patients after lung transplantation with severe AKI requiring RRT; Figure S5: Funnel plot evaluating for publication bias evaluating mortality risk of AKI in patients after lung transplant with AKI; Figure S6: Funnel plot evaluating for publication bias evaluating mortality risk of AKI in patients after lung transplant with severe AKI requiring RRT.

Author Contributions: Conceptualization, W.C., N.S., T.B., K.W. (Kanramon Watthanasuntorn), N.R.A., S.A.S., E.A.G., (K.W.) Karn Wijarnpreecha, M.A.M. and W.K.; data curation, P.L., C.T. and O.A.O.; formal analysis, W.C.; funding acquisition, T.B.; investigation, P.L., C.T., W.C., E.A.G. and W.K.; methodology, C.T, O.A.O., N.R.A., S.A.S., P.U., K.W. (Karn Wijarnpreecha), M.A.M. and W.K.; project administration, W.C., T.B. and K.W. (Kanramon Watthanasuntorn); resources, W.C., T.B., K.W. (Kanramon Watthanasuntorn) and W.K.; software, K.W. (Kanramon Watthanasuntorn); supervision, N.S., N.R.A., S.A.S., P.U., E.A.G., K.W. (Karn Wijarnpreecha), M.A.M. and W.K.; validation, P.L., W.C., N.S., T.B., P.U. and W.K.; visualization, O.A.O., P.U. and W.K.; writing—original draft, P.L. and W.K.; writing—review and editing, C.T., W.C., O.A.O., N.S., T.B., K.W. (Kanramon Watthanasuntorn), N.R.A., S.A.S., P.U., E.A.G., K.W. (Karn Wijarnpreecha), M.A.M. and W.K.

Acknowledgments: None. All authors had access to the data and had important roles in the writing of the manuscript.

References

1. Gameiro, J.; Agapito Fonseca, J.; Jorge, S.; Lopes, J.A. Acute Kidney Injury Definition and Diagnosis: A Narrative Review. *J. Clin. Med.* **2018**, *7*, 307. [CrossRef] [PubMed]
2. Thongprayoon, C.; Cheungpasitporn, W.; Mao, M.A.; Harrison, A.M.; Erickson, S.B. Elevated admission serum calcium phosphate product as an independent risk factor for acute kidney injury in hospitalized patients. *Hosp Pract (1995)* **2019**, *47*, 73–79. [CrossRef] [PubMed]
3. Thongprayoon, C.; Cheungpasitporn, W.; Mao, M.A.; Sakhuja, A.; Kashani, K. U-shape association of serum albumin level and acute kidney injury risk in hospitalized patients. *PLoS ONE* **2018**, *13*, e0199153. [CrossRef]
4. Kashani, K.; Cheungpasitporn, W.; Ronco, C. Biomarkers of acute kidney injury: The pathway from discovery to clinical adoption. *Clin. Chem. Lab. Med.* **2017**, *55*, 1074–1089. [CrossRef] [PubMed]
5. Wang, Y.; Fang, Y.; Teng, J.; Ding, X. Acute Kidney Injury Epidemiology: From Recognition to Intervention. *Contrib. Nephrol.* **2016**, *187*, 1–8. [PubMed]
6. Negi, S.; Koreeda, D.; Kobayashi, S.; Yano, T.; Tatsuta, K.; Mima, T.; Shigematsu, T.; Ohya, M. Acute kidney injury: Epidemiology, outcomes, complications, and therapeutic strategies. *Semin. Dial.* **2018**, *31*, 519–527. [CrossRef] [PubMed]
7. Hoste, E.A.J.; Bagshaw, S.M.; Bellomo, R.; Cely, C.M.; Colman, R.; Cruz, D.N.; Edipidis, K.; Forni, L.G.; Gomersall, C.D.; Govil, D.; et al. Epidemiology of acute kidney injury in critically ill patients: The multinational AKI-EPI study. *Intensiv. Care Med.* **2015**, *41*, 1411–1423. [CrossRef]
8. Cheungpasitporn, W.; Kashani, K. Electronic Data Systems and Acute Kidney Injury. *Contrib. Nephrol.* **2016**, *187*, 73–83.

9.   Sawhney, S.; Marks, A.; Fluck, N.; Levin, A.; McLernon, D.; Prescott, G.; Black, C. Post-discharge kidney function is associated with subsequent ten-year renal progression risk among survivors of acute kidney injury. *Kidney Int.* **2017**, *92*, 440–452. [CrossRef]

10. Nguyen, A.P.; Gabriel, R.A.; Golts, E.; Kistler, E.B.; Schmidt, U. Severity of Acute Kidney Injury in the Post-Lung Transplant Patient Is Associated with Higher Healthcare Resources and Cost. *J. Cardiothorac. Vasc. Anesth.* **2017**, *31*, 1361–1369. [CrossRef]

11. Arnaoutakis, G.J.; George, T.J.; Robinson, C.W.; Gibbs, K.W.; Orens, J.B.; Merlo, C.A.; Shah, A.S. Severe acute kidney injury according to the RIFLE (risk, injury, failure, loss, end stage) criteria affects mortality in lung transplantation. *J. Heart Lung Transplant.* **2011**, *30*, 1161–1168. [CrossRef] [PubMed]

12. Puttarajappa, C.M.; Bernardo, J.F.; Kellum, J.A. Renal Complications Following Lung Transplantation and Heart Transplantation. *Crit. Care Clin.* **2019**, *35*, 61–73. [CrossRef] [PubMed]

13. Rocha, P.N.; Rocha, A.T.; Palmer, S.M.; Davis, R.D.; Smith, S.R. Acute renal failure after lung transplantation: Incidence, predictors and impact on perioperative morbidity and mortality. *Am. J. Transplant.* **2005**, *5*, 1469–1476. [CrossRef] [PubMed]

14. Fidalgo, P.; Ahmed, M.; Meyer, S.R.; Lien, D.; Weinkauf, J.; Cardoso, F.S.; Jackson, K.; Bagshaw, S.M. Incidence and outcomes of acute kidney injury following orthotopic lung transplantation: A population-based cohort study. *Nephrol. Dial. Transplant.* **2014**, *29*, 1702–1709. [CrossRef]

15. Fidalgo, P.; Ahmed, M.; Meyer, S.R.; Lien, D.; Weinkauf, J.; Kapasi, A.; Cardoso, F.S.; Jackson, K.; Bagshaw, S.M. Association between transient acute kidney injury and morbidity and mortality after lung transplantation: A retrospective cohort study. *J. Crit. Care* **2014**, *29*, 1028–1034. [CrossRef]

16. Wehbe, E.; Duncan, A.E.; Dar, G.; Budev, M.; Stephany, B. Recovery from AKI and short- and long-term outcomes after lung transplantation. *Clin. J. Am. Soc. Nephrol.* **2013**, *8*, 19–25. [CrossRef]

17. Chambers, D.C.; Yusen, R.D.; Cherikh, W.S.; Goldfarb, S.B.; Kucheryavaya, A.Y.; Khusch, K.; Levvey, B.J.; Lund, L.H.; Meiser, B.; Rossano, J.W.; et al. The Registry of the International Society for Heart and Lung Transplantation: Thirty-fourth Adult Lung and Heart-Lung Transplantation Report—2017; Focus Theme: Allograft ischemic time. *J. Heart Lung Transplant.* **2017**, *36*, 1047–1059. [CrossRef]

18. Bloom, R.; Doyle, A. Kidney Disease after Heart and Lung Transplantation. *Arab. Archaeol. Epigr.* **2006**, *6*, 671–679. [CrossRef]

19. George, T.J.; Arnaoutakis, G.J.; Beaty, C.A.; Pipeling, M.R.; Merlo, C.A.; Conte, J.V.; Shah, A.S. Acute kidney injury increases mortality after lung transplantation. *Ann. Thorac. Surg.* **2012**, *94*, 185–192. [CrossRef]

20. Lafrance, J.P.; Miller, D.R. Acute kidney injury associates with increased long-term mortality. *J. Am. Soc. Nephrol. JASN* **2010**, *21*, 345–352. [CrossRef]

21. Jacques, F.; El-Hamamsy, I.; Fortier, A.; Maltais, S.; Perrault, L.P.; Liberman, M.; Noiseux, N.; Ferraro, P. Acute renal failure following lung transplantation: Risk factors, mortality, and long-term consequences. *Eur. J. Cardiothorac. Surg.* **2012**, *41*, 193–199. [CrossRef] [PubMed]

22. Jardel, S.; Reynaud, Q.; Durieu, I. Long-term extrapulmonary comorbidities after lung transplantation in cystic fibrosis: Update of specificities. *Clin. Transplant.* **2018**, *32*, e13269. [CrossRef] [PubMed]

23. Yusen, R.D.; Edwards, L.B.; Kucheryavaya, A.Y.; Benden, C.; Dipchand, A.I.; Goldfarb, S.B.; Levvey, B.J.; Lund, L.H.; Meiser, B.; Rossano, J.W.; et al. The Registry of the International Society for Heart and Lung Transplantation: Thirty-second Official Adult Lung and Heart-Lung Transplantation Report—2015; Focus Theme: Early Graft Failure. *J. Heart Lung Transplant.* **2015**, *34*, 1264–1277. [CrossRef] [PubMed]

24. Balci, M.; Vayvada, M.; Salturk, C.; Kutlu, C.; Ari, E. Incidence of Early Acute Kidney Injury in Lung Transplant Patients: A Single-Center Experience. *Transplant. Proc.* **2017**, *49*, 593–598. [CrossRef]

25. De La Morena, M.P.; Bravos, M.D.L.T.; Prado, R.F.; Roel, M.D.; Salcedo, J.G.; Costa, E.F.; Rivas, D.G.; Maté, J.B. Chronic Kidney Disease After Lung Transplantation: Incidence, Risk Factors, and Treatment. *Transplant. Proc.* **2010**, *42*, 3217–3219. [CrossRef]

26. Hornum, M.; Iversen, M.; Steffensen, I.; Hovind, P.; Carlsen, J.; Andersen, L.W.; Steinbrüchel, D.A.; Feldt-Rasmussen, B.; Feldt-Rasmussen, B.; Feldt-Rasmussen, B. Rapid Decline in51Cr-EDTA Measured Renal Function During the First Weeks Following Lung Transplantation. *Arab. Archaeol. Epigr.* **2009**, *9*, 1420–1426. [CrossRef]

27. Castro, A.G.; Llorca, J.; Cañas, B.S.; Fernández-Miret, B.; Zurbano, F.; Miñambres, E. Acute renal failure in lung transplantation: Incidence, correlation with subsequent kidney disease, and prognostic value. *Arch. Bronconeumol.* **2008**, *44*, 353–359. [CrossRef]

28. Xue, J.; Wang, L.; Chen, C.-M.; Chen, J.-Y.; Sun, Z.-X. Acute kidney injury influences mortality in lung transplantation. *Ren. Fail.* **2014**, *36*, 541–545. [CrossRef]
29. Ishikawa, S.; Griesdale, D.E.; Lohser, J. Acute Kidney Injury within 72 Hours After Lung Transplantation: Incidence and Perioperative Risk Factors. *J. Cardiothorac. Vasc. Anesth.* **2014**, *28*, 931–935. [CrossRef]
30. Bagshaw, S.M.; George, C.; Bellomo, R. A comparison of the RIFLE and AKIN criteria for acute kidney injury in critically ill patients. *Nephrol. Dial. Transplant.* **2008**, *23*, 1569–1574. [CrossRef]
31. Uchino, S.; Bellomo, R.; Goldsmith, D.; Bates, S.; Ronco, C. An assessment of the RIFLE criteria for acute renal failure in hospitalized patients. *Crit. Care Med.* **2006**, *34*, 1913–1917. [CrossRef] [PubMed]
32. Palevsky, P.M.; Liu, K.D.; Brophy, P.D.; Chawla, L.S.; Parikh, C.R.; Thakar, C.V.; Tolwani, A.J.; Waikar, S.S.; Weisbord, S.D. KDOQI US Commentary on the 2012 KDIGO Clinical Practice Guideline for Acute Kidney Injury. *Am. J. Kidney Dis.* **2013**, *61*, 649–672. [CrossRef] [PubMed]
33. Moher, D.; Liberati, A.; Tetzlaff, J.; Altman, D.G. Preferred reporting items for systematic reviews and meta-analyses: The PRISMA statement. *PLoS Med.* **2009**, *6*, e1000097. [CrossRef] [PubMed]
34. DerSimonian, R.; Laird, N. Meta-analysis in clinical trials. *Control. Clin. Trials* **1986**, *7*, 177–188. [CrossRef]
35. Higgins, J.P.T.; Thompson, S.G.; Deeks, J.J.; Altman, D.G. Measuring inconsistency in meta-analyses. *BMJ* **2003**, *327*, 557–560. [CrossRef]
36. Easterbrook, P.; Gopalan, R.; Berlin, J.; Matthews, D. Publication bias in clinical research. *Lancet* **1991**, *337*, 867–872. [CrossRef]
37. Machuca, T.N.; Schio, S.M.; Camargo, S.M.; Lobato, V.; Costa, C.D.O.; Felicetti, J.C.; Moreira, J.S.; Camargo, J.J. Prognostic Factors in Lung Transplantation: The Santa Casa de Porto Alegre Experience. *Transplantation* **2011**, *91*, 1297–1303. [CrossRef]
38. Wehbe, E.; Brock, R.; Budev, M.; Xu, M.; Demirjian, S.; Schreiber, M.J.; Stephany, B. Short-term and long-term outcomes of acute kidney injury after lung transplantation. *J. Heart Lung Transplant.* **2012**, *31*, 244–251. [CrossRef]
39. Hennessy, S.A.; Gillen, J.R.; Hranjec, T.; Kozower, B.D.; Jones, D.R.; Kron, I.L.; Lau, C.L. Influence of hemodialysis on clinical outcomes after lung transplantation. *J. Surg. Res.* **2013**, *183*, 916–921. [CrossRef]
40. Shigemura, N.; D'Cunha, J.; Bhama, J.K.; Shiose, A.; El Ela, A.A.; Hackmann, A.; Zaldonis, D.; Toyoda, Y.; Pilewski, J.M.; Luketich, J.D.; et al. Lobar Lung Transplantation: A Relevant Surgical Option in the Current Era of Lung Allocation Score. *Ann. Thorac. Surg.* **2013**, *96*, 451–456. [CrossRef]
41. Silhan, L.L.; Shah, P.D.; Chambers, D.C.; Snyder, L.D.; Riise, G.C.; Wagner, C.L.; Hellström-Lindberg, E.; Orens, J.B.; Mewton, J.F.; Danoff, S.K.; et al. Lung transplantation in telomerase mutation carriers with pulmonary fibrosis. *Eur. Respir. J.* **2014**, *44*, 178–187. [CrossRef] [PubMed]
42. Tokman, S.; Singer, J.P.; Devine, M.S.; Westall, G.P.; Aubert, J.-D.; Tamm, M.; Snell, G.I.; Lee, J.S.; Goldberg, H.J.; Kukreja, J.; et al. Clinical outcomes of lung transplant recipients with telomerase mutations. *J. Heart Lung Transplant.* **2015**, *34*, 1318–1324. [CrossRef] [PubMed]
43. Carillo, C.; Pecoraro, Y.; Anile, M.; Mantovani, S.; Oliva, A.; D'Abramo, A.; Amore, D.; Pagini, A.; De Giacomo, T.; Pugliese, F.; et al. Evaluation of Renal Function in Patients Undergoing Lung Transplantation. *Transplant. Proc.* **2017**, *49*, 699–701. [CrossRef] [PubMed]
44. Sikma, M.A.; Hunault, C.C.; Van De Graaf, E.A.; Verhaar, M.C.; Kesecioglu, J.; De Lange, D.W.; Meulenbelt, J. High tacrolimus blood concentrations early after lung transplantation and the risk of kidney injury. *Eur. J. Clin. Pharmacol.* **2017**, *73*, 573–580. [CrossRef]
45. Newton, C.A.; Kozlitina, J.; Lines, J.R.; Kaza, V.; Torres, F.; Garcia, C.K. Telomere length in patients with pulmonary fibrosis associated with chronic lung allograft dysfunction and post-lung transplantation survival. *J. Heart Lung Transplant.* **2017**, *36*, 845–853. [CrossRef]
46. Banga, A.; Mohanka, M.; Mullins, J.; Bollineni, S.; Kaza, V.; Tanriover, B.; Torres, F. Characteristics and outcomes among patients with need for early dialysis after lung transplantation surgery. *Clin. Transplant.* **2017**, *31*, e13106. [CrossRef]
47. Cosgun, T.; Tomaszek, S.; Opitz, I.; Wilhelm, M.; Schuurmans, M.M.; Weder, W.; Inci, I. Single-center experience with intraoperative extracorporeal membrane oxygenation use in lung transplantation. *Int. J. Artif. Organs* **2017**. [CrossRef]
48. Ahmad, O.; Shafii, A.E.; Mannino, D.M.; Choate, R.; Baz, M.A. Impact of donor lung pathogenic bacteria on patient outcomes in the immediate post-transplant period. *Transpl. Infect. Dis.* **2018**, *20*, e12986. [CrossRef]

49. Iyengar, A.; Kwon, O.J.; Sanaiha, Y.; Eisenring, C.; Biniwale, R.; Ross, D.; Ardehali, A. Lung transplantation in the Lung Allocation Score era: Medium-term analysis from a single center. *Clin. Transplant.* **2018**, *32*, e13298. [CrossRef]

50. Ri, H.S.; Son, H.J.; Oh, H.B.; Kim, S.Y.; Park, J.Y.; Kim, J.Y.; Choi, Y.J. Inhaled nitric oxide therapy was not associated with postoperative acute kidney injury in patients undergoing lung transplantation: A retrospective pilot study. *Medicine* **2018**, *97*, e10915. [CrossRef]

51. Calabrese, D.R.; Florez, R.; Dewey, K.; Hui, C.; Torgerson, D.; Chong, T.; Faust, H.; Rajalingam, R.; Hays, S.R.; Golden, J.A.; et al. Genotypes associated with tacrolimus pharmacokinetics impact clinical outcomes in lung transplant recipients. *Clin. Transplant.* **2018**, *32*, e13332. [CrossRef] [PubMed]

52. Bennett, D.; Fossi, A.; Marchetti, L.; Lanzarone, N.; Sisi, S.; Refini, R.M.; Sestini, P.; Luzzi, L.; Paladini, P.; Rottoli, P. Postoperative acute kidney injury in lung transplant recipients. *Interact. Cardiovasc. Thorac. Surg.* **2019**, *28*, 929–935. [CrossRef] [PubMed]

53. Shashaty, M.G.S.; Forker, C.M.; Miano, T.A.; Wu, Q.; Yang, W.; Oyster, M.L.; Porteous, M.K.; Cantu, E.E., III; Diamond, J.M.; Christie, J.D. The association of post-lung transplant acute kidney injury with mortality is independent of primary graft dysfunction: A cohort study. *Clin. Transplant.* **2019**, e13678. [CrossRef]

54. Sharma, P.; Welch, K.; Eikstadt, R.; Marrero, J.A.; Fontana, R.J.; Lok, A.S. Renal outcomes after liver transplantation in the model for end-stage liver disease era. *Liver Transplant.* **2009**, *15*, 1142–1148. [CrossRef] [PubMed]

55. Chatila, W.M.; Furukawa, S.; Gaughan, J.P.; Criner, G.J. Respiratory failure after lung transplantation. *Chest* **2003**, *123*, 165–173. [CrossRef] [PubMed]

56. Husain-Syed, F.; Slutsky, A.S.; Ronco, C. Lung–Kidney Cross-Talk in the Critically Ill Patient. *Am. J. Respir. Crit. Care Med.* **2016**, *194*, 402–414. [CrossRef] [PubMed]

57. Sharkey, R.; Mulloy, E.; O'Neill, S. Acute effects of hypoxaemia, hyperoxaemia and hypercapnia on renal blood flow in normal and renal transplant subjects. *Eur. Respir. J.* **1998**, *12*, 653–657. [CrossRef]

58. Hemlin, M.; Ljungman, S.; Carlson, J.; Maljukanovic, S.; Mobini, R.; Bech-Hanssen, O.; Skoogh, B.-E.; Skoogh, B. The effects of hypoxia and hypercapnia on renal and heart function, haemodynamics and plasma hormone levels in stable COPD patients. *Clin. Respir. J.* **2007**, *1*, 80–90. [CrossRef]

59. Sharkey, R.A.; Mulloy, E.M.; O'Neill, S.J. The Acute Effects of Oxygen and Carbon Dioxide on Renal Vascular Resistance in Patients with an Acute Exacerbation of COPD. *Chest* **1999**, *115*, 1588–1592. [CrossRef]

60. Anand, I.S.; Chandrashekhar, Y.; Ferrari, R.; Sarma, R.; Guleria, R.; Jindal, S.K.; Wahi, P.L.; Poole-Wilson, P.A.; Harris, P. Pathogenesis of congestive state in chronic obstructive pulmonary disease. Studies of body water and sodium, renal function, hemodynamics, and plasma hormones during edema and after recovery. *Circulation* **1992**, *86*, 12–21. [CrossRef]

61. Sharkey, R.A.; Mulloy, E.M.; Kilgallen, I.A.; O'Neill, S.J. Renal functional reserve in patients with severe chronic obstructive pulmonary disease. *Thorax* **1997**, *52*, 411–415. [CrossRef] [PubMed]

62. MacNee, W. Pathophysiology of cor pulmonale in chronic obstructive pulmonary disease. Part One. *Am. J. Respir. Crit. Care Med.* **1994**, *150*, 833–852. [CrossRef] [PubMed]

63. Magouliotis, D.E.; Tasiopoulou, V.S.; Svokos, A.A.; Svokos, K.A.; Zacharoulis, D. Extracorporeal membrane oxygenation versus cardiopulmonary bypass during lung transplantation: A meta-analysis. *Gen. Thorac. Cardiovasc. Surg.* **2018**, *66*, 38–47. [CrossRef] [PubMed]

64. Cheungpasitporn, W.; Thongprayoon, C.; Kittanamongkolchai, W.; Srivali, N.; O'corragain, O.A.; Edmonds, P.J.; Ratanapo, S.; Spanuchart, I.; Erickson, S.B. Comparison of Renal Outcomes in Off-Pump Versus On-Pump Coronary Artery Bypass Grafting: A Systematic Review and Meta-analysis of Randomized Controlled Trials. *Nephrology* **2015**, *20*, 727–735. [CrossRef]

65. Thongprayoon, C.; Cheungpasitporn, W.; Lertjitbanjong, P.; Aeddula, N.R.; Bathini, T.; Watthanasuntorn, K.; Srivali, N.; Mao, M.A.; Kashani, K. Incidence and Impact of Acute Kidney Injury in Patients Receiving Extracorporeal Membrane Oxygenation: A Meta-Analysis. *J. Clin. Med.* **2019**, *8*, 981. [CrossRef]

66. Thongprayoon, C.; Kaewput, W.; Thamcharoen, N.; Bathini, T.; Watthanasuntorn, K.; Lertjitbanjong, P.; Sharma, K.; Salim, S.A.; Ungprasert, P.; Wijarnpreecha, K.; et al. Incidence and Impact of Acute Kidney Injury after Liver Transplantation: A Meta-Analysis. *J. Clin. Med.* **2019**, *8*, 372. [CrossRef]

67. Ojo, A.O.; Held, P.J.; Port, F.K.; Wolfe, R.A.; Leichtman, A.B.; Young, E.W.; Arndorfer, J.; Christensen, L.; Merion, R.M. Chronic Renal Failure after Transplantation of a Nonrenal Organ. *N. Engl. J. Med.* **2003**, *349*, 931–940. [CrossRef]

68. Grimm, J.C.; Lui, C.; Kilic, A.; Valero, V., 3rd; Sciortino, C.M.; Whitman, G.J.; Shah, A.S. A risk score to predict acute renal failure in adult patients after lung transplantation. *Ann. Thorac. Surg.* **2015**, *99*, 251–257. [CrossRef]

69. Imai, Y.; Parodo, J.; Kajikawa, O.; De Perrot, M.; Fischer, S.; Edwards, V.; Cutz, E.; Liu, M.; Keshavjee, S.; Martin, T.R.; et al. Injurious Mechanical Ventilation and End-Organ Epithelial Cell Apoptosis and Organ Dysfunction in an Experimental Model of Acute Respiratory Distress Syndrome. *JAMA* **2003**, *289*, 2104–2112. [CrossRef]

70. Koyner, J.L.; Murray, P.T. Mechanical ventilation and the kidney. *Blood Purif.* **2010**, *29*, 52–68. [CrossRef]

71. Brower, R.G.; Matthay, M.A.; Morris, A.; Schoenfeld, D.; Thompson, B.T.; Wheeler, A. Ventilation with lower tidal volumes as compared with traditional tidal volumes for acute lung injury and the acute respiratory distress syndrome. *N. Engl. J. Med.* **2000**, *342*, 1301–1308. [CrossRef] [PubMed]

72. Ojo, A.O. Renal Disease in Recipients of Nonrenal Solid Organ Transplantation. *Semin. Nephrol.* **2007**, *27*, 498–507. [CrossRef] [PubMed]

73. Clajus, C.; Hanke, N.; Gottlieb, J.; Stadler, M.; Weismüller, T.J.; Strassburg, C.P.; Bröcker, V.; Bara, C.; Lehner, F.; Drube, J.; et al. Renal Comorbidity After Solid Organ and Stem Cell Transplantation. *Arab. Archaeol. Epigr.* **2012**, *12*, 1691–1699. [CrossRef] [PubMed]

9

Complement and Complement Targeting Therapies in Glomerular Diseases

Sofia Andrighetto [1,2], **Jeremy Leventhal** [1], **Gianluigi Zaza** [2] and **Paolo Cravedi** [1,*]

[1]   Department of Medicine, Division of Nephrology, Icahn School of Medicine at Mount Sinai, 1 Levy Place, New York, NY 10029, USA; sofia.andrighetto@gmail.com (S.A.); jeremy.leventhal@mssm.edu (J.L.)

[2]   Renal Unit, Department of Medicine, University/Hospital of Verona, 37126 Verona, Italy; gianluigi.zaza@univr.it

*   Correspondence: paolo.cravedi@mssm.edu

Abstract: The complement cascade is part of the innate immune system whose actions protect hosts from pathogens. Recent research shows complement involvement in a wide spectrum of renal disease pathogenesis including antibody-related glomerulopathies and non-antibody-mediated kidney diseases, such as C3 glomerular disease, atypical hemolytic uremic syndrome, and focal segmental glomerulosclerosis. A pivotal role in renal pathogenesis makes targeting complement activation an attractive therapeutic strategy. Over the last decade, a growing number of anti-complement agents have been developed; some are approved for clinical use and many others are in the pipeline. Herein, we review the pathways of complement activation and regulation, illustrate its role instigating or amplifying glomerular injury, and discuss the most promising novel complement-targeting therapies.

Keywords: complement; alternative complement pathway; complement-targeting therapies; C3 glomerulopathy; hemolytic uremic syndrome; focal segmental glomerulosclerosis

1. Complement Cascade

The complement system consists of soluble or membrane-bound molecules, mostly zymogens, activated through a tightly regulated proteolytic cascade [1,2]. Current understanding of complement immune mechanisms include (1) functioning as opsonins; (2) producing chemoattractants to recruit immune cells thereby enhancing site specific angiogenesis, vasodilation and coagulation cascade regulator; and (3) functioning as an enhancing bridge to adaptive T and B lymphocyte responses [3]. Current research suggests that abnormal complement activation plays a role in autoimmune inflammatory diseases and particularly in those targeting the kidney.

2. Complement Cascade Activation and Regulation

Complement activation proceeds via three pathways: the classical, alternative, and mannitol-binding lectin (MBL). The pathways have both unique and overlapping proteins, activated by a proteolytic cascade, that respond to pathogenic insults [3,4] (Figure 1). The classical and MBL pathways are initiated by antibodies and bacterial mannose motifs binding to C1q and mannose-associated serine proteases (MASPs), respectively [5,6]. Conversely, spontaneous hydrolysis of C3 on cell surfaces produces constitutive alternative pathway (AP) activation [7], and is tightly controlled by a number of regulators [8]. Decay accelerating factor (DAF) and membrane cofactor protein (MCP) (CD46, murine homolog Crry) are cell surface-expressed complement regulators that accelerate the decay of surface-assembled C3 convertases, thereby limiting amplification of the downstream cascade. DAF restrains convertase-mediated C3 cleavage; MCP and factor H (fH) also have a cofactor activity: together with soluble factor I (fI), they irreversibly cleave C3b into iC3b, thereby preventing reformation of the C3 convertase.

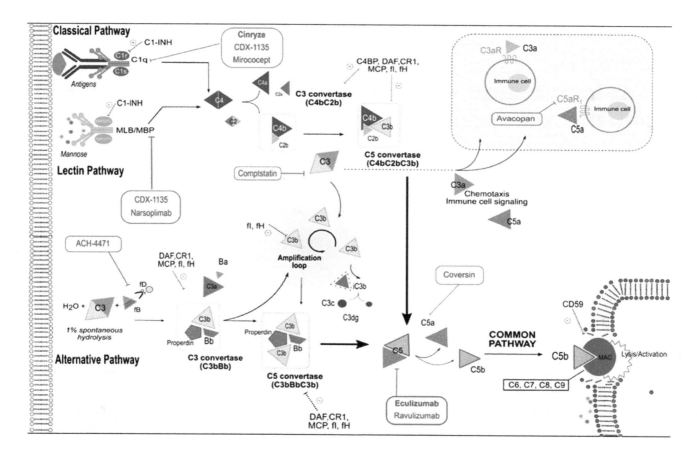

Figure 1. Overview of the complement cascade and principal complement targeting molecules. Three pathways can initiate complement cascade: (1) The classical, (2) the mannose-binding lectin (MBL), and (3) the alternative pathway. They all converge on C3 convertases formation which continuously cleave C3; after they are activated, the C3 convertase from alternative pathway dominates within an amplification loop that sustains the production of C3b (circular arrow). The three C3 convertases associate with an additional C3b to form the C5 convertases, which cleave C5 into C5a + C5b. C5b fragments recruits C6, C7, C8, and multiple C9 molecules to generate the terminal membrane attack complex (MAC); MAC inserts pores into cell membranes to induce cell lysis or activation. Anaphilotoxins C3a and C5a through their G protein-coupled receptors C3aR and C5aR, respectively, can promote signaling, inflammation, chemotaxis of leukocytes, vasodilation, cytokine and chemokine release, and activation of adaptive immunity. Dotted black arrows: inhibitor function of a complement effector on its target. Red arrows emerging from balloons: inhibitor function of anti complement drug on its target (bold drugs' names are the FDA approved ones). Full arrow: consequential interaction between complement fractions leads to the subsequent cascade step. Full bold arrow: final convergence of the three complement pathways on same final target. MBL: Mannose binding lectin; MASP: Mannose-binding lectin-associated serine protease; C4BP: C4 binding protein; C1-INH: C1 inhibitor; DAF: Decay accelerating factor; CR1: Surface complement receptor 1; MCP: Membrane cofactor protein; CD59: Protectin; fD: Factor D; fB: Factor B; fI: Factor I; fH: Factor H. Red balloons highlights complement target drugs' points of action (see Table 1).

Table 1. Summary of complement blocking agents.

Name.	Class	Pharmacodinamics	Disease	Status	Additional Info
Eculizumab	Humanized monoclonal antibody	Binds C5 preventing MAC generation	aHUS, DDD, C3GN	Available for use in PHN and aHUS	First USA FDA-approved among anti-complement drugs
Ravulizumab ALXN1210	Humanized monoclonal antibody	Binds C5 preventing MAC generation	aHUS	Phase III for PHN	Induces prolonged decease of C5 plasmatic levels allowing longer dosing intervals compared to Eculizumab
Coversin	Small dimension recombinant protein	Prevents cleavage of C5 into C5a/C5b by C5 convertase	aHUS	Phase II for PHN	Valid alternative for patients bearer of C5 molecule polymorphisms which interferes with correct binding of Eculizumab
Avacopan CCX168	Small dimension anti-inflammatory molecule	Inhibits selectively C5aR	aHUS ANCA-vasculitides	Phanse III for ANCA vasculitides. Phase II for aHUS	Effective replacing high-dose glucocorticoids in treating vasculitis
CDX-1135	C1R-based molecule	Inhibits CR1	DDD	Phase I for DDD	
Mirococept APT070	CR1-based molecule	Inhibits CR1	IRI in Tx	Phase I for DDD, C3GN	
Cinryze	C1 estarase	Inhibits CR1	Antibody-mediated rejection in renal transplant	Available for use in HAE. Phase III for prevention of DGF in cadaveric allograft	FDA approved for hereditary angioedema
Narsoplimab OMS721	Humanized monoclonal antibody	Binds the mannan-binding lectin-associated serinprotease-2	aHUS, TTP IgAN	Phase II for aHUS, IgA, LES, MN, C3G	Multi-dose administration is needed
ACH-4471	Small dimension molecule	Inhibits factor D	aHUS	Phase II for IC-MPGN, DDD, C3GN	Oral assumption with delivery advantage over intravenously infused agents

aHUS: Atypical hemolytic uremic syndrome, DDD: Dense deposit disease, C3GN: C3 glomerular disease, MAC: Membrane attack complex, ANCA: Antineutrophilic cystoplasmic antibody, IRI: Ischemia riper fusion injury, TTP: Thrombotic thrombocytopenia, IgAN: IgA Nephropathy, HAE: Hereditary angioedema, DGF: Delayed graft function.

The three activation pathways converge in C3 convertases that continuously cleave C3 into C3a and C3b. C3a signals on cell surface G protein-coupled receptor (GPCR) C3aR, while C3b forms additional alternative pathways C3 convertases (even if initiated via the other pathways), as well as C5 convertases. C5 convertases produce the split products C5a and C5b. While C5a functions similarly to C3a (but signals via C5aR) C5b, in conjunction with C6–C9, forms the membrane attack complex (MAC) leading to cell lysis/activation [9]. Countering distal complement MAC formation is CD59, a circulating complement inhibitor.

3. Effector Functions

Complement proteins promote inflammation and immune cell activity in multiple ways. C3a and C5a ligate their transmembrane-spanning receptors, C3aR and C5aR, on immune cells, leading to the production of proinflammatory cytokines and chemokines and promoting vasodilation. They also mediate neutrophil and macrophage chemoattraction, activate macrophages to promote intracellular killing of engulfed organisms, and contribute to T-cell and antigen-presenting cell (APC) activation, expansion, and survival [10–13]. The more distal complement proteins (C5b-9) form MAC complexes on cell membranes, promoting lysis of non-nucleated cells, such as red blood cells, or pathogens lacking cell surface complement inhibitors, such as bacteria. MAC insertion into nucleated eukaryotic cells generally does not result in lysis, but rather induces immune activation [14] and/or promotes tissue injury [15]. C3b and other bound cleavage products function as opsonins binding to specific surface-expressed receptors (complement receptors CR1, CR2, CR3, and CR4).

4. Complement in Glomerular Diseases

4.1. Diseases with Antibody-Mediated Complement Activation

The majority of circulating, or fluid-phase, complement components are produced by the liver. Liver produced complement components are involved in auto-antibody initiated glomerulonephritis (GN) through the classical and/or MBL pathways. Inadequate regulation of alternative pathway activity, due to inherited and/or acquired abnormalities of complement regulators, can result in glomerular injury from persistent C3 convertase activity with consequent excessive MAC activity. Complement can also be produced by parenchymal (e.g., tubular cells in the kidney [16] and resident/infiltrating immune cells, (e.g., T cells and APCs) [17–19]. The relative contributions of systemic or locally produced complement in GN pathogenesis remains unclear.

4.2. IgA Nephropathy

IgA nephropathy (IgAN) is the most common form of GN worldwide [20,21]; its clinical presentation varies, but it often includes proteinuria and hematuria. The disease is associated with aberrant O-glycosylation of mucosal IgA1 with galactose-deficient IgA1 (Gd-IgA1) which plays a pivotal role in the progression of IgAN [22]. They deposit in glomeruli and, subsequently, development of circulating/in situ immunoglobulins (IgA or IgG) targeting glycosylated IgA takes place [23,24]. Mesangial IgA and immune complexes deposits are often observed and initiate glomerular injury.

In vitro and in vivo studies showed that polymeric mucosal IgA activates the complement system through the alternative or MBL pathway [25], and glomerular MBL correlates with greater disease severity and a worse prognosis [26]. Although C3 levels in plasma are usually normal, glomerular C3 deposits can be detected in approximately 85% of biopsies, with C5b-9 also often present along with C3 during infections [27]. MAC generated from complement activation attack on mesangial cells inducing them to proliferate and over-produce oxidants, proteases, cytokines, growth factors (e.g., transforming growth factor β and platelet-derived growth factor) and extracellular matrix material that together result in the typical focal proliferative GN with mesangial matrix expansion characteristic of IgA nephropathy [28].

A genomic wide association study (GWAS) of IgAN in a cohort of 3144 cases of Chinese and European ancestry, linked allele deletion polymorphisms of complement factor H-related proteins one and three (*CFHR1* and *CFHR3*) with less severe IgA nephropathy [29,30]. Since CFHR proteins interfere with factor H complement regulation (Figure 1) their deficiency might reduce complement activation and lessen IgAN. CFHR1, CFHR3, and CFHR5 especially have been studied for their role in IgAN [29,31]; another study of 1126 Chinese patients concluded that circulating CFHR5 levels are an independent risk factor for the disease: levels were higher in IgAN subjects compared to heathy controls, and correlated directly with worst Oxford MEST pathology score, a lower glomerular filtration rate (GFR), and hypertension [32].

4.3. Membranous Nephropathy

Membranous nephropathy (MN) is the second most commonly diagnosed GN, and the most common cause for nephrotic syndrome in adults (20–50%) [33]. Disease progression varies greatly with ~1/3 of patients undergoing spontaneous remission, ~1/3 developing progressive renal insufficiency, and ~1/3 maintaining normal GFR despite persistent proteinuria. MN is characterized by presence of anti-podocyte antibodies in the subepithelial space of glomerular capillary loops and granular deposits of IgG4 and C3. M-type phospholipase A2 receptor (PLA$_2$R) has been found as the main target podocyte antigen for autoantibodies in 70–80% of patients with primary MN, while antibodies against thrombospondin type 1 domain-containing 7A (THSD7A) are detected in a minority of patients [34]. Although antibodies from IgG4 subclass are poor classical complement pathway activators, deposition of C3 and breakdown of C4b products are detectable in almost all patients with a primary form of MN [27]. Mannose binding lectin and MBL-associated serine protease expression (MASP-1, MASP-2) are detected in PLA$_2$R positive patients' glomeruli, suggesting that complement activation proceeds through this pathway [35]. Hypogalactosylated IgG (including IgG4) binds MBL and activates the complement providing a possible explanation to the IgG4 conundrum [36]. Animal studies also indicate a role for MAC insertion into podocytes; blocking their formation prevents disease [37]. Sublytic activation alters podocyte cytoskeletal structure crucial for slit diaphragm integrity and function, leading to proteinuria [38,39].

4.4. Post Infectious Glomerulonephritis

Post infectious GN is a common cause of nephritic syndrome that develops after self-limited bacterial infections (most commonly from *streptococcal* or *staphylococcal* species). It occurs mainly in childhood, but can also be seen in adults. It is characterized by hypercellularity within the capillary loops (caused by neutrophils infiltration and endothelial proliferation) and strong C3 staining, usually in addition to IgG. Post infectious GN occurs due to passive glomerular trapping of circulating immune complexes composed of nephritogenic bacterial antigens and IgG, complement activation, and attraction of neutrophils responsible for glomerular injury [28]. However, levels of C1q and C4 deposition are lacking or low in most of the cases [40,41], suggesting contributions from lectin and alternative pathway. This is eventually triggered from specific pathogens' components; for example, streptococcal pyrogenic exotoxin B is a possible alternative pathway activation [42]. Autoantibodies with C3 nephritic factor (C3nef), activity that binds to and stabilizes C3 convertases, has also been reported in post-infectious GN and may be associated with an enhanced cleavage of C3 [28]. In some patients underlying genetic defects in the regulation of the alternative pathway, including mutations in complement regulators (fH or CFHR5) and presence of C3Nef, lead to persistent glomerular deposition of complement factors within the glomeruli and inflammatory infiltrates that resemble features of a persistent proliferative glomerulonephritis [43]. Interestingly, in few cases, post infectious GN evolved into C3 glomerulopathy (C3G) [44]: recent reports document repeat biopsies demonstrating transformation of post infectious GN to C3G, including identical appearing early lesions of C3G and initiation of C3G by streptococcal infection. Sethi et al. [43] described that most of the cases with biopsy-proven persistent post-infectious GN had underlying genetic mutations and/or auto-antibodies affecting regulation of the alternative complement pathway. These findings indicate that glomerular injuries initiated by infection may transfer to C3G by imbalanced alternative complement pathway activation: C3G is initiated by heterogeneous insults, leading to a final common pathway of alternative complement dysregulation.

4.5. Immune Complex-Mediated Membranoproliferative Glomerulonephritis (MPGN)

Membranoproliferative glomerulonephritis (MPGN) is a histopathological pattern of glomerular injury characterized by mesangial hypercellularity, capillary wall changes (i.e., "tram-tracking"), and endocapillary proliferation found in 7–10% of biopsy-diagnosed glomerulonephritis [45]. MPGN classification was based on electron micrograph ultrastructural findings but advances in our understanding of underlying pathomechanisms produced a rethinking of MPGN and a classification schema based on immunofluorescence findings; MPGN is caused by immune complex deposition, C3 dysregulation, or thrombotic microangiopathy (TMA) [45]. Immune complex-mediated MPGN is caused by immune complex deposition in the subendothelial space activating complement classical pathways and causing glomerular injury. When not linked to a systemic disease, it is termed 'idiopathic' but secondary forms more commonly occur in association with infections (e.g., hepatitis B, C, or tuberculosis), autoimmune diseases (e.g., Sjogren's Syndrome or systemic lupus erythematosus SLE), or monoclonal gammopathy. Clinical evidence of classical complement activation in immune complex-mediated MPGN includes preferential consumption of plasma C4 (although C3 is often low as well) and detection of C1q and terminal C5b-9 complex in glomeruli. This phase is followed by an influx of leukocytes, promoted by formation of the C3a and C5a anaphylatoxins, leading to capillary damage and proteinuria [46]. Activation of classical pathway through immunoglobulins is the most prominent pathogenic process, but heterozygous mutations in alternative pathway complement regulators and the presence of circulating C3nef factor are also identified in some patients with immune complex-mediated MPGN, suggesting additional contributions from the alternative pathway [47]. These findings raise the possibility that in individuals with genetic or acquired complement alternative pathway dysregulation, immune complex deposition initially triggers injury through the classical pathway but chronic kidney injury is sustained through the enhanced alternative pathway [46]. The complement also features prominently in the two other dominant etiologies of MPGN: C3 glomerulopathies and TMA from atypical Hemolytic Uremic Syndrome (aHUS), and these are discussed in detail later in this paper.

4.6. Anti-GBM Glomerulonephritis

Anti-glomerular basement membrane (GBM) is a rare life-threatening autoimmune disease, caused by IgG autoantibodies against alpha 3 NC1 domain of collagen IV of the GBM. Antibody binding to the GBM leads to injury characterized by strong complement activation, leukocyte infiltration, and proteinuria; leading to crescent formation, scarring, and, frequently, end-stage renal disease (ESRD). Evidence of complement pathogenic role comes from detection of complement components MBL, C1q, factor B (fB), properdin, C3d/C4d, and C5b-9 in GBM, and circulating MAC levels that correlate with kidney injury severity [48]. Local complement activation produces C3a- and C5a-mediated inflammation, as well as MAC-dependent sublytic activation of glomerular cells, which together enhance inflammation and extracellular matrix formation [49]. Pathways of complement activation in anti-GBM disease have been studied in murine models by injection of heterologous antibodies against GBM, where C3 and C4 deficiency prevented full manifestation of renal disease [46,50,51]. This evidence supports involvement of, at least, both classical and alternative pathways in anti-GBM disease.

4.7. ANCA Induced Renal Vasculitis

Antineutrophil cytoplasmic antibody (ANCA) associated vasculitides commonly target the kidney, with abundant complement component deposition in vessels and glomeruli without immunoglobulin (pauci-immune). Current research supports that vascular injury is due to cytokine-primed neutrophils displaying surface ANCA-binding antigens (myeloperoxidase and proteinase-3) that undergo degranulation while simultaneously activating alternative complement pathways which potentiates neutrophil recruitment via C5a [8]. C5a generation functions as an amplification loop for ANCA-mediated neutrophil activation, eventually culminating in the severe necrotizing inflammation of the vessel walls. Studies in animal models have also shown complement contributes to pathogenesis, and agents blocking C5 cleavage/C5a signaling or C5 and fB deficiency themselves are protective; conversely, preventing MAC formation is ineffective, supporting the importance of C5a in ANCA-mediated pathogenesis [52,53]. A recent trial of patients with ANCA vasculitis compared the use of rituximab/cyclophosphamide in addition to either placebo and high-dose steroids, avacopan (C5aR antagonist) plus reduced dose steroids, or avacopan and no steroids. Regimens with low or absent steroids were non-inferior to traditional regimens; this illustrates complement's essential role in ANCA vasculitis and suggests C5aR antagonism as a feasible alternative in patients where steroids are contraindicated [54].

4.8. Lupus Nephritis

Systemic lupus erythematosus (SLE) is an autoimmune disorder characterized by antibodies to self-antigens (e.g., anti-nuclear) leading to the formation of immune complexes that deposit in target organs. Lupus nephritis (LN) is one severe complication of SLE. Up to 50% of patients with SLE have clinically evident kidney disease at presentation, and up to 75% develop it during the course of the disease [55]. The hallmark of renal pathology is simultaneous glomerular deposition of IgG, IgM, IgA, C4, and C3, referring to the poker hand ranking, the "full house pattern" [55]. Complement deposition is not merely a biomarker of LN, as it mediates direct glomerular injury: Immune complex-mediated classical pathway plays a key pathogenic role through both intra capillary generation of neutrophil and macrophage chemotactic factors (class II–IV) and formation of MAC (class V) [56]. Circulating C3 and C4 levels are reduced in more than 90% of patients with diffuse proliferative LN and their decline often reflects a worsening in disease activity [57]. Extensive data from animal models also indicate a significant role for alternative pathway activation: Deletion of regulators (i.e., fH) or activators (i.e., fB and fD) worsen or ameliorate, respectively, experimental LN [58–60]. In humans, plasma Bb levels (but not C3) are associated with LN outcome and strongly correlated with MAC levels. In addition, Bb co-localized with MAC in the glomeruli with LN, overall supporting the concept that activation of MAC in LN reflects alternative pathway activation [57]. Experimental LN can be prevented by blockade of all complement pathways through the administration of CR2-*Crry* fusion protein [61]. Data also show that the disease severity can be ameliorated by C5aR blockade [62] or anti-C5 mAb [63], which suggests the potential clinical relevance of complement pathway intervention. A phase 1 human trial with eculizumab (anti-C5) suggested preliminary efficacy, but the treatment period was too short to draw definitive conclusions [64]. The complement system seems to have a paradoxical role in SLE: genetically determined complement deficiencies or development of anti-complement antibodies involving components of the classical pathway (anti-C1q or C1-INH) [65], are strong risk factors. Susceptibility is likely due to a defective clearance of nuclear antigens released by injured and apoptotic cells since experimental studies have shown that such deficiencies lead to autoantibody production and glomerular injury [66].

5. Disease with Complement Activation in the Absence of Detectable Serum Antibodies

5.1. Atypical Hemolytic Uremic Syndrome

Hemolytic uremic syndrome (HUS) is defined by the triad of mechanical hemolytic anemia, thrombocytopenia and acute kidney injury. Renal pathology shows typically diffuse fibrin thrombi, endothelial swelling and capillary lumens narrowed/collapsed (acute features), or reduplication of GMB, mesangiolysis, and vessels recanalization (chronic phase). Typical forms of HUS are related to infection by Shiga toxin (Stx) producing *Escherichia coli* (STEC), while aHUS) is a condition due to defects in alternative complement activation. It has been associated with a predisposing genotype, usually an inherited heterozygous mutation [67,68], rather than an acquired mutation or loss of complement proteins (e.g., fI, fH, MCP).

The first identified mutant gene encodes for fH [28], the most important alternative pathway regulator in plasma and on cell surfaces. Subsequently, over 100 mutations were identified and most commonly lead to normal levels of a protein that is unable to bind and regulate complement components on endothelial cells [69].

Most complement genes mutations associated with aHUS result in an altered cell surface regulation: MCP mutation and fI mutation prevent effective degradation of C3 convertase. Although rarer, factors C3/C3b or fB gain of function mutations have been described [28]. Formation of blocking antibodies direct against fH is also another possible pathogenic mechanism [46,68]. 3–5% of patients with aHUS also carry heterozygous mutation of thrombomodulin (THBD), a molecule that normally enhances fI function [70]. As discussed below, complement targeting therapies have been extremely effective in treating this condition.

5.2. C3 Nephropathy

C3 nephropathy (C3N) is a rare nephritic disease, with a poor long-term outcome. The membranoproliferative pattern is the most common (not unique) histological presentation of C3 nephropathy and is further divided in the two entities of: Dense deposit disease (DDD), with typical ultrastructural evidence of intramembranous highly electron-dense osmophilic deposits with or without IgG and C3 on immunofluorescence, and C3 glomerulonephritis (C3GN) diagnosed with C3 positive on IF while all others immunoglobulins are negative [71,72]. Low serum C3 and glomerular deposits of C3 are emblematic of alternative pathway dysregulation.

A major subset of C3 glomerulopathies arises from C3Nef autoantibodies (present in 40% of C3GN and 80% of DDD) stabilizing C3 convertases against complement regulatory proteins (CRegs), or from other antibodies (former anti-fB, anti-fH) targeting directly CRegs [47]. C3 glomerulopathy can be due to genetic missense or non-sense mutations, affecting genes that encode for complement components or regulators [46,73]. The most important seems to involve fH, fI, and CFHR proteins with loss of function [74]; C3 mutation with gain of function and resistance to fH is uncommon [75] and when C5 genes are affected a less severe form of GN occurs [76]. fH/fI deficiency/resistance play a critical role in developing the disease because the GBM does not express CRegs and therefore relies on circulating ones (i.e., fH/fI) to prevent excessive local fluid phase AP activation.

Several cases of familiar C3 glomerulopathy have also been described when mutation of CFHR gene cluster occurs; recently an autosomal dominant inheritance among some Cypriote families has been described. In this nephropathy, CFHR5 has reduced affinity for surface-bound complement [77], the glomeruli present with C3GN features but C3 levels in the serum tend to be normal suggesting that improper complement activation occurs in the glomerulus rather than plasma [46,78–81].

6. Other Glomerular Diseases

Focal Segmental Glomerulosclerosis

Focal segmental glomerulosclerosis (FSGS), is one of the leading causes of nephrotic syndrome in adults. Patients with non-nephrotic proteinuria have good prognosis and about 15% progress to ESRD over the course of 10 years, whereas 50% of patients with nephrotic-range proteinuria progress to ESRD over 5–10 years [82]. In patients with massive proteinuria (10–14 g/d), the course is malignant, resulting in ESRD by 2–3 years on average [82]. It is characterized by focal and segmental obliteration of glomerular capillary tufts, with an increase in matrix. The sources of podocyte damage are varied and not altogether known, but include circulating factors, genetic abnormalities, viral infection, and medications that produce common deleterious effects on podocytes. C3 and IgM glomerular deposition is typical, suggesting complement activation contributes to FSGS pathogenesis [83]. Sclerotic lesions are significantly higher in patients with C3 deposition combined with IgM; they have worse renal dysfunction and limited response to therapy [84]. Murine models of FSGS clarified that glomerular IgM deposits activate complement, suggesting that glomerular injury simultaneously increases classical pathway activation by natural IgM, which binds to injury associated epitopes, while also decreasing glomerular alternative complement regulating abilities [85]. Consistent with a pathogenic role for IgM, B cell absence in murine FSGS models prevents IgM deposition and albuminuria [85]. In humans, mutations in fH and C3 have been described in literature cases of biopsy documented FSGS [86] and FSGS patient urine and plasma are enriched with complement fragments C3a, C3b, Ba, Bb, C4a, sC5b-9 compared to samples from patients with other renal diseases [87].

7. Complement Inhibitory Drugs in Kidney Diseases

Identification of complement component contributions to renal pathogenesis recently spurred pharmaceutical industry efforts to therapeutically target complement

Many available agents target terminal complement molecules and more proximal roles, such as opsonization, remains preserved. Even so, since these agents are immunosuppressants, they convey increased infection risk. More importantly, relevant to kidney diseases, many upstream elements (e.g., C3a, C5a, and C3b) contribute to pathogenesis and are not effectively targeted by available compounds. Currently, Food and Drug Administration (FDA) approved complement inhibitors include the monoclonal anti-C5 antibody Eculizumab, and Cynrize an inhibitor of fragment C1 (C1-INH) [88–90].

7.1. Eculizumab

Eculizumab is a humanized murine monoclonal antibody to complement C5 that acts on the terminal complement cascade preventing the formation of C5a, C5b, and C5b-9. The drug use has been approved by European Medicines Agency's (EMA) and FDA for treatment of paroxysmal nocturnal hemoglobinuria (PNH) and aHUS [91]. The major side effect is predisposition to infections, especially from gram-negative bacteria; as such, all patients are advised to be immunized for *meningococcus* before receiving eculizumab. Eculizumab approval for aHUS treatment was given based on results from two prospective trials: one involving 17 aHUS patients with thrombocytopenia and the other with 20 aHUS patients requiring persistent plasma exchange (PE) [92]. Whole patients from these cohorts no longer required PE and 88% reached normal hematological values after median of 63 weeks of Eculizumab treatment. This medication has dramatically improved renal morbidity, with consistent decreases in ESRD risk, but its clinical use is still limited by uncertainty over patient selection, timing, and duration of treatment. An ongoing multi center single-arm trial is now testing the safety Eculizumab discontinuation in patients with aHUS (NCT02574403). Eculizumab has also been successfully used to prevent or treat recurrence of aHUS after kidney transplant [93–95], but appears ineffective in preventing delayed graft function (NCT01919346) [96] in sensitized kidney transplant recipients (NCT00670774, NCT01095887, NCT01327573) [97,98].

Eculizumab has successfully treated patients with DDD and C3GN highlighting its potential with these rare diseases. Treatment of six patients (three C3GN and three DDD) resulted in complete to partial remission in four patients at one year of follow-up [99]. This positive effect was limited to patients with crescentic rapidly progressive C3 glomerulopathy as opposed to a more insidious C3GN suggesting that it is specific to disease pathogenesis. Moreover, advantages are not seen so far in C3GN recurrence after kidney transplantation [100]. Eculizumab use in patients with glomerular diseases other than aHUS or C3GN/DDD is limited to case reports and of uncertain efficacy. The price of eculizumab is a factor that limits its use. Competitors have in clinical development both similar agents targeting C5 (e.g., Ravulizumab), as well as agents that affect complement component C5a (i.e., Avacoban).

7.2. C1 Inhibitor

Despite the potential advantages of terminal complement inhibition, these approaches may not be sufficient in conditions stemming from more proximal complement activation. Classical complement pathway activation occurs when C1q binds the Fc portion of antigen bound immunoglobulin. Preventing this process is C1-esterase inhibitor and its absence or mutated function produces the condition hereditary angioedema. *Cinryze,* a human serum derived C1 inhibitor (C1-INH) is FDA approved for treatment of hereditary angioedema. C1-INH does not have approved indications for kidney disease, but a phase I/II study was conducted on highly sensitized renal transplant recipients randomized to C1INH or placebo. Antibody mediated rejection was prevented in all 10 patients receiving C1INH group and 9/10 only receiving placebo. Efficacy and safety of C1INH for treatment of acute antibody mediated rejection in kidney transplantation is being evaluated in a randomized double-blind study of donor-sensitized kidney transplants recipients (NCT02052141, NCT02547220) [101]. Results may broaden its use to patients with antibody mediated rejection.

8. Conclusions

The complement system is a complex network of proteins that augment immune system function and, in many cases, contribute to kidney disease pathogenesis. Increasing research suggests that selective interventions to stop cascade activation can halt or even reverse renal disease. Ongoing research, both translational and in animal models, will help delineate which pathway(s), and at what level, intervention could be effective. Although infrequently a primary insult, common mutations affecting complement regulation synergize with other pathological features perpetuating inflammation and, ultimately, nephron loss. The advent of selective complement-targeting therapeutics offers the opportunity for new treatment strategies for renal disease, an area in desperate need of new options.

Author Contributions: S.A. and J.L. searched the literature and wrote the manuscript. G.Z. and P.C. contributed to the literature search and literature analysis. P.C. revised the manuscript. All authors read and approved the final manuscript.

References

1. Walport, M.J. Complement—First of Two Parts. *N. Engl. J. Med.* **2001**, *344*, 1058–1066. [CrossRef] [PubMed]
2. Walport, M.J. Complement: Second of two parts: Complement at the interface between innate and adaptive immunity. *N. Engl. J. Med.* **2001**, *344*, 1140–1144. [CrossRef] [PubMed]
3. Mizuno, M.; Suzuki, Y.; Ito, Y. Complement regulation and kidney diseases: Recent knowledge of the double-edged roles of complement activation in nephrology. *Clin. Exp. Nephrol.* **2018**, *22*, 3–14. [CrossRef] [PubMed]
4. Hourcade, D.E.; Spitzer, D.; Mitchell, L.M.; Atkinson, J.P. Properdin Can Initiate Complement Activation by Binding Specific Target Surfaces and Providing a Platform for De Novo. *J. Immunol. Ref.* **2007**, *179*, 2600–2608.
5. Holmskov, U.; Thiel, S.; Jensenius, J.C. Collectin and Ficolins: Humoral Lectins of the Innate Immune Defense. *Annu. Rev. Immunol.* **2003**, *21*, 547–578. [CrossRef]
6. Endo, Y.; Matsushita, M.; Fujita, T. The role of ficolins in the lectin pathway of innate immunity. *Int. J. Biochem. Cell Biol.* **2011**, *43*, 705–712. [CrossRef]
7. Forneris, F.; Ricklin, D.; Wu, J.; Tzekou, A.; Wallace, R.S.; Lambris, J.D.; Gros, P. Structures of C3b in Complex with Factors B and D Give Insight into Complement Convertase Formation. *Science* **2010**, *330*, 1816–1820. [CrossRef]
8. Mathern, D.R.; Heeger, P.S. Molecules Great and Small: The Complement System. *Clin. J. Am. Soc. Nephrol.* **2015**, *10*, 1636–1650. [CrossRef]
9. Ricklin, D.; Hajishengallis, G.; Yang, K.; Lambris, J.D. Complement-a key system for immune surveillance and homeostasis. *Nat. Immunol.* **2010**, *11*, 785. [CrossRef]

10.   Guo, R.-F.; Ward, P.A. Role of C5a in inflamatory response. *Annu. Rev. Immunol.* **2005**, *23*, 821–852. [CrossRef]

11.   Kwan, W.H.; van der Touw, W.; Paz-Artal, E.; Li, M.O.; Heeger, P.S. Signaling through C5a receptor and C3a receptor diminishes function of murine natural regulatory T cells. *J. Exp. Med.* **2013**, *210*, 257–268. [CrossRef] [PubMed]

12.   Van Der Touw, W.; Cravedi, P.; Kwan, W.-H.; Paz-Artal, E.; Merad, M.; Heeger, P.S. Receptors for C3a and C5a modulate stability of alloantigen-reactive induced regulatory T cells. *J. Immunol.* **2013**, *190*, 5921–5925. [CrossRef] [PubMed]

13.   Klos, A.; Tenner, A.J.; Johswich, K.-O.; Ager, R.R.; Reis, E.S.; Köhl, J. The Role of the Anaphylatoxins in Health and Disease. *Mol. Immunol.* **2009**, *46*, 2753–2766. [CrossRef] [PubMed]

14.   Jane-wit, D.; Manes, T.D.; Yi, T.; Qin, L.; Clark, P.; Kirkiles-Smith, N.C.; Abrahimi, P.; Devalliere, J.; Moeckel, G.; Kulkarni, S.; et al. Alloantibody and Complement Promote T Cell-Mediated Cardiac Allograft Vasculopathy through Non-Canonical NF-κB Signaling in Endothelial Cells. *Circulation* **2013**, *128*, 2504–2516. [CrossRef]

15.   Adler, S.; Baker, P.J.; Johnson, R.J.; Ochi, R.F.; Pritzl, P.; Couser, W.G. Complement Membrane Attack Complex. Stimulates Production of Reactive Oxygen Metabolites by Cultured Rat Mesangial Cells. *J. Clin. Investig.* **1996**, *77*, 762–767. [CrossRef]

16.   Peake, P.W.; O'Grady, S.; Pussell, B.A.; Charlesworth, J.A. C3a is made by proximal tubular HK-2 cells and activates them via the C3a receptor. *Kidney Int.* **1999**, *56*, 1729–1736. [CrossRef]

17.   Lalli, P.N.; Strainic, M.G.; Yang, M.; Lin, F.; Medof, M.E.; Heeger, P.S. Locally produced C5a binds to T cell-expressed C5aR to enhance effector T-cell expansion by limiting antigen-induced apoptosis. *Blood* **2008**, *11*, 1759–1766. [CrossRef]

18.   Strainic, M.G.; Liu, J.; Huang, D.; An, F.; Lalli, P.N.; Muqim, N.; Shapiro, V.S.; Dubyak, G.R.; Heeger, P.S.; Medof, M.E. Locally Produced Complement Fragments C5a and C3a Provide Both Costimulatory and Survival Signals to Naive CD4 + T. Cells. *Immunity* **2008**, *28*, 425–435. [CrossRef]

19.   Heeger, P.S.; Lalli, P.N.; Lin, F.; Valujskikh, A.; Liu, J.; Muqim, N.; Xu, Y.; Medof, M.E. Decay-accelerating factor modulates induction of T cell immunity. *J. Exp. Med.* **2005**, *201*, 1523–1530. [CrossRef]

20.   Hanko, J.B.; Mullan, R.N.; O'rourke, D.M.; Mcnamee, P.T.; Maxwell, A.P.; Courtney, A.E. The changing pattern of adult primary glomerular disease. *Nephrol. Dial. Transpl.* **2009**, *24*, 3050–3054. [CrossRef]

21.   Nair, R.; Walker, P.D. Is IgA nephropathy the commonest primary glomerulopathy among young adults in the USA? *Kidney Int.* **2006**, *69*, 1455–1458. [CrossRef] [PubMed]

22.   Wada Id, Y.; Matsumoto, K.; Suzuki, T.; Saito, T.; Kanazawa, N.; Tachibanaid, S.; Iseri, K.; Sugiyama, M.; Iyoda, M.; Shibata, T. Clinical significance of serum and mesangial galactose-deficient IgA1 in patients with IgA nephropathy. *PLoS ONE* **2018**, *13*, e0206865. [CrossRef] [PubMed]

23.   Mestecky, J.; Raska, M.; Julian, B.A.; Gharavi, A.G.; Renfrow, M.B.; Moldoveanu, Z.; Novak, L.; Matousovic, K.; Novak, J. IgA Nephropathy: Molecular Mechanisms of the Disease. *Annu. Rev. Pathol: Mech. Dis.* **2012**, *8*, 217–240. [CrossRef] [PubMed]

24.   Lafayette, R.A.; Kelepouris, E.; Lafayette, R. Immunoglobulin A Nephropathy: Advances in Understanding of Pathogenesis and Treatment. *Rev. Artic. Am. J. Nephrol* **2018**, *47*, 43–52. [CrossRef] [PubMed]

25.   Oortwijn, B.D.; Eijgenraam, J.W.; Rastaldi, M.P.; Roos, A.; Daha, M.R.; van Kooten, C. The Role of Secretory IgA and Complement in IgA Nephropathy. *Semin. Nephrol.* **2008**, *28*, 58–65. [CrossRef] [PubMed]

26.   Roos, A.; Rastaldi, M.P.; Calvaresi, N.; Oortwijn, B.D.; Schlagwein, N.; Van Gijlswijk-Janssen, D.J.; Stahl, G.L.; Matsushita, M.; Fujita, T.; Van Kooten, C.; et al. Glomerular Activation of the Lectin Pathway of Complement in IgA Nephropathy Is Associated with More Severe Renal Disease. *J. Am. Soc. Nephrol.* **2006**, *17*, 1724–1734. [CrossRef] [PubMed]

27.   Thurman, J.M. Complement in Kidney Disease: Core Curriculum. *Am. J. Kidney Dis.* **2015**, *65*, 156–168. [CrossRef]

28.   Couser, W.G. Pathogenesis and treatment of glomerulonephritis-an update. *J. Bras. Nefrol.* **2016**, *38*, 107–122. [CrossRef]

29.   Gharavi, A.G.; Kiryluk, K.; Choi, M.; Li, Y.; Hou, P.; Xie, J.; Sanna-Cherchi, S.; Men, C.J.; Julian, B.A.; Wyatt, R.J.; et al. Genome-wide association study identifies susceptibility loci for IgA nephropathy. *Nat. Genet.* **2011**, *43*, 321–329. [CrossRef]

30.   Xie, J.; Kiryluk, K.; Li, Y.; Mladkova, N.; Zhu, L.; Hou, P.; Ren, H.; Wang, W.; Zhang, H.; Chen, N.; et al. Fine Mapping Implicates a Deletion of CFHR1 and CFHR3 in Protection from IgA Nephropathy in Han Chinese. *J. Am. Soc. Nephrol.* **2016**, *27*, 3187–3194. [CrossRef]

31. Medjeral-Thomas, N.R.; Lomax-Browne, H.J.; Beckwith, H.; Willicombe, M.; McLean, A.G.; Brookes, P.; Pusey, C.D.; Falchi, M.; Cook, H.T.; Pickering, M.C. Circulating complement factor H–related proteins 1 and 5 correlate with disease activity in IgA nephropathy. *Kidney Int.* **2017**, *92*, 942–952. [CrossRef]

32. Zhu, L.; Guo, W.Y.; Shi, S.F.; Liu, L.J.; Lv, J.C.; Medjeral-Thomas, N.R.; Lomax-Browne, H.J.; Pickering, M.C.; Zhang, H. Circulating complement factor H–related protein 5 levels contribute to development and progression of IgA nephropathy. *Kidney Int.* **2018**, *94*, 150–158. [CrossRef] [PubMed]

33. Akiyama, S.I.; Imai, E.; Maruyama, S. Immunology of membranous nephropathy. *F1000 Res.* **2019**, *8*. [CrossRef] [PubMed]

34. Wang, Z.; Wen, L.; Dou, Y.; Zhao, Z. Human anti-thrombospondin type 1 domain-containing 7A antibodies induce membranous nephropathy through activation of lectin complement pathway. *Biosci. Rep.* **2018**, 38. [CrossRef] [PubMed]

35. Yang, Y.; Wang, C.; Jin, L.; He, F.; Li, C.; Gao, Q.; Chen, G.; He, Z.; Song, M.; Zhou, Z.; et al. IgG4 anti-phospholipase A2 receptor might activate lectin and alternative complement pathway meanwhile in idiopathic membranous nephropathy: An inspiration from a cross-sectional study. *Immunol. Res.* **2016**, *64*, 919–930. [CrossRef] [PubMed]

36. Ma, H.; Sandor, D.G.; Beck, L.H., Jr. The role of complement inmembranous nephropathy. *Semin. Nephrol.* **2013**, *33*, 531–542. [CrossRef]

37. Baker, P.J.; Ochi, R.F.; Schulze, M.; Johnson, R.J.; Campbell, C.; Couser, W.G. Depletion of C6 Prevents Development of Proteinuria in Experimental Membranous Nephropathy in Rats. *Am. J. Pathol.* **1989**, *135*, 185–194.

38. Saran, A.M.; Yuan, H.; Takeuchi, E.; McLaughlin, M.; Salant, D.J. Complement mediates nephrin redistribution and actin dissociation in experimental membranous nephropathy. *Kidney Int.* **2003**, *64*, 2072–2078. [CrossRef]

39. Yuan, H.; Takeuchi, E.; Taylor, G.A.; Mclaughlin, M.; Brown, D.; Salant, D.J. Nephrin Dissociates from Actin, and Its Expression Is Reduced in Early Experimental Membranous Nephropathy. *J. Am. Soc. Nephrol.* **2002**, *13*, 946–956.

40. Morel-Maroger, L.; Leathem, A.; Richet, G. Glomerular abnormalities in nonsystemic diseases. Relationship between findings by light microscopy and immunofluorescence in 433 renal biopsy specimens. *Am. J. Med.* **1972**, *53*, 170–184. [CrossRef]

41. Verroust, P.J.; Wilson, C.B.; Cooper, N.R.; Edgington, T.S.; Dixon, F.J. Glomerular Complement Components in Human Glomerulonephritis. *J. Clin. Investig.* **1974**, *53*, 77–84. [CrossRef] [PubMed]

42. Hisano, S.; Matsushita, M.; Fujita, T.; Takeshita, M.; Iwasaki, H. Activation of the lectin complement pathway in post-streptococcal acute glomerulonephritis. *Pathol. Int.* **2007**, *57*, 351–357. [CrossRef] [PubMed]

43. Sethi, S.; Fervenza, F.C.; Zhang, Y.; Zand, L.; Meyer, N.C.; Borsa, N.; Nasr, S.H.; Smith, R.J.H. Atypical post-infectious glomerulonephritis is associated with abnormalities in the alternative pathway of complement. *Kidney Int.* **2013**, *83*, 293–299. [CrossRef] [PubMed]

44. Ito, N.; Ohashi, R.; Nagata, M. C3 glomerulopathy and current dilemmas. *Clin. Exp. Nephrol.* **2017**, *21*, 541–551. [CrossRef]

45. Masani, N.; Jhaveri, K.D.; Fishbane, S. Update on membranoproliferative GN. *Clin. J. Am. Soc. Nephrol.* **2014**, *9*, 600–608. [CrossRef]

46. Noris, M.; Remuzzi, G. Glomerular Diseases Dependent on Complement Activation, Including Atypical Hemolytic Uremic Syndrome, Membranoproliferative Glomerulonephritis, and C3 Glomerulopathy: Core Curriculum 2015. *Am. J. Kidney Dis.* **2015**, *66*, 359–375. [CrossRef]

47. Servais, A.; Ne Noël, L.-H.; Roumenina, L.T.; Le Quintrec, M.; Ngo, S.; -Agnès Dragon-Durey, M.; Macher, M.-A.; Zuber, J.; Karras, A.; Provot, F.; et al. Acquired and genetic complement abnormalities play a critical role in dense deposit disease and other C3 glomerulopathies. *Kidney Int.* **2012**, *82*, 454–464. [CrossRef]

48. Ma, R.; Cui, Z.; Hu, S.-Y.; Jia, X.-Y.; Yang, R. The Alternative Pathway of Complement Activation May Be Involved in the Renal Damage of Human Anti-Glomerular Basement Membrane Disease. *PLoS ONE* **2014**, *9*, 91250. [CrossRef]

49. Minto, A.W.; Kalluri, R.; Togawa, M.; Bergijk, E.C.; Killen, P.D.; Salant, D.J. Augmented expression of glomerular basement membrane specific type IV collagen isoforms (alpha3-alpha5) in experimental membranous nephropathy. *Proc. Assoc. Am. Physicians* **1998**, *110*, 207–217.

50.   Sheerin, N.S.; Springall, T.; Carroll, M.C.; Hartley, B.; Sacks, S.H. Protection against anti-glomerular basement membrane (GBM)-mediated nephritis in C3-and C4-deficient mice. *Clin. Exp. Immunol.* **1997**, *110*, 403–409. [CrossRef]

51.   Fischer, E.G.; Lager, D.J. Anti-glomerular basement membrane glomerulonephritis: A morphologic study of 80 cases. *Am. J. Clin. Pathol.* **2006**, *125*, 445–450. [CrossRef] [PubMed]

52.   Xiao, H.; Dairaghi, D.J.; Powers, J.P.; Ertl, L.S.; Baumgart, T.; Wang, Y.; Seitz, L.C.; Penfold, M.E.; Gan, L.; Hu, P.; et al. C5a Receptor (CD88) Blockade Protects against MPO-ANCA GN Necrotizing and crescentic GN (NCGN) and vasculitis are associated with ANCA. *J. Am. Soc. Nephrol.* **2014**, *25*, 225–231. [CrossRef] [PubMed]

53.   Xiao, H.; Schreiber, A.; Heeringa, P.; Falk, R.J.; Jennette, J.C. Alternative complement pathway in the pathogenesis of disease mediated by anti-neutrophil cytoplasmic autoantibodies. *Am. J. Pathol.* **2007**, *170*, 52–64. [CrossRef] [PubMed]

54.   Jayne, D.R.W.; Bruchfeld, A.N.; Harper, L.; Schaier, M.; Venning, M.C.; Hamilton, P.; Burst, V.; Grundmann, F.; Jadoul, M.; Szombati, I.; et al. Randomized trial of C5a receptor inhibitor avacopan in ANCA-associated vasculitis. *J. Am. Soc. Nephrol.* **2017**, *28*, 2756–2767. [CrossRef] [PubMed]

55.   Markowitz, G.S.; D'Agati, V.D. Classification of lupus nephritis. *Curr. Opin. Nephrol. Hypertens.* **2009**, *18*, 220–225. [CrossRef] [PubMed]

56.   Couser, W.G. Basic and Translational Concepts of Immune-Mediated Glomerular Diseases. *J. Am. Soc. Nephrol.* **2012**, *23*, 381–399. [CrossRef] [PubMed]

57.   Song, D.; Guo, W.Y.; Wang, F.M.; Li, Y.Z.; Song, Y.; Yu, F.; Zhao, M.H. Complement Alternative Pathway's Activation in Patients with Lupus Nephritis. *Am. J. Med. Sci.* **2017**, *353*, 247–257. [CrossRef]

58.   Pickering, M.C.; Botto, M. Are anti-C1q antibodies different from other SLE autoantibodies? *Nat. Publ. Gr.* **2010**, *6*, 490–493. [CrossRef]

59.   Bao, L.; Haas, M.; Quigg, R.J. Complement Factor H Deficiency Accelerates Development of Lupus Nephritis. *J. Am. Soc. Nephrol.* **2011**, *22*, 285–295. [CrossRef]

60.   Bao, L.; Quigg, R.J. Complement in Lupus Nephritis: The Good, the Bad, and the Unknown. *Semin. Nephrol.* **2007**, *27*, 69–80. [CrossRef]

61.   Tomlinson, S.; Atkinson, C.; Qiao, F.; Song, H.; Gilkeson, G.S. Mice lpr MRL/ Manifestations of Autoimmune Disease in Protects against Renal Disease and Other Low-Dose Targeted Complement Inhibition. *J. Immunol. Ref.* **2019**, *180*, 1231–1238.

62.   Bao, L.; Osawe, I.; Puri, T.; Lambris, J.D.; Haas, M.; Quigg, R.J. C5a promotes development of experimental lupus nephritis which can be blocked with a specific receptor antagonist. *Eur. J. Immunol.* **2005**, *35*, 2496–2506. [CrossRef] [PubMed]

63.   Wang, Y.; Hu, Q.; MADRIt, J.A.; Rollins, S.A.; Chodera, A.; Matis, L.A.; Talmage, D.W. Amelioration of lupus-like autoimmune disease in NZB/W F1 mice after treatment with a blocking monoclonal antibody specific for complement component C5. *Proc. Natl. Acad. Sci. USA* **1996**, *93*, 8563–8568. [CrossRef] [PubMed]

64.   Murdaca, G.; Colombo, B.M.; Puppo, F. Emerging biological drugs: A new therapeutic approach for Systemic Lupus Erythematosus. An update upon efficacy and adverse events. *Autoimmun. Rev.* **2011**, *11*, 56–60. [CrossRef] [PubMed]

65.   Mészáros, T.; Füst, G.; Farkas, H.; Jakab, L.; Temesszentandrási, G.; Nagy, G.; Kiss, E.; Gergely, P.; Zeher, M.; Griger, Z.; et al. C1-inhibitor autoantibodies in SLE. *Lupus* **2010**, *19*, 634–638.

66.   Al-Mayouf, S.M.; Abanomi, H.; Eldali, A. Impact of C1q deficiency on the severity and outcome of childhood systemic lupus erythematosus. *Int. J. Rheum. Dis.* **2011**, *14*, 81–85. [CrossRef]

67.   Heurich, M.; Martínez-Barricarte, R.; Francis, N.J.; Roberts, D.L.; Rodríguez De Córdoba, S.; Morgan, B.P.; Harris, C.L. Common polymorphisms in C3, factor B, and factor H collaborate to determine systemic complement activity and disease risk. *Proc. Natl. Acad. Sci. USA* **2011**, *108*, 8761–8766. [CrossRef]

68.   Noris, M.; Caprioli, J.; Bresin, E.; Mossali, C.; Pianetti, G.; Gamba, S.; Daina, E.; Fenili, C.; Castelletti, F.; Sorosina, A.; et al. Relative Role of Genetic Complement Abnormalities in Sporadic and Familial aHUS and Their Impact on Clinical Phenotype. *Clin. J. Am. Soc. Nephrol.* **2010**, *5*, 1844–1859. [CrossRef]

69.   Manuelian, T.; Hellwage, J.; Meri, S.; Caprioli, J.; Noris, M.; Heinen, S.; Jozsi, M.; Neumann, H.P.H.; Remuzzi, G.; Zipfel, P.F. Mutations in factor H reduce binding affinity to C3b and heparin and surface attachment to endothelial cells in hemolytic uremic syndrome. *J. Clin. Invest.* **2003**, *111*, 1181–1190. [CrossRef]

70. Caprioli, J.; Noris, M.; Brioschi, S.; Pianetti, G.; Castelletti, F.; Bettinaglio, P.; Mele, C.; Bresin, E.; Cassis, L.; Gamba, S.; et al. Genetics of HUS: The impact of MCP, CFH, and IF mutations on clinical presentation, response to treatment, and outcome. *Blood* **2006**, *108*, 1267–1279. [CrossRef]

71. Sethi, S.; Haas, M.; Markowitz, G.S.; D'agati, V.D.; Rennke, H.G.; Jennette, J.C.; Bajema, I.M.; Alpers, C.E.; Chang, A.; Cornell, L.D.; et al. Mayo Clinic/Renal Pathology Society Consensus Report on Pathologic Classification, Diagnosis, and Reporting of GN. *J. Am. Soc. Nephrol.* **2016**, *27*, 1278–1287. [CrossRef] [PubMed]

72. Sethi, S.; Fervenza, F.C. Pathology of Renal Diseases Associated with Dysfunction of the Alternative Pathway of Complement: C3 Glomerulopathy and Atypical Hemolytic Uremic Syndrome (aHUS). *Semin. Thromb. Hemost.* **2014**, *40*, 416–421. [PubMed]

73. Łukawska, E.; Polcyn-Adamczak, M.; Niemir, Z.I. The role of the alternative pathway of complement activation in glomerular diseases. *Clin. Exp. Med.* **2018**, *18*, 297–318. [CrossRef] [PubMed]

74. Barbour, T.D.; Pickering, M.C.; Cook, H.T. Recent insights into C3 glomerulopathy. *Nephrol. Dial. Transpl.* **2013**, *28*, 1685–1693. [CrossRef] [PubMed]

75. Schramm, E.C.; Roumenina, L.T.; Rybkine, T.; Chauvet, S.; Vieira-Martins, P.; Hue, C.; Maga, T.; Valoti, E.; Wilson, V.; Jokiranta, S.; et al. Mapping interactions between complement C3 and regulators using mutations in atypical hemolytic uremic syndrome. *Blood* **2015**, *125*, 2359–2369. [CrossRef]

76. Pickering, M.C.; Warren, J.; Rose, K.L.; Carlucci, F.; Wang, Y.; Walport, M.J.; Cook, H.T.; Botto, M. Prevention of C5 activation ameliorates spontaneous and experimental glomerulonephritis in factor H-deficient mice. *Proc. Natl. Acad. Sci. USA* **2006**, *103*, 9649–9654. [CrossRef]

77. Gale, D.P.; De Jorge, E.G.; Cook, H.T.; Martinez-Barricarte, R.; Hadjisavvas, A.; McLean, A.G.; Pusey, C.D.; Pierides, A.; Kyriacou, K.; Athanasiou, Y.; et al. Identification of a mutation in complement factor H-related protein 5 in patients of Cypriot origin with glomerulonephritis. *Lancet* **2010**, *376*, 794–801. [CrossRef]

78. Xiao, X.; Ghossein, C.; Tortajadam, A.; Zhang, Y.; Meyer, N.; Jones, M.; Borsa, N.G.; Nester, C.M.; Thomas, C.P.; de Córdoba, S.R.; et al. Familial C3 glomerulonephritis caused by a novel CFHR5-CFHR2 fusion gene. *Mol. Immunol.* **2016**, *77*, 89–96. [CrossRef]

79. Chen, Q.; Wiesener, M.; Eberhardt, H.U.; Hartmann, A.; Uzonyi, B.; Kirschfink, M.; Amann, K.; Buettner, M.; Goodship, T.; Hugo, C.; et al. Complement factor H-related hybrid protein deregulates complement in dense deposit disease. *J. Clin. Investig.* **2014**, *124*, 145–155. [CrossRef]

80. Kościelska-Kasprzak, K.; Bartoszek, D.; Myszka, M.; Zabińska, M.; Klinger, M. The Complement Cascade and Renal Disease. *Arch. Immunol. Ther. Exp.* **2014**, *62*, 47–57. [CrossRef]

81. Kim, M.-K.; Maeng, Y.-I.; Lee, S.-J.; Lee, I.H.; Bae, J.; Kang, Y.-N.; Park, B.-T.; Park, K.-K. Pathogenesis and significance of glomerular C4d deposition in lupus nephritis: Activation of classical and lectin pathways. *Int. J. Clin. Exp. Pathol.* **2013**, *6*, 2157–2167. [PubMed]

82. Korbet, S.M. Treatment of Primary FSGS in Adults. *J. Am. Soc. Nephrol.* **2012**, *23*, 1769–1776. [CrossRef] [PubMed]

83. D'Agati, V.D.; Fogo, A.B.; Bruijn, J.A.; Jennette, J.C. Pathologic Classification of Focal Segmental Glomerulosclerosis: A Working Proposal. *Am. J. Kidney Dis.* **2004**, *43*, 368–382. [CrossRef] [PubMed]

84. Zhang, Y.; Gu, Q.; Huang, J.; Qu, Z.; Wang, X.; Meng, L.; Wang, F.; Liu, G.; Cui, Z.; Zhao, M. Article Clinical Significance of IgM and C3 Glomerular Deposition in Primary Focal Segmental Glomerulosclerosis. *Clin. J. Am. Soc. Nephrol.* **2016**, *11*, 1582–1589. [CrossRef]

85. Strassheim, D.; Renner, B.; Panzer, S.; Fuquay, R.; Kulik, L.; Ljubanovi, D.; Holers, V.M.; Thurman, J.M. IgM Contributes to Glomerular Injury in FSGS. *J. Am. Soc. Nephrol.* **2013**, *24*, 393–406. [CrossRef]

86. Sethi, S.; Fervenza, F.C.; Zhang, Y.; Smith, R.J. Secondary Focal and Segmental Glomerulosclerosis Associated with Single-Nucleotide Polymorphisms in the Genes Encoding Complement Factor H and C3 HHS Public Access. *Am. J. Kidney Dis.* **2012**, *60*, 316–321. [CrossRef]

87. Thurman, J.M.; Wong, M.; Renner, B.; Frazer-Abel, A.; Giclas, P.C.; Joy, M.S.; Jalal, D.; Radeva, M.K.; Gassman, J.; Gipson, D.S.; et al. Complement Activation in Patients with Focal Segmental Glomerulosclerosis. *PLoS ONE* **2015**, *10*, e0136558. [CrossRef]

88. Tomlinson, S.; Thurman, J.M. Tissue-targeted complement therapeutics. *Mol. Immunol.* **2018**, *102*, 120–128. [CrossRef]

89. Horiuchi, T.; Tsukamoto, H. Complement-targeted therapy: Development of C5-and C5a-targeted inhibition. *Inflamm. Regen.* **2016**, *36*, 11. [CrossRef]

90.   Cicardi, M.; Aberer, W.; Banerji, A.; Bas, M.; Bernstein, J.A.; Bork, K.; Caballero, T.; Farkas, H.; Grumach, A.; Kaplan, A.P.; et al. Classification, diagnosis, and approach to treatment for angioedema: Consensus report from the Hereditary Angioedema International Working Group. *Allergy* **2014**, *69*, 602–616. [CrossRef]

91.   Rother, R.P.; Rollins, S.A.; Mojcik, C.F.; Brodsky, R.A.; Bell, L. Discovery and development of the complement inhibitor eculizumab for the treatment of paroxysmal nocturnal hemoglobinuria. *Nat. Biotechnol.* **2007**, *25*, 1256–1264. [CrossRef] [PubMed]

92.   Legendre, C.M.; Licht, C.; Muus, P.; Greenbaum, L.A.; Babu, S.; Bedrosian, C.; Bingham, C.; Cohen, D.J.; Delmas, Y.; Douglas, K.; et al. Terminal complement inhibitor eculizumab in atypical hemolytic-uremic syndrome. *N. Engl. J. Med.* **2013**, *368*, 2169–2181. [CrossRef] [PubMed]

93.   Chatelet, V.; Frémeaux, V.; Frémeaux-Bacchi, F.; Lobbedez, T.; Ficheux, M.; Hurault De Ligny, B. Safety and Long-Term Efficacy of Eculizumab in a Renal Transplant Patient with Recurrent Atypical Hemolytic-Uremic Syndrome. *Am. J. Transpl.* **2009**, *9*, 2644–2645. [PubMed]

94.   Wong, E.K.S.; Goodship, T.H.J.; Kavanagh, D. Complement therapy in atypical haemolytic uraemic syndrome (aHUS). *Mol. Immunol.* **2013**, *56*, 199–212. [CrossRef]

95.   Kaabak, M.; Babenko, N.; Shapiro, R.; Zokoyev, A. A prospective randomized, controlled trial of eculizumab to prevent ischemia-reperfusion injury in pediatric kidney transplantation. *Pediatr. Transpl.* **2018**, *22*. [CrossRef]

96.   Marks, W.H.; Mamode, N.; Montgomery, R.A.; Stegall, M.D.; Ratner, L.E.; Cornell, L.D.; Rowshani, A.T.; Colvin, R.B.; Dain, B.; Boice, J.A.; et al. Safety and efficacy of eculizumab in the prevention of antibody-mediated rejection in living-donor kidney transplant recipients requiring desensitization therapy: A randomized trial. *Am. J. Transpl.* **2019**, 1–13. [CrossRef]

97.   Glotz, D.; Russ, G.; Rostaing, L.; Legendre, C.; Tufveson, G.; Chadban, S.; Grinyó, J.; Mamode, N.; Rigotti, P.; Couzi, L.; et al. Safety and efficacy of eculizumab for the prevention of antibody-mediated rejection after deceased-donor kidney transplantation in patients with preformed donor-specific antibodies. *Am. J. Transpl.* **2019**, *19*, 2865–2875. [CrossRef]

98.   Bomback, A.S.; Smith, R.J.; Barile, G.R.; Zhang, Y.; Heher, E.C.; Herlitz, L.; Stokes, B.M.; Markowitz, G.S.; D'agati, V.D.; Canetta, P.A.; et al. Article Eculizumab for Dense Deposit Disease and C3 Glomerulonephritis. *Clin. J. Am. Soc. Nephrol.* **2012**, *7*, 748–756. [CrossRef]

99.   Radhakrishnan, S.; Lunn, A.; Kirschfink, M.; Thorner, P.; Hebert, D.; Langlois, V.; Pluthero, F.; Licht, C. Eculizumab and refractory membranoproliferative glomerulonephritis. *N. Engl. J. Med.* **2012**, *366*, 1165–1166. [CrossRef]

100. Mccaughan, J.A.; O'rourke, D.M.; Courtney, A.E. Recurrent Dense Deposit Disease After Renal Transplantation: An Emerging Role for Complementary Therapies. *Am. J. Transpl.* **2012**, *12*, 1046–1051. [CrossRef]

101. Thurman, J.M.; Le Quintrec, M. Targeting the complement cascade: Novel treatments coming down the pike. *Kidney Int.* **2016**, *90*, 746–752. [CrossRef] [PubMed]

10

Fluctuations in Serum Chloride and Acute Kidney Injury among Critically Ill Patients

Tak Kyu Oh [1], In-Ae Song [1,*], Young-Tae Jeon [1] and You Hwan Jo [2]

[1]   Department of Anesthesiology and Pain Medicine, Seoul National University Bundang Hospital, Seoul 13620, Korea; airohtak@hotmail.com (T.K.O.); ytjeon@snubh.org (Y.-T.J.)

[2]   Department of Emergency Medicine, Seoul National University Bundang Hospital, Seoul 13620, Korea; drakejo@snubh.org

*   Correspondence: songoficu@outlook.kr

Abstract: Exposure to dyschloremia among critically ill patients is associated with an increased risk of acute kidney injury (AKI). We aimed to investigate how fluctuations in serum chloride (Cl^-) are associated with the development of AKI in critically ill patients. We retrospectively analyzed medical records of adult patients admitted to the intensive care unit (ICU) between January 2012 and December 2017. Positive and negative fluctuations in Cl^- were defined as the difference between the baseline Cl- and maximum Cl- levels and the difference between the baseline Cl^- and minimum Cl^- levels measured within 72 h after ICU admission, respectively. In total, 19,707 patients were included. The odds of developing AKI increased 1.06-fold for every 1 mmol L^{-1} increase in the positive fluctuations in Cl^- (odds ratio: 1.06; 95% confidence interval: 1.04 to 1.08; $p < 0.001$) and 1.04-fold for every 1 mmol L^{-1} increase in the negative fluctuations in Cl^- (odds ratio: 1.04; 95% confidence interval: 1.02 to 1.06; $p < 0.001$). Increases in both the positive and negative fluctuations in Cl- after ICU admission were associated with an increased risk of AKI. Furthermore, these associations differed based on the functional status of the kidneys at ICU admission or postoperative ICU admission.

Keywords: acute kidney injury; critical care; intensive care units

1. Introduction

Acute kidney injury (AKI) is defined as an impairment of renal function [1], and is reported to occur in 2–18% of all inpatients, and 35.7–57% of all critically ill patients [2–5]. AKI that affects patients in intensive care units (ICUs) not only increases the duration of hospitalization and medical costs [6], but also increases in-hospital mortality [7]. Therefore, adequate prevention of AKI in ICUs is an important challenge in ICU patient management [8].

Serum chloride (Cl^-) is the most common anion in the human body. Dyschloremia is a collective term for hypochloremia, in which the Cl^- level is below the normal range, and hyperchloremia, in which the Cl^- level is above the normal range [9]. Increased Cl^- levels induce hyperchloremic metabolic acidosis through physiologic compensation, whereas decreased Cl^- levels induce hypochloremic metabolic alkalosis. Both conditions are associated with increased risks of AKI [10,11]. It is important to understand the association between dyschloremia and AKI in the ICU because the Cl^- level can provide important information in the planning of a fluid management strategy [12].

It is well known that increases in Cl^- levels after ICU admission are associated with the development of AKI [13–15], while the association between a decrease in Cl^- levels and the development of AKI has not been extensively studied. Critically ill patients may experience a reduction in Cl^- levels after ICU admission due to the active loss of Cl^- in the gastrointestinal tract, impaired renal Cl^- reabsorption, hypotonic fluid infusion, excessive diuretics therapy, and malnutrition [16,17]. These conditions may be associated with the development of AKI. Thus, when studying the association between Cl$^-$ levels and the incidence of AKI among critically ill patients, fluctuations of Cl$^-$ levels (increases and decreases) must be considered.

Therefore, this study aimed to investigate the association between the total, positive, and negative fluctuations in Cl$^-$ levels and the incidence of AKI.

2. Materials and Methods

2.1. Study Design and Subjects

This retrospective observational study was approved by the Institutional Review Board (IRB) of Seoul National University Bundang Hospital (IRB approval number B-1806/474-105). The IRB exempted the need for informed consent, considering the retrospective study design. The medical records of adult patients aged ≥18 years admitted to the ICU between January 2012 and December 2017 were analyzed. For single patients admitted to the ICU twice or more during the study period, only the last ICU admission in which the patient could be in the most critical condition was included in the analysis. Patients whose medical records, regarding Cl$^-$ and creatinine, were incomplete or missing were excluded from the analysis. Patients with an estimated glomerular filtration rate (eGFR) <15 mL min^{-1} 1.73 m^{-2}, patients with end-stage renal disease (ESRD) who underwent chronic renal replacement therapy (RRT) before ICU admission, and patients with undiagnosed AKI before ICU admission were also excluded.

This study succeeds a previous study [18] that analyzed the medical records of patients in the surgical ICU at our institution from 2011 to 2016. The previous study reported that exposure to hyperchloremia in the postoperative period in the surgical ICU was not associated with the incidence of AKI. This study differs from the previous study that analyzed the positive or negative fluctuations in Cl$^-$ within 72 h after ICU admission; previous studies have analyzed the increases in the preoperative Cl$^-$ to the maximum Cl$^-$ in 0–3 days postoperatively.

2.2. Fluctuations in Cl- Levels (Independent Variables)

For the purpose of this study, the Cl- level on ICU admission (baseline Cl-) was defined as that measured within 24 h after ICU admission, and the Cl- level closest to the ICU admission time. Positive fluctuations in Cl- were defined as the difference between the baseline Cl- and the maximum Cl- levels measured within 72 h after ICU admission, while negative fluctuations in Cl- were defined as the difference between the baseline Cl- and the minimum Cl- levels measured within 72 h after ICU admission. Lastly, the total fluctuations in Cl- were defined as the difference between the minimum and maximum Cl- levels measured within 72 h after ICU admission. For example, if baseline Cl-, maximum Cl-, and minimum Cl- levels were 107 mmol L^{-1}, 111 mmol L^{-1}, and 105 mmol L^{-1}, respectively, the total positive and negative fluctuations were 6 mmol L^{-1} (111–105 mmol L^{-1}), 4 mmol L^{-1} (111–107 mmol L^{-1}), and 2 mmol L^{-1} (107–105 mmol L^{-1}), respectively. In situations where no maximum or minimum value of Cl- within 72 h after ICU admission was noted, the positive or negative fluctuation of Cl-, respectively, was considered as 0. In those cases, the total fluctuation was calculated using baseline Cl- level. For example, if baseline Cl-, maximum Cl-, and minimum Cl- levels were 105 mmol L^{-1}, 111 mmol L^{-1}, and 107 mmol L^{-1}, respectively, the total, positive, and negative fluctuations were 6 mmol L^{-1} (111–105 mmol L^{-1}), 6 mmol L^{-1} (111–105 mmol L^{-1}), and 0 mmol L^{-1} (no minimum Cl- level), respectively.

2.3. Potential Covariates

Data regarding demographics (sex, age, and body mass index), Acute Physiology, Chronic Health Evaluation II, comorbidities at ICU admission (eGFR, mL min^{-1} 1.73 m^{-2}, hypertension, diabetes mellitus, history of ischemic heart disease and cerebrovascular disease, chronic obstructive lung disease, liver disease (liver cirrhosis, hepatitis, and fatty liver), anemia (hemoglobin <10 g dL^{-1}), cancer status regarding hospital admission through the emergency department, postoperative admission status, and the admission department (internal medicine/neurologic center/postcardiothoracic surgery/post-other surgery) at the time of ICU admission were collected. Information regarding fluid administration (i.e., NaCl 0.9%, balanced crystalloid, and hydroxyethyl starch (all in mL)) for 72 h after ICU admission was collected. Additionally, the maximum value of the cystatin c level (mg dL^{-1}) for 72 h after ICU admission was collected. Finally, the number of Cl- level measurements taken for 72 h after ICU admission were collected. The Modification of Diet in Renal Disease equation was used to calculate the eGFR before ICU admission [19]: eGFR (mL min^{-1} 1.73 m^{-2}) = 186 × (Creatinine)$^{-1.154}$ × (Age)$^{-0.203}$ × (0.742 if female).

2.4. Acute Kidney Injury within 72 h after ICU Admission (Dependent Variable)

The Kidney Disease: Improving Global Outcomes (KDIGO) criteria and grading method were used to diagnose AKI (Appendix A) [20]. Considering the differences in the duration of urinary catheterization among the patients, only the serum creatinine (mg dL^{-1}) level was used to diagnose AKI. The serum creatinine value measured within 1 month before ICU admission closest to the time of ICU admission was used as the baseline creatinine concentration for AKI diagnosis. The serum creatinine level measured within 72 h after ICU admission was used to diagnose AKI.

2.5. Endpoint

This study investigated the associations between total, positive, and negative fluctuations in Cl- within 72 h after ICU admission and the total incidence of AKI and AKI stage ≥2. In addition, we investigated relationships between total, positive, and negative fluctuations in serum Cl$^-$ with the maximum serum cystatin C level for 72 h after ICU admission.

2.6. Statistical Analysis

The patients' baseline characteristics were expressed as means and standard deviations (SDs) or numbers and proportions. The log odds of AKI occurrence and fluctuations in Cl$^-$ were presented as restricted cubic splines (RCSs). After confirming a linear relationship between the fluctuation in Cl$^-$ and log odds of developing AKI in RCSs, the fluctuation in Cl$^-$ was included in the logistic regression model as a continuous variable. A univariable logistic regression analysis was performed to investigate the association of each covariate with the incidence of the dependent variable (AKI). Covariates with $p < 0.1$ were selected from the univariable logistic regression model, and were controlled for in the final multivariable logistic regression analysis. In the multivariable logistic regression analysis, total fluctuations in Cl$^-$ were included in another multivariable logistic regression model with positive and negative fluctuations in Cl$^-$ to avoid multicollinearity within variables.

Next, considering that baseline kidney function is a major risk factor of AKI [21], the interaction between fluctuations in Cl$^-$ and eGFR and the incidence of AKI before ICU admission were investigated. After confirming that there was a significant interaction between fluctuations in Cl$^-$ and eGFR with the incidence of AKI, we performed a subgroup analysis with four eGFR groups (eGFR ≥90, <90, <60, and <30 mL min^{-1} 1.73 m^{-2}). Lastly, the interaction between fluctuations in Cl$^-$ and postoperative ICU admission for the incidence of AKI were investigated, and the significant interactions were also confirmed. Therefore, we performed a subgroup analysis based on postoperative ICU admission. To reduce type I errors due to multiple comparisons in the subgroup analysis, the Bonferroni correction was used [22]. The same method was used in the analysis of stage ≥2 as a dependent variable. The results of the logistic regression analysis were expressed as odds ratios (ORs) and 95% confidence intervals (CIs). Additionally, considering that the serum cystatin C was a marker of renal function in the detection of early AKI [23], we performed a generalized linear regression analysis to investigate the association between fluctuation in serum Cl$^-$ and the maximum serum cystatin C level for 72 h after ICU admission. In this generalized linear model (GLM), gamma distribution and the log link function were assumed for the dependent variable (maximum cystatin C level within 72 h after ICU admission). All covariates were included in the GLM. The results of GLM were expressed as the exponentiated (exp) regression coefficient (coef) with 95% CIs. All analyses were performed using SPSS version 24.0 (IBM Corp., Armonk, NY) and R program (version 3.5.2 with R packages), with the level of statistical significance set at $p < 0.05$.

3. Results

There was a total of 40,533 ICU admissions between 2012 and 2017. Of these, 10,135 admission cases in which a single patient was admitted twice or more were excluded. Next, 5440 patients younger than 17 years, 44 ESRD patients who received RRT before ICU admission, 4730 patients with incomplete medical records regarding serum Cl- or creatinine levels, and 477 patients with undiagnosed AKI before admission were excluded, and the remaining 19,707 patients were finally included. There was a total of 5284 (26.8%) AKI cases within 72 h after ICU admission; 2233 (11.4%) patients had AKI stage ≥2 (Figure 1). Table 1 shows the baseline characteristics of these patients. The mean (SD) values of the total, positive, and negative fluctuations in Cl- were 7.0 (5.7), 4.4 (4.1), and 2.9 (4.6), respectively.

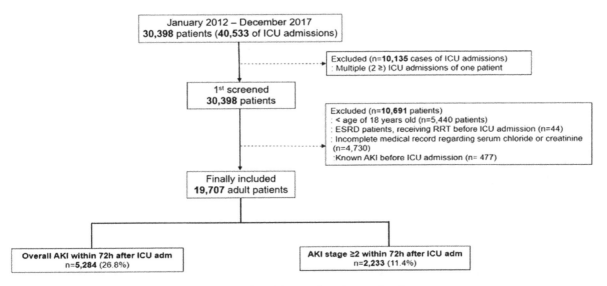

Figure 1. Flow chart of patient selection.

Table 1. Baseline characteristics of adult patients admitted to the ICU between 2012 and 2017.

Variable	Total (19,707)	Mean	SD
Sex: male	11,412 (57.9%)		
Age, year		63.8	15.9
Body mass index, kg m^{-2}		23.6	3.9
Comorbidities at ICU admission			
APACHE II		20.3	10.0
eGFR [a]: ≥90	12,164 (61.7%)		
60–90	4079 (20.7%)		
30–60	2163 (11.0%)		
<30	1301 (6.6%)		
Hypertension	8511 (43.2%)		
Diabetes mellitus	1775 (9.0%)		
Ischemic heart disease	481 (2.4%)		
Cerebrovascular disease	886 (4.5%)		
Chronic obstructive lung disease	868 (4.4%)		
Liver disease (LC, hepatitis, fatty liver)	649 (3.3%)		
Anemia (Hb <10 g dL^{-1})	7266 (36.9%)		
Cancer	4137 (21.0%)		

Table 1. *Cont.*

Variable	Total (19,707)	Mean	SD
Sex: male	11,412 (57.9%)		
Age, year		63.8	15.9
Body mass index, kg m^{-2}		23.6	3.9
Characteristics of ICU admission			
Admission through emergency department	11,435 (58.0%)		
Postoperative admission	8728 (44.3%)		
Admission department			
Internal medicine	4231 (21.5%)		
Neurologic center	4805 (24.4%)		
Cardiothoracic surgical department	6093 (30.9%)		
Other surgical departments	4578 (23.2%)		
Length of ICU stay, day		3.2	10.4
Length of hospital stay, day		13.3	20.5
Fluid administration for 72 h after ICU admission			
NaCl 0.9%, mL		1745.5	2124.1
Balanced crystalloid, mL		505.5	862.5
Hydroxyethyl starch, mL		79.4	270.1
Transfusion of packed RBC	8530 (43.3%)		
Serum chloride (Cl$^-$) in ICU, mmol L^{-1}			
Cl$^-$ on ICU admission		106.4	6.2
The number of measurements for 72 h after ICU admission		3.2	1.0
Total fluctuation of Cl$^-$ for 72 h after ICU admission [b]		7.0	5.7
Positive fluctuation of Cl$^-$ for 72 h after ICU admission [c]		4.4	4.1
Negative fluctuation of Cl$^-$ for 72 h after ICU admission [d]		2.9	4.6
Max cystatin C level mg dL^{-1} for 72 h after ICU adm ($n = 2,021$)		2.0	1.2
Total AKI within 72 h after ICU admission	5284 (26.8%)		
AKI stage $\geq$2 within 72 h after ICU admission	2233 (11.4%)		
RRT after ICU admission (within 72 h)	468 (2.4%)		

[a] eGFR (mL min $^{-1}$ 1.73 m^{-2}): $186 \times$ (Creatinine)$^{-1.154} \times$ (Age)$^{-0.203} \times$ (0.742 if female). [b] Total fluctuation of Cl$^-$: (Maximum Cl$^-$ − Minimum Cl$^-$) for 72 h after ICU admission. [c] Positive fluctuation of Cl$^-$: (Maximum Cl$^-$ − Preadmission Cl$^-$) for 72 h after ICU admission. [d] Negative fluctuation of Cl$^-$: (Preadmission Cl$^-$ − Minimum Cl$^-$) for 72 h after ICU admission. ICU, intensive care unit; APACHE, acute physiology and chronic health evaluation; eGFR, estimated glomerular filtration rate; LC, liver cirrhosis; Hb, hemoglobin; RBC, red blood cell; Max, maximum; AKI, acute kidney injury; RRT, renal replacement therapy.

3.1. AKI within 72 h after ICU Admission Based on Cl- Fluctuations

The RCSs in Figure 2 show that the log odds of developing AKI had positive and linear relationships with total (A), positive (B), and negative fluctuations (C) in Cl$^-$ levels. Appendix B shows the results of the univariable logistic regression analysis of the associations between the individual covariates and AKI. Table 2 shows the results of the multivariable logistic regression analysis adjusted for the covariates selected from the univariable logistic regression analysis. The odds of developing AKI increased 1.05-fold for every 1 mmol L^{-1} increase in the total fluctuations in Cl$^-$ (OR: 1.05; 95% CI: 1.03 to 1.06; $p < 0.001$), 1.06-fold for every 1 mmol L^{-1} increase in the positive fluctuations in Cl$^-$ (OR: 1.06; 95% CI: 1.04 to 1.08; $p < 0.001$), and 1.04-fold for every 1 mmol L^{-1} increase in the negative fluctuations in Cl$^-$ (OR: 1.04; 95% CI: 1.02 to 1.06; $p < 0.001$). The results of the subgroup analysis for total AKI based on the preadmission eGFR status and the postoperative ICU admission status are shown in Tables 3 and 4, respectively.

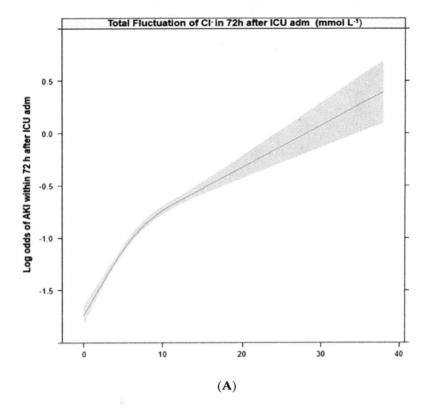

(**A**)

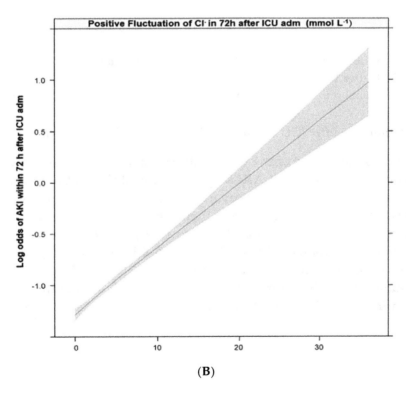

(**B**)

Figure 2. *Cont.*

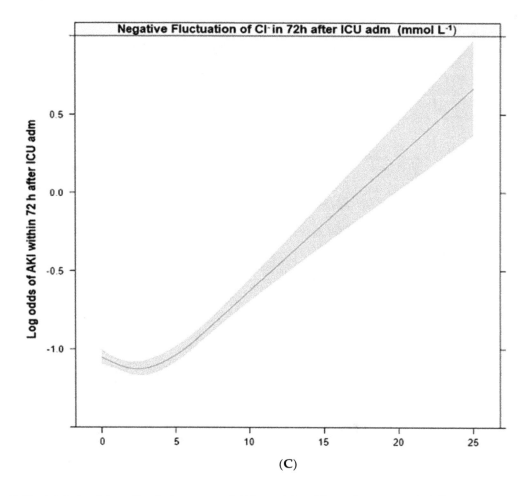

(C)

Figure 2. Restricted cubic spline between total (**A**), positive (**B**), and negative (**C**) fluctuations in serum chloride within 72 h after ICU admission and occurrence of AKI. ICU, intensive care unit; AKI, acute kidney injury. RRT, renal replacement therapy.

3.2. AKI Stage ≥2 within 72 h after ICU Admission According to Cl⁻ Fluctuation

Appendix B shows the results of the univariable logistic regression analysis of the associations between the individual covariates and AKI stage ≥2. Table 2 shows the results of the multivariable logistic regression analysis adjusted for the covariates selected from the univariable logistic regression analysis. The odds of developing stage ≥2 AKI increased 1.08-fold for every 1 mmol L^{-1} increase in the total fluctuations in Cl⁻ (OR: 1.08; 95% CI: 1.06 to 1.10; $p < 0.001$), 1.09-fold for every 1 mmol L^{-1} increase in the positive fluctuations in Cl⁻ (OR: 1.09; 95% CI: 1.07 to 1.11; $p < 0.001$), and 1.09-fold for every 1 mmol L^{-1} increase in the negative fluctuations in Cl⁻ (OR: 1.09; 95% CI: 1.06 to 1.11; $p < 0.001$). The results of the subgroup analysis for AKI stage ≥2 according to preadmission eGFR grouping and postoperative ICU admission status are shown in Tables 3 and 4, respectively.

Table 2. Multivariable logistic regression analysis for total AKI and AKI stage ≥ 2 after ICU admission according to fluctuations of serum chloride (mmol L^{-1}).

Variables	Odds Ratio (95% CI)	p-Value
Dependent variables: Total AKI		
Total fluctuation of Cl^- [a] (model 1)	**1.05** (1.03, 1.06)	**<0.001**
Interaction: Total fluctuation of Cl^- [a],* eGFR [b] ≥ 90	1	(<0.001)
Total fluctuation of Cl^- [a],* eGFR [b]: 60–90	1.02 (1.00, 1.04)	0.114
Total fluctuation of Cl^- [a],* eGFR [b]: 30–60	1.02 (1.00, 1.05)	0.153
Total fluctuation of Cl^- [a],* eGFR [b]: <30	0.90 (0.88, 0.93)	<0.001
Interaction: Total fluctuation of Cl^- [a],* postoperative admission	0.96 (0.95, 0.98)	<0.001
Positive fluctuation of Cl^- [c] (model 2)	**1.06** (1.04, 1.08)	**<0.001**
Interaction: Positive fluctuation of Cl^- [a],*eGFR [b] ≥ 90	1	(<0.001)
Positive fluctuation of Cl^- [a],* eGFR [b]:60–90	1.02 (0.99, 1.04)	0.259
Positive fluctuation of Cl^- [a],* eGFR [b]:30–60	1.00 (0.97, 1.03)	0.812
Positive fluctuation of Cl^- [a],* eGFR [b]:<30	0.87 (0.84, 0.90)	<0.001
Interaction: Positive fluctuation of Cl^- [a],* postoperative admission	0.98 (0.96, 1.00)	0.095
Negative fluctuation of Cl^- [c] (model 2)	**1.04** (1.02, 1.06)	**<0.001**
Interaction: Negative fluctuation of Cl^- [a],*eGFR [b] ≥ 90	1	(<0.001)
Negative fluctuation of Cl^- [a],* eGFR [b]: 60–90	1.02 (0.99, 1.06)	0.145
Negative fluctuation of Cl^- [a],* eGFR [b]: 30–60	1.05 (1.01, 1.09)	0.006
Negative fluctuation of Cl^- [a],* eGFR [b]: <30	0.94 (0.91, 0.98)	0.003
Interaction: Negative fluctuation of Cl^- [a],* postoperative admission	0.94 (0.92, 0.97)	<0.001
Dependent variables: AKI stage ≥ 2		
Total fluctuation of Cl^- [a]	**1.08** (1.06, 1.10)	**<0.001**
Interaction: Total fluctuation of Cl^- [a],* eGFR [b]: ≥ 90	1	(<0.001)
Total fluctuation of Cl^- [a],* eGFR [b]: 60–90	1.00 (0.97, 1.03)	0.853
Total fluctuation of Cl^- [a],* eGFR [b]: 30–60	0.96 (0.92, 0.99)	0.022
Total fluctuation of Cl^- [a],* eGFR [b]: <30	0.89 (0.86, 0.92)	<0.001
Interaction: Total fluctuation of Cl^- [a],* postoperative admission	0.96 (0.93, 0.98)	<0.001
Positive fluctuation of Cl^- [c]	**1.09** (1.07, 1.11)	**<0.001**
Interaction: Positive fluctuation of Cl^- [a],*eGFR [b] ≥ 90	1	(<0.001)
Positive fluctuation of Cl^- [a],* eGFR [b]: 60–90	1.00 (0.96, 1.03)	0.881
Positive fluctuation of Cl^- [a],* eGFR [b]: 30–60	0.92 (0.88, 0.96)	<0.001
Positive fluctuation of Cl^- [a],* eGFR [b]: <30	0.87 (0.84, 0.91)	<0.001
Interaction: Positive fluctuation of Cl^- [a],* postoperative admission		
Negative fluctuation of Cl^- [d]	**1.09** (1.06, 1.11)	**<0.001**
Interaction: Negative fluctuation of Cl^- [a],*eGFR [b] ≥ 90	1	(<0.001)
Negative fluctuation of Cl^- [a],* eGFR [b]: 60–90	0.99 (0.95, 1.04)	0.789
Negative fluctuation of Cl^- [a],* eGFR [b]: 30–60	1.00 (0.95, 1.04)	0.853
Negative fluctuation of Cl^- [a],* eGFR [b]: <30	0.91 (0.87, 0.95)	<0.001
Interaction: Negative fluctuation of Cl^- [a],* postoperative admission	0.91 (0.89, 0.94)	<0.001

Covariates of $p < 0.1$ in univariable logistic regression analysis (Appendix B) were included to adjust the multivariable logistic regression model. [a] Total fluctuation of Cl^- (mmol L^{-1}): (Maximum Cl^- − Minimum Cl^-) for 72 h after ICU admission. [b] eGFR (mL min^{-1} 1.73 m^{-2}): 186 × $(Creatinine)^{-1.154}$ × $(Age)^{-0.203}$ × (0.742 if female). [c] Positive fluctuation of Cl^- (mmol L^{-1}): (Maximum Cl^- − Preadmission Cl^-) for 72 h after ICU admission. [d] Negative fluctuation of Cl^- (mmol L^{-1}): (Preadmission Cl^- − Minimum Cl^-) for 72 h after ICU admission. AKI, acute kidney injury; ICU, intensive care unit; eGFR, estimated glomerular filtration rate.

Table 3. Multivariable logistic regression analysis for total AKI and AKI stage ≥2 after ICU admission according to preadmission eGFR [a] group.

Variables	Odds Ratio (95% CI)	p *
Dependent variable: Total AKI		
eGFR [a] ≥90 ($n = 12,164$)		
Total fluctuation of Cl[-] [b] (per 1 mmol L^{-1})	**1.04** (1.02, 1.05)	**<0.001**
Positive fluctuation of Cl[-] [c] (per 1 mmol L^{-1})	**1.05** (1.03, 1.06)	**<0.001**
Negative fluctuation of Cl[-] [d] (per 1 mmol L^{-1})	1.01 (0.99, 1.03)	0.204
eGFR [a] <90 ($n = 7,543$)		
Total fluctuation of Cl[-] [b] (per 1 mmol L^{-1})	**1.02** (1.01, 1.04)	**0.002**
Positive fluctuation of Cl[-] [c] (per 1 mmol L^{-1})	**1.02** (1.00, 1.04)	**0.024**
Negative fluctuation of Cl[-] [d] (per 1 mmol L^{-1})	**1.03** (1.01, 1.05)	**0.004**
eGFR [a]: <60 ($n = 3,464$)		
Total fluctuation of Cl[-] [b] (per 1 mmol L^{-1})	1.01 (0.99, 1.03)	0.239
Positive fluctuation of Cl[-] [c] (per 1 mmol L^{-1})	0.99 (0.97, 1.01)	0.529
Negative fluctuation of Cl[-] [d] (per 1 mmol L^{-1})	**1.03** (1.01, 1.06)	**0.004**
eGFR [a]: <30 ($n = 1,301$)		
Total fluctuation of Cl[-] [b] (per 1 mmol L^{-1})	0.98 (0.95, 1.01)	0.150
Positive fluctuation of Cl[-] [c] (per 1 mmol L^{-1})	0.99 (0.91, 1.01)	0.052
Negative fluctuation of Cl[-] [d] (per 1 mmol L^{-1})	1.01 (0.98, 1.05)	0.469
Dependent variables: AKI stage ≥2		
eGFR [a] ≥90 ($n = 12,164$)		
Total fluctuation of Cl[-] [b] (per 1 mmol L^{-1})	**1.06** (1.04, 1.08)	**<0.001**
Positive fluctuation of Cl[-] [c] (per 1 mmol L^{-1})	**1.07** (1.05, 1.09)	**<0.001**
Negative fluctuation of Cl[-] [d] (per 1 mmol L^{-1})	**1.04** (1.02, 1.06)	**0.001**
eGFR [a] <90 ($n = 7,543$)		
Total fluctuation of Cl[-] [b] (per 1 mmol L^{-1})	**1.03** (1.01, 1.05)	**0.002**
Positive fluctuation of Cl[-] [c] (per 1 mmol L^{-1})	1.02 (1.00, 1.04)	0.059
Negative fluctuation of Cl[-] [d] (per 1 mmol L^{-1})	**1.04** (1.02, 1.06)	**0.001**
eGFR [a]: <60 ($n = 3,464$)		
Total fluctuation of Cl[-] [b] (per 1 mmol L^{-1})	1.01 (0.99, 1.03)	0.317
Positive fluctuation of Cl[-] [c] (per 1 mmol L^{-1})	0.99 (0.96, 1.01)	0.280
Negative fluctuation of Cl[-] [d] (per 1 mmol L^{-1})	**1.04** (1.01, 1.07)	**0.003**
eGFR [a]: <30 ($n = 1,301$)		
Total fluctuation of Cl[-] [b] (per 1 mmol L^{-1})	1.00 (0.97, 1.04)	0.788
Positive fluctuation of Cl[-] [c] (per 1 mmol L^{-1})	0.99 (0.95, 1.03)	0.489
Negative fluctuation of Cl[-] [d] (per 1 mmol L^{-1})	1.02 (0.98, 1.06)	0.247

* $p < 0.013$ was considered as statistically significant after Bonferroni correction. Covariates of $p < 0.1$ in univariable logistic regression analysis (Appendix B) were included to adjust the multivariable logistic regression model. [a] eGFR (mL min^{-1} 1.73m^{-2}): $186 \times (Creatinine)^{-1.154} \times (Age)^{-0.203} \times (0.742$ if female). [b] Total fluctuation of Cl[-] (mmol L^{-1}): (Maximum Cl[-] – Minimum Cl[-]) for 72 h after ICU admission. [c] Positive fluctuation of Cl[-] (mmol L^{-1}): (Maximum Cl[-] – Preadmission Cl[-]) for 72 h after ICU admission. [d] Negative fluctuation of Cl[-] (mmol L^{-1}): (Preadmission Cl[-] – Minimum Cl[-]) for 72 h after ICU admission.

Table 4. Multivariable logistic regression analysis for total AKI and AKI (stage ≥2) after ICU admission according to postoperative admission.

Variables	Odds ratio (95% CI)	p *
Dependent variable: Total AKI		
Postoperative admission (n = 8,728)		
Total fluctuation of Cl$^-$ [a] (per 1 mmol L^{-1})	1.01 (1.00, 1.02)	0.170
Positive fluctuation of Cl$^-$ [b] (per 1 mmol L^{-1})	**1.03** (1.01, 1.04)	**0.002**
Negative fluctuation of Cl$^-$ [c] (per 1 mmol L^{-1})	0.99 (0.97, 1.01)	0.254
Non-postoperative admission (n = 10,992)		
Total fluctuation of Cl$^-$ [a] (per 1 mmol L^{-1})	**1.04** (1.02, 1.05)	**<0.001**
Positive fluctuation of Cl$^-$ [b] (per 1 mmol L^{-1})	**1.04** (1.02, 1.05)	**<0.001**
Negative fluctuation of Cl$^-$ [c] (per 1 mmol L^{-1})	**1.04** (1.02, 1.05)	**<0.001**
Dependent variables: AKI stage ≥2		
Postoperative admission (n = 8,728)		
Total fluctuation of Cl$^-$ [a] (per 1 mmol L^{-1})	1.01 (0.99, 1.03)	0.300
Positive fluctuation of Cl$^-$ [b] (per 1 mmol L^{-1})	**1.03** (1.00, 1.05)	**0.023**
Negative fluctuation of Cl$^-$ [c] (per 1 mmol L^{-1})	0.99 (0.96, 1.02)	0.396
Non-postoperative admission (n = 10,992)		
Total fluctuation of Cl$^-$ [a] (per 1 mmol L^{-1})	**1.05** (1.04, 1.07)	**<0.001**
Positive fluctuation of Cl$^-$ [b] (per 1 mmol L^{-1})	**1.05** (1.03, 1.07)	**<0.001**
Negative fluctuation of Cl$^-$ [c] (per 1 mmol L^{-1})	**1.06** (1.04, 1.08)	**<0.001**

* $p < 0.025$ was considered as statistically significant after Bonferroni correction. Covariates of $p < 0.1$ in univariable logistic regression analysis (Appendix B) were included to adjust the multivariable logistic regression model. [a] Total fluctuation of Cl$^-$ (mmol L^{-1}): (Maximum Cl$^-$ − Minimum Cl$^-$) for 72 h after ICU admission. [b] Positive fluctuation of Cl$^-$ (mmol L^{-1}): (Maximum Cl$^-$ − Preadmission Cl$^-$) for 72 h after ICU admission. [c] Negative fluctuation of Cl$^-$ (mmol L^{-1}): (Preadmission Cl$^-$ − Minimum Cl$^-$) for 72 h after ICU admission. AKI, acute kidney injury; ICU, intensive care unit; eGFR, estimated glomerular filtration rate.

3.3. Fluctuation in Cl$^-$ and Maximum Serum Cystatin Level during the 72 h after ICU Admission

Serum cystatin C was measured in the 2021 patients at least once within 72 h after ICU admission. In these patients, generalized linear regression analysis was performed, and the results of the GLM are presented in Table 5. A 1 mmol L^{-1} increase in the negative fluctuation in Cl$^-$ was associated with a 1.4% increase of maximum cystatin C level (exp coef: 0.014, 95% CI: 0.002 to 0.026; $p = 0.026$), while total fluctuation of Cl$^-$ ($p = 0.374$) and positive fluctuation of Cl$^-$ (0.682) were not associated with the maximum cystatin C level.

Table 5. Generalized linear regression model for maximum cystatin C level within 72 h after ICU admission according to fluctuation of Cl$^-$ (n = 2,021).

Variables	Exp Coef (95% CI)	p *
Dependent variable: maximum cystatin C level (mmol L^{-1})		
Total fluctuation of Cl$^-$ [a] (per 1 mmol L^{-1}, model 1)	0.004 (−0.005, 0.013)	0.374
Positive fluctuation of Cl$^-$ [b] (per 1 mmol L^{-1}, model 2)	−0.002 (−0.012, 0.008)	0.682
Negative fluctuation of Cl$^-$ [c] (per 1 mmol L^{-1}, model 2)	**0.014** (0.002, 0.026)	0.026

* In the generalized linear model, gamma distribution and the log link function were assumed for the dependent variable (maximum cystatin C level within 72 h after ICU admission). All covariates were included in the model. [a] Total fluctuation of Cl$^-$ (mmol L^{-1}): (maximum Cl$^-$ − minimum Cl$^-$) for 72 h after ICU admission. [b] Positive fluctuation of Cl$^-$ (mmol L^{-1}): (maximum Cl$^-$ − preadmission Cl$^-$) for 72 h after ICU admission. [c] Negative fluctuation of Cl$^-$ (mmol L^{-1}): (preadmission Cl$^-$ − minimum Cl$^-$) for 72 h after ICU admission. Exp, exponentiated; Coef, coefficient; APACHE, acute physiology and chronic health evaluation; eGFR, estimated glomerular filtration rate.

4. Discussion

This study showed that both positive and negative fluctuations in Cl$^-$ within 72 h after ICU admission were significantly associated with the potential risk of AKI in a mixed ICU adult population. This association was also observed for AKI stage ≥2. In the subgroup analysis based on preadmission eGFR grouping, the association between positive fluctuations in Cl$^-$ and AKI was more evident in the eGFR $\geq$90 mL min^{-1} 1.73 m^{-2} group, while the association between negative fluctuations in Cl$^-$ and AKI was more evident in the eGFR <90 or <60 mL min^{-1} 1.73 m^{-2} group. Additionally, both positive and negative fluctuations in Cl$^-$ were associated with the risk of AKI in patients without postoperative ICU admission, while only positive fluctuations in Cl$^-$ were significantly associated with the risk of AKI in patients with postoperative admissions.

The most novel finding of this study is that we reported that the negative fluctuations in Cl$^-$ could also be associated with the risk of AKI in critically ill patients. While the association between positive fluctuations in Cl$^-$ and AKI were reported in previous studies [13–15], the association regarding the negative fluctuations has yet to be reported. While positive fluctuations in Cl$^-$ could be caused by fluid resuscitation [24], negative fluctuations in Cl$^-$ could be caused by a loss of active Cl$^-$ from the gastrointestinal tract, impaired renal Cl$^-$ reabsorption, and an infusion of hypotonic fluid [16,17], which might be related to AKI [25]. Additionally, hypochloremia might be caused by negative fluctuations in Cl$^-$, which is a common and independent poor prognostic factor in critically ill patients [26]. Although our findings regarding positive fluctuations in Cl$^-$ were consistent with those of a meta-analysis published in 2015 [27], there was another meta-analysis, published in 2018, which concluded that the relationship between the use of chloride-rich solution and AKI remains controversial [28]. Therefore, future studies should investigate the effect of positive or negative fluctuations in Cl$^-$ on AKI.

Another interesting finding was that the interactions related to AKI existed between the eGFR status at the time of ICU admission and total fluctuations in Cl$^-$. The results of the subgroup analysis based on eGFR grouping showed that the positive fluctuations in Cl$^-$ tended to be more frequently associated with AKI in patients with normal kidney function (eGFR $\geq$90 mL min^{-1} 1.73 m^{-2}). In contrast, negative fluctuations in Cl$^-$ tended to be more frequently associated with AKI in patients with CKD (eGFR <90 or 60 mL min^{-1} 1.73 m^{-2}). There are several potential explanations for our findings. First, patients with normal kidney function at ICU admission might have received more chloride-rich fluid resuscitation than CKD patients; this might have impacted the positive fluctuations in Cl$^-$. Secondly, since CKD patients often had disruptions in their acid–base balance [25], the negative fluctuations in Cl$^-$ might have had a greater impact on the patients with CKD. Lastly, the impact of both positive and negative fluctuations in Cl$^-$ was not significant in patients with CKD 4 or 5 (<30). There is a possibility that the fluctuations in Cl$^-$ were minimized by physicians for such severe CKD patients, thus impacting these results in patients with CKD 4 or 5.

The difference in the results regarding positive fluctuations in Cl$^-$ between this study and our previous study is also interesting [18]. In our previous study, we found that hyperchloremia (>110 mmol L^{-1}) was not associated with postoperative AKI in the surgical ICU, and there was a positive association in the increase from the preoperative Cl$^-$ (which was measured within 1 month prior to surgery) to the maximum Cl$^-$ measured 0–3 days postoperatively in patients with a CKD stage $\geq$3. The differences between two studies might be caused by the study designs. Our previous study might have been affected by fluid resuscitation or blood loss during surgery, while the present study was not affected by these factors. In general, more fluid administration is required to replace ongoing bleeding or insensible loss of fluid during surgery [29], so that the impact of the Cl$^-$ load on AKI would be different from that in the ICU.

Although the serum cystatin C level was measured in only 2021 patients (10.2%) for 72 h after ICU admission in this study, our results regarding the relationship between Cl$^-$ fluctuation and cystatin level were also notable. In this study, only the negative Cl$^-$ fluctuation was associated with an increase in serum cystatin level during the 72 h after ICU admission. Considering that cystatin C is known as a marker of renal function in AKI [23], our results suggest that a decrease of Cl$^-$ level might be an associated factor for development of AKI after ICU admission. In addition, the relationship between AKI and the increase of Cl$^-$ could be caused by fluid administration. Furthermore, the significant relationship between the positive fluctuation and development of AKI could be related to clinical situations that require fluid administration. However, a decrease of Cl$^-$ was more related to kidney damage via hypochloremic metabolic alkalosis [10] than to an increase in Cl$^-$. Considering the relatively small sample size of patients who had their serum cystatin C measured for 72 h after ICU admission in this study, more studies should be performed in the future to confirm the relationship between dyschloremia, cystatin C levels, and AKI.

This study had a number of limitations. First, due to the retrospective cohort design, selection bias may have occurred during the data collection process. To minimize this bias, all data were collected by a medical record technician blinded from the purpose of this study. Second, this study was performed at a single center, and therefore its results may have limited generalizability. Third, Cl^- levels were not measured during the same period, using the same method for all patients included in this study. Fourth, since patients who developed AKI were much more likely to develop dyschloremia due to the inability of their kidneys to effectively regulate Cl^- levels, there is a possibility that AKI may precede changes in Cl^-, and thus might confound our study conclusions. Fifth, we could only use serum creatinine concentrations for the accurate diagnosis of AKI in accordance with the KDIGO criteria due to a lack of accurate urine output data. The exclusion of urine output data may reduce the accuracy and sensitivity of AKI diagnosis, especially for the diagnosis of more severe stages of AKI (stage 2 or 3) [30,31]. Lastly, in this study, we did not evaluate various biomarkers for AKI such as beta-2 microglobulin, liver-type fatty acid binding protein, and neutrophil gelatinase-associated lipocalin. Considering there are many biomarkers for the early detection of AKI [32], more biomarkers are needed to evaluate the direct effect of Cl^- fluctuation on AKI development.

5. Conclusions

This study showed that an increase in both the positive and negative fluctuations in Cl- after ICU admission were associated with an increased risk of AKI after ICU admission. Furthermore, these associations differed based on the kidney functionality at ICU admission or postoperative ICU admission. However, the results should be interpreted carefully considering the retrospective design, and future studies should be performed using biomarkers for AKI.

Author Contributions: T.K.O. and I.A.S. designed the study, analyzed and interpreted the data, and drafted the manuscript. Y.T.J. and Y.H.J. contributed to the acquisition of data. All authors have given approval of the final version of the manuscript.

Appendix A

Table A1. Staging of postoperative acute kidney injury (KDIGO).

Stage	Serum Creatinine
1	1.5–1.9 times baseline or ≥0.3 mg dL^{-1} increase within 72 h after ICU admission
2	2.0–2.9 times baseline within 72 h after ICU admission
3	3.0 times baseline or increase in serum creatinine to ≥4.0 mg dL^{-1} or initiation of RRT within 72 h after ICU admission

KDIGO, kidney disease: improving global outcomes; RRT, renal replacement therapy.

Appendix B

Table A2. Univariable logistic regression analysis of covariates for occurrence of total AKI and AKI stage ≥2 during 72 h after ICU admission.

Variables	Total AKI		AKI Stage ≥2	
	OR (95% CI)	*p*-Value	OR (95% CI)	*p*-Value
Sex: male	1.09 (1.02–1.16)	0.012	1.08 (0.99–1.18)	0.093
Age, year	1.02 (1.02–1.02)	<0.001	1.01 (1.01–1.02)	<0.001
Body mass index, kg m^{-2}	0.96 (0.95–0.97)	<0.001	0.93 (0.92–0.95)	<0.001
APACHE II	1.04 (1.04–1.04)	<0.001	1.04 (1.03–1.04)	<0.001

Table A2. *Cont.*

Variables	Total AKI		AKI Stage ≥2	
	OR (95% CI)	*p*-Value	OR (95% CI)	*p*-Value
Comorbidities at ICU admission				
Hypertension	1.30 (1.22–1.38)	<0.001	1.16 (1.06–1.26)	0.001
Diabetes mellitus	1.51 (1.36–1.67)	<0.001	1.42 (1.23–1.63)	<0.001
Ischemic heart disease	1.20 (0.98–1.46)	0.076	1.01 (0.76–1.34)	0.942
Cerebrovascular disease	1.31 (1.14–1.52)	<0.001	1.13 (0.92–1.38)	0.250
Chronic obstructive lung disease	1.12 (0.97–1.30)	0.131	0.96 (0.77–1.19)	0.713
Liver disease	2.46 (2.10–2.88)	<0.001	3.21 (2.68–3.83)	<0.001
Anemia (Hb <10 g dL^{-1})	3.73 (3.49–4.00)	<0.001	4.77 (4.33–5.25)	<0.001
Cancer	1.83 (1.70–1.97)	<0.001	2.06 (1.88–2.27)	<0.001
eGFR mL min^{-1} 1.73 m^{-2}				
≥90	1	(<0.001)	1	(<0.001)
60–90	1.04 (0.96–1.13)	0.343	0.77 (0.68–0.88)	<0.001
30–60	2.21 (2.01–2.44)	<0.001	1.17 (1.02–1.35)	0.029
<30	5.33 (4.73–6.00)	<0.001	3.69 (3.24–4.22)	<0.001
Admission through ED	1.51 (1.41–1.61)	<0.001	1.91 (1.73–2.10)	<0.001
Postoperative admission	0.86 (0.81, 0.92)	<0.001	0.68 (0.62, 0.74)	<0.001
Fluid administration for 72 h				
NaCl 0.9%, per 100 ml increase	1.00 (1.00, 1.00)	0.018	1.01 (1.00, 1.01)	0.001
Balanced crystalloid, per 100 mL	0.99 (0.99, 1.00)	0.014	0.98 (0.97, 0.98)	<0.001
Hydroxyethyl starch, per 100 mL	0.98 (0.97, 0.99)	0.002	0.96 (0.95, 0.98)	<0.001
Transfusion of packed RBC	2.43 (2.28, 2.60)	<0.001	2.34 (2.14, 2.57)	<0.001
The number of measurements of Cl$^-$	1.93 (1.86, 2.01)	<0.001	1.63 (1.54, 1.72)	<0.001
Admission department				
Internal medicine	1	(<0.001)	1	(<0.001)
Neurologic center	0.23 (0.21–0.26)	<0.001	0.19 (0.16–0.22)	<0.001
Cardiothoracic surgical department	0.79 (0.73–0.86)	<0.001	0.52 (0.47–0.59)	<0.001
Other surgical departments	0.77 (0.71–0.85)	<0.001	0.64 (0.57–0.72)	<0.001

AKI, acute kidney injury; ICU, intensive care unit; APACHE, acute physiology and chronic health evaluation; eGFR, estimated glomerular filtration rate; ED, emergency department; Hb, hemoglobin; RBC, red blood cell; RRT, renal replacement therapy.

References

1. Waikar, S.S.; Bonventre, J.V. Creatinine kinetics and the definition of acute kidney injury. *J. Am. Soc. Nephrol.* **2009**, *20*, 672–679. [CrossRef] [PubMed]
2. Bellomo, R.; Kellum, J.A.; Ronco, C. Acute kidney injury. *Lancet* **2012**, *380*, 756–766. [CrossRef]
3. Lewington, A.J.; Cerda, J.; Mehta, R.L. Raising awareness of acute kidney injury: A global perspective of a silent killer. *Kidney Int.* **2013**, *84*, 457–467. [CrossRef] [PubMed]
4. Nash, K.; Hafeez, A.; Hou, S. Hospital-acquired renal insufficiency. *Am. J. Kidney Dis.* **2002**, *39*, 930–936. [CrossRef] [PubMed]
5. Ostermann, M.; Chang, R.W. Acute kidney injury in the intensive care unit according to rifle. *Crit. Care Med.* **2007**, *35*, 1837–1843, quiz 1852. [CrossRef] [PubMed]
6. Rewa, O.; Bagshaw, S.M. Acute kidney injury-epidemiology, outcomes and economics. *Nat. Rev. Nephrol.* **2014**, *10*, 193–207. [CrossRef] [PubMed]
7. Thakar, C.V.; Christianson, A.; Freyberg, R.; Almenoff, P.; Render, M.L. Incidence and outcomes of acute kidney injury in intensive care units: A veterans administration study. *Crit. Care Med.* **2009**, *37*, 2552–2558. [CrossRef]
8. Macedo, E.; Mehta, R.L. Preventing acute kidney injury. *Crit. Care Clin.* **2015**, *31*, 773–784. [CrossRef]
9. Pfortmueller, C.A.; Uehlinger, D.; von Haehling, S.; Schefold, J.C. Serum chloride levels in critical illness-the hidden story. *Intensive Care Med. Exp.* **2018**, *6*, 10. [CrossRef]
10. Shao, M.; Li, G.; Sarvottam, K.; Wang, S.; Thongprayoon, C.; Dong, Y.; Gajic, O.; Kashani, K. Dyschloremia is a risk factor for the development of acute kidney injury in critically ill patients. *PLoS ONE* **2016**, *11*, e0160322. [CrossRef]
11. Toyonaga, Y.; Kikura, M. Hyperchloremic acidosis is associated with acute kidney injury after abdominal surgery. *Nephrology* **2017**, *22*, 720–727. [CrossRef] [PubMed]
12. Yunos, N.M.; Bellomo, R.; Glassford, N.; Sutcliffe, H.; Lam, Q.; Bailey, M. Chloride-liberal vs. Chloride-restrictive intravenous fluid administration and acute kidney injury: An extended analysis. *Intensive Care Med.* **2015**, *41*, 257–264. [CrossRef]

13. De Vasconcellos, K.; Skinner, D.L. Hyperchloraemia is associated with acute kidney injury and mortality in the critically ill: A retrospective observational study in a multidisciplinary intensive care unit. *J. Crit. Care* **2018**, *45*, 45–51. [CrossRef]

14. Jaynes, M.P.; Murphy, C.V.; Ali, N.; Krautwater, A.; Lehman, A.; Doepker, B.A. Association between chloride content of intravenous fluids and acute kidney injury in critically ill medical patients with sepsis. *J. Crit. Care* **2018**, *44*, 363–367. [CrossRef] [PubMed]

15. Sadan, O.; Singbartl, K.; Kandiah, P.A.; Martin, K.S.; Samuels, O.B. Hyperchloremia is associated with acute kidney injury in patients with subarachnoid hemorrhage. *Crit. Care Med.* **2017**, *45*, 1382–1388. [CrossRef]

16. Berend, K.; van Hulsteijn, L.H.; Gans, R.O. Chloride: The queen of electrolytes? *Eur. J. Intern. Med.* **2012**, *23*, 203–211. [CrossRef] [PubMed]

17. Yunos, N.M.; Bellomo, R.; Story, D.; Kellum, J. Bench-to-bedside review: Chloride in critical illness. *Crit. Care* **2010**, *14*, 226. [CrossRef] [PubMed]

18. Oh, T.K.; Song, I.-A.; Kim, S.J.; Lim, S.Y.; Do, S.-H.; Hwang, J.-W.; Kim, J.; Jeon, Y.-T. Hyperchloremia and postoperative acute kidney injury: A retrospective analysis of data from the surgical intensive care unit. *Crit. Care* **2018**, *22*, 277. [CrossRef] [PubMed]

19. Hallan, S.; Asberg, A.; Lindberg, M.; Johnsen, H. Validation of the modification of diet in renal disease formula for estimating gfr with special emphasis on calibration of the serum creatinine assay. *Am. J. Kidney Dis.* **2004**, *44*, 84–93. [CrossRef] [PubMed]

20. Kellum, J.A.; Lameire, N.; Group, K.A.G.W. Diagnosis, evaluation, and management of acute kidney injury: A kdigo summary (part 1). *Crit. Care* **2013**, *17*, 204. [CrossRef]

21. Chawla, L.S.; Eggers, P.W.; Star, R.A.; Kimmel, P.L. Acute kidney injury and chronic kidney disease as interconnected syndromes. *N. Engl. J. Med.* **2014**, *371*, 58–66. [CrossRef] [PubMed]

22. Armstrong, R.A. When to use the bonferroni correction. *Ophthalmic Physiol. Opt.* **2014**, *34*, 502–508. [CrossRef] [PubMed]

23. Murty, M.S.; Sharma, U.K.; Pandey, V.B.; Kankare, S.B. Serum cystatin c as a marker of renal function in detection of early acute kidney injury. *Indian J. Nephrol.* **2013**, *23*, 180–183. [CrossRef]

24. Nagami, G.T. Hyperchloremia—Why and how. *Nefrologia* **2016**, *36*, 347–353. [CrossRef] [PubMed]

25. Bank, N.; Better, O.S. Acid-base balance and acute renal failure. *Miner Electrolyte Metab.* **1991**, *17*, 116–123.

26. Tani, M.; Morimatsu, H.; Takatsu, F.; Morita, K. The incidence and prognostic value of hypochloremia in critically ill patients. *Sci. World J.* **2012**, *2012*, 474185. [CrossRef]

27. Krajewski, M.L.; Raghunathan, K.; Paluszkiewicz, S.M.; Schermer, C.R.; Shaw, A.D. Meta-analysis of high- versus low-chloride content in perioperative and critical care fluid resuscitation. *Br. J. Surg.* **2015**, *102*, 24–36. [CrossRef] [PubMed]

28. Kawano-Dourado, L.; Zampieri, F.G.; Azevedo, L.C.P.; Correa, T.D.; Figueiro, M.; Semler, M.W.; Kellum, J.A.; Cavalcanti, A.B. Low- versus high-chloride content intravenous solutions for critically ill and perioperative adult patients: A systematic review and meta-analysis. *Anesth. Analg.* **2018**, *126*, 513–521. [CrossRef]

29. Chappell, D.; Jacob, M.; Hofmann-Kiefer, K.; Conzen, P.; Rehm, M. A rational approach to perioperative fluid management. *Anesthesiology* **2008**, *109*, 723–740. [CrossRef]

30. Bagshaw, S.M.; George, C.; Bellomo, R.; Committee, A.D.M. Changes in the incidence and outcome for early acute kidney injury in a cohort of australian intensive care units. *Crit. Care* **2007**, *11*, R68. [CrossRef]

31. Kellum, J.A.; Sileanu, F.E.; Murugan, R.; Lucko, N.; Shaw, A.D.; Clermont, G. Classifying aki by urine output versus serum creatinine level. *J. Am. Soc. Nephrol.* **2015**, *26*, 2231–2238. [CrossRef] [PubMed]

32. Vaidya, V.S.; Ferguson, M.A.; Bonventre, J.V. Biomarkers of acute kidney injury. *Annu. Rev. Pharmacol. Toxicol.* **2008**, *48*, 463–493. [CrossRef] [PubMed]

11

Utilizing the Patient Care Process to Minimize the Risk of Vancomycin-Associated Nephrotoxicity

Ashley R. Selby [1,2,*] and Ronald G. Hall II [1,2,3,4]

[1] Department of Pharmacy Practice, Texas Tech University Health Sciences Center Jerry H. Hodge School of Pharmacy, Dallas, TX 75235, USA; Ronald.Hall@ttuhsc.edu
[2] VA North Texas Health Care System, Dallas, TX 75216, USA
[3] Department of Surgery, University of Texas Southwestern Medical Center, Dallas, TX 75390, USA
[4] Dose Optimization and Outcomes Research (DOOR) Program, Dallas, TX 75235, USA
* Correspondence: Ashley.Selby@ttuhsc.edu

Abstract: Vancomycin-associated acute kidney injury (AKI) is a popular topic in the medical literature with few clear answers. While many studies evaluate the risk of AKI associated with vancomycin, few data are high quality and/or long in duration of follow-up. This review takes the clinician through an approach to evaluate a patient for risk of AKI. This evaluation should include patient assessment, antibiotic prescription, duration, and monitoring. Patient assessment involves evaluating severity of illness, baseline renal function, hypotension/vasopressor use, and concomitant nephrotoxins. Evaluation of antibiotic prescription includes evaluating the need for methicillin-resistant *Staphylococcus aureus* (MRSA) coverage and/or vancomycin use. Duration of therapy has been shown to increase the risk of AKI. Efforts to de-escalate vancomycin from the antimicrobial regimen, including MRSA nasal swabs and rapid diagnostics, should be used to lessen the likelihood of AKI. Adequate monitoring includes therapeutic drug monitoring, ongoing fluid status evaluations, and a continual reassessment of AKI risk. The issues with serum creatinine make the timely evaluation of renal function and diagnosis of the cause of AKI problematic. Most notably, concomitant piperacillin-tazobactam can increase serum creatinine via tubular secretion, resulting in higher rates of AKI being reported. The few studies evaluating the long-term prognosis of AKI in patients receiving vancomycin have found that few patients require renal replacement therapy and that the long-term risk of death is unaffected for patients surviving after the initial 28-day period.

Keywords: vancomycin; MRSA; nephrotoxicity; acute kidney injury; piperacillin-tazobactam; creatinine; KIM-1; AKIN; KDIGO; RIFLE

1. Introduction

Vancomycin has been a mainstay of empiric therapy for gram-positive pathogens, particularly methicillin-resistant *Staphylococcus aureus* (MRSA), for over 50 years. The history of vancomycin has also been littered with safety concerns since the days of "Mississippi Mud", which the impure formulations of vancomycin were affectionately called. In the 1980s, nephrotoxicity concerns rose again. These concerns largely went away as studies found that this nephrotoxicity was generally reversible and randomized; controlled trials of one gram of vancomycin every 12 h reported nephrotoxicity rates of 0–5% [1–3].

Efficacy concerns prompted the development of the vancomycin consensus document. The 2009 consensus statement recommended trough concentrations of 15–20 mg/L for severe infections in an attempt to overcome increasing vancomycin minimum inhibitory concentrations (MICs) in MRSA [4]. The unintended consequence of this recommendation was a significant increase in the rate of nephrotoxicity reported in the literature. However, it is unclear how much of this increase was due to increased trough concentrations versus the more stringent nephrotoxicity definitions that were being adopted into routine use for research.

Vancomycin use rose by 32% from 2006 to 2012 in the US despite increasing fears regarding nephrotoxicity [5]. Therefore, many clinicians still have faith in vancomycin as a relatively safe antimicrobial despite multiple observational reports and one randomized, controlled trial suggesting otherwise [1,4,5].

The discordance between the data associating vancomycin with nephrotoxicity (including unclear dosing and monitoring requirements) and routine antibiotic prescribing patterns for MRSA infections leave the reasonable clinician debating the best course of action regarding how to incorporate this literature into practice. This review aims to walk the reader through the patient care process (Table 1), analyzing potential factors associated with the development of vancomycin-associated nephrotoxicity or its outcomes during each step.

Table 1. Summary of the patient care process to assess the risk of nephrotoxicity in patients being considered for vancomycin therapy.

Stage of Patient Care Process	Characteristic	Measures	Notes
Patient assessment	Severity of illness	APACHE II Pitt bacteremia score ICU residence	Increased severity of illness has been associated with nephrotoxicity
	Concomitant disease states	Renal dysfunction	Nephrotoxicity increased whether as a cutpoint for serum creatinine or creatinine clearance. Also serum creatinine as a continuous variable.
		Increased creatinine clearance	Only found as a risk factor in one cohort to date.
	Concomitant nephrotoxins	Hypotension and/or vasopressor use	No data regarding the impact of the duration of hypotension.
		ACE inhibitor, amphotericin B, tacrolimus, loop diuretics, and tenofovir	Information regarding the impact of dose and/or duration is lacking
		Piperacillin/tazobactam	Increases diagnosis of nephrotoxicity, but may be renal-protective
Antibiotic prescription	Patient need for an antibiotic	Clinical and microbiologic assessment	Tension exists between the need for rapid adequate empiric therapy and providing antibiotics to patients with non-infectious diseases
	Patient need for vancomycin	Clinical and microbiologic assessment	Assess for risk of MRSA. Further advances in risk scores for assessing risk are needed.
Duration of therapy	Vancomycin duration	Days of vancomycin therapy	Nephrotoxicity risk increases with longer durations of therapy. Most clinical guidelines recommend seven days of vancomycin. Notable exceptions include endocarditis and osteomyelitis.
	Vancomycin discontinuation	Microbiologic assessment	Use of rapid diagnostics, nasal PCR swabs can help aid in discontinuation of vancomycin.
Monitoring	Therapeutic drug monitoring	Vancomycin concentrations	AUC goal should be 400–650 mg·h/L If a trough approach is utilized, please hold at least one dose for a trough ≥25 mg/L
	Fluid status	Intake and output reporting	Both fluid overload and hypovolemia are associated with nephrotoxicity. Accurate intake and output charting can be difficult in some practice environments.
	Reassessment of nephrotoxicity risk	See patient assessment section	

ICU: intensive care unit; ACE: angiotensin converting enzyme; MRSA: methicillin-resistant *Staphylococcus aureus*; PCR: polymerase chain reaction; AUC: area under the curve.

2. Patient Assessment

Every patient that receives vancomycin is not the same. The baseline risk of nephrotoxicity varies based on several factors. These factors include the patient's baseline severity of illness, concomitant disease states, and concomitant nephrotoxins. This means that the patients are likely to have a higher or lower baseline risk of nephrotoxicity based on the presence or absence of the factors that will be discussed in this section.

Several patient characteristics can be utilized to indicate a patient's severity of illness. These variables are not routinely evaluated together in a multivariable model due to concerns regarding collinearity. Multiple studies have found that the risk of nephrotoxicity increases as the baseline APACHE II score increases [6,7]. We have also found that an increased Pitt bacteremia score was associated with nephrotoxicity in patients with MRSA bacteremia [8]. The impact of increasing Sequential Organ Failure Assessmentscores on nephrotoxicity has not been studied, to our knowledge. Intensive care unit residence has also been associated with vancomycin-associated nephrotoxicity in two retrospective studies by Lodise and colleagues [9,10].

Renal dysfunction at baseline has also been associated with nephrotoxicity in multiple studies. Baseline serum creatinine levels ≥1.7 or 2.0 mg/dL were found to be independent predictors of nephrotoxicity in retrospective analyses [11,12]. We have also found that evaluating baseline serum creatinine as a continuous variable (1 mg/dL increments) is also associated with nephrotoxicity [13]. A computer-guided cutpoint of an estimated CrCl ≤ 86.6 mL/min was also associated with time to nephrotoxicity (adjusted odds ratio (OR) 3.7; 95% confidence interval (CI) 1.2–11.5) [9]. The mechanism of why impaired renal function would play a role in the development of nephrotoxicity has yet to be fully elucidated. Some potential reasons would include increased drug exposure through decreased baseline renal function as well the pre-existing kidney damage noted by an increased serum creatinine (and possible diagnosis of chronic kidney disease). The finding by Rutter and colleagues of increased creatinine clearance being associated with nephrotoxicity further adds to the uncertainty regarding this potential factor [14].

Several studies have also reported the association between vasopressor use and nephrotoxicity. These studies do not report information regarding the duration of hypotension prior to vasopressor use [6,12,15,16]. This means that vasopressor use is sometimes used as a surrogate marker of hypotension. It is unknown whether the hypotensive episode or vasopressor use has a greater impact on the development of nephrotoxicity. The majority of studies that have evaluated the impact of hypotensive events on nephrotoxicity have had limited numbers of patients having hypotensive events [17–19]. Rutter and colleagues found hypotensive events to be significantly associated with nephrotoxicity in the largest study to evaluate the impact of hypotensive events in patients receiving vancomycin [14].

Receipt of other nephrotoxic agents may also contribute to nephrotoxicity. A systematic review demonstrated that patients receiving concomitant nephrotoxins were more likely to develop nephrotoxicity (OR 3.30; 95% CI 1.30–8.39) [20]. The role of individual agents, including dose and/or duration, is more difficult to ascertain given that most currently available data have very few events and only allow for the evaluation of a few select covariates. Models that attempt to evaluate too many variables compared to the number of events in the study suffer from overfitting issues, compromising their external validity.

Nephrotoxicity is a known risk associated with the use of aminoglycosides and amphotericin B [21,22]. The use of concomitant aminoglycoside or amphotericin B in addition to vancomycin was the only factor independently associated with nephrotoxicity in one multivariate analysis [23]. Aminoglycosides were also the only concomitant medication associated with nephrotoxicity in a study specifically evaluating critically ill patients [24].

Two large, retrospective cohort studies of hospitalized patients suggest that nephrotoxicity is associated with concomitant angiotensin converting enzyme inhibitor, amphotericin B, tacrolimus, loop diuretics, and tenofovir [14,25]. The concomitant use of a loop diuretic in patients receiving vancomycin and an antipseudomonal beta-lactam was associated with nephrotoxicity in a multicenter observational study (OR 3.27; 95% CI 1.42–7.53) [16].

The concomitant receipt of piperacillin-tazobactam has been the focus of most recent studies regarding vancomycin-associated nephrotoxicity. Several studies have highlighted the increased risk of acute kidney injury (AKI) associated with concomitant receipt of piperacillin-tazobactam with vancomycin [16,26–28]. Some studies focused on patients admitted to the intensive care unit have not found this association [29,30]. Schreier and colleagues demonstrated that the empiric use of this combination is not associated with nephrotoxicity when de-escalation occurs within the first 48–72 h [31].

The mechanisms for the increased rates of nephrotoxicity with piperacillin-tazobactam have been unclear. Data suggest that the association is not due to the beta-lactamase inhibitor or the infusion strategy [32]. Some have even suggested that the increase in serum creatinine with piperacillin-tazobactam does not represent nephrotoxicity in these patients. Piperacillin-tazobactam is known to increase serum creatinine through inhibition of creatinine tubular secretion without decreasing glomerular filtration rate [33]. There are also clinical data suggesting that the addition of piperacillin-tazobactam to vancomycin lowers dialysis rates even in the face of increased rates of AKI as measured by increases in serum creatinine [29]. Data from a benchtop animal study suggest that the concomitant use of piperacillin/tazobactam may delay the increase in kidney injury molecule-1 (KIM-1) in animals receiving vancomycin [34]. Therefore, piperacillin-tazobactam may be renal-protective even though it increases serum creatinine.

3. Antibiotic Prescription

Up to 50% of inpatient antimicrobial use has been shown to be inappropriate [35]. A recent study has also shown that vancomycin remains one of the most commonly used antimicrobials in hospitals [5]. This is in part due to the high prevalence of methicillin-resistance amongst *S. aureus* isolates as well as the pressures to ensure adequate empiric coverage for the suspected infection. Adding to the concern are diagnostic dilemmas including inconclusive radiographic evidence of infection and the era of health-care associated pneumonia that dramatically increased vancomycin use. A patient-by-patient assessment MRSA risk is needed to avoid the overprescribing of empiric MRSA coverage, which will hopefully be aided in the future by better risk scores and/or rapid diagnostics beyond nasal swabs.

Given the high prevalence of methicillin-resistance amongst *S. aureus* isolates, empiric therapy with vancomycin is common. This is in part due to its inclusion as a first-line option for MRSA in Infectious Diseases Society of America (IDSA) guidelines for skin and soft-tissue infections, diabetic foot infections, endocarditis, febrile neutropenia, meningitis, pneumonia, and surgical prophylaxis [36–43].

However, there are clinical scenarios where vancomycin is not the optimal agent for definitive therapy. There are currently seven oral and 11 intravenous agents that are approved by the U.S. Food and Drug Administration that are active against MRSA. Vancomycin should be evaluated against these other options to determine the optimal agent for a particular patient. Vancomycin is not the optimal agent for a patient that is eligible for oral antimicrobial therapy, as multiple studies have shown the non-inferiority of oral antimicrobials for serious infections [44,45].

4. Duration of Therapy

Several studies have demonstrated that the risk of nephrotoxicity is associated with the duration of vancomycin therapy [27]. Multiple studies have shown that the risk of nephrotoxicity increases after four days of therapy [9,10,15,19,20]. Others have found that a duration of therapy of seven or 14–15 days is associated with nephrotoxicity [6,8,11]. Another study found that the rates of nephrotoxicity increased when the duration was extended from seven or fewer days (6%) to 8–14 days (21%), and to 30% when extended >14 days [23]. Most patients should not require vancomycin for more than seven days [36,39,41–43]. Some notable exceptions include osteomyelitis and endocarditis [37,38].

De-escalation is a sound antimicrobial strategy for several reasons, including reducing vancomycin duration and possibly the risk of nephrotoxicity. A retrospective study found that the de-escalation of anti-MRSA agents in culture-negative nosocomial pneumonia within the first four days of empiric therapy was associated with a lower rate of AKI (36% vs. 50%; difference, −13.8%; 95% CI −26.9 to −0.4) [46]. Rapid diagnostic tests may further assist with de-escalation due to their strong negative predictive value [47,48]. The use of MRSA polymerase chain reaction (PCR) testing shortened the duration of anti-MRSA coverage in a small retrospective study by approximately two days and was associated with decreased rates of AKI (26% vs. 3%; $p = 0.02$) [49].

5. Monitoring

5.1. Vancomycin Concentrations

The IDSA/Society for Healthcare Epidemiology of America (SHEA) antimicrobial stewardship guidelines provide a weak recommendation for the therapeutic drug monitoring of vancomycin based on low-quality evidence [50]. To date, only one randomized controlled trial has evaluated the impact of vancomycin therapeutic drug monitoring on the development of nephrotoxicity (serum creatinine increase of 0.5 mg/dL or more) [51]. This trial did observe that vancomycin therapeutic drug monitoring was independently inversely associated with nephrotoxicity (adjusted OR 0.04; 95% CI 0.01–0.30) in 70 patients with hematologic malignancies. However, the generalizability of this study is somewhat limited given the patient population and routine concomitant administration of amikacin (~80%) and amphotericin B (~30%).

The 2009 version of the vancomycin consensus guidelines recommended using 30–45 mg/kg/day based on total body weight to achieve vancomycin serum trough concentrations of 15–20 mg/L [4]. The authors stated that this approach should extrapolate to an area under the curve (AUC) of ~400 mg·h/L. There were several reports of increased nephrotoxicity associated with the implementation of these guideline recommendations. The vast majority of these reports discussed the increased risk of nephrotoxicity being associated with vancomycin trough concentrations (either 15 or 20 mg/L or greater). A meta-analysis of these studies documented that a vancomycin trough of 15 mg/L or greater was associated with nephrotoxicity (OR 2.67; 95% CI 1.95–3.65) [20]. However, the authors note that nephrotoxicity was reversible in the majority of cases and that short-term dialysis was only required in 3% of nephrotoxic episodes. A case series of nine patients found obstructive tubular casts containing vancomycin in the presence of elevated serum vancomycin concentrations [52]. Eight of the nine patients had serum vancomycin concentrations of at least 35 mg/L. The authors confirmed the clinical observations by administrating vancomycin to four mice. The vancomycin-containing casts also occurred in the mice in the presence of elevated vancomycin concentrations. Vancomycin therapy should be held for at least one dosing interval if the true vancomycin trough is greater than 25 mg/L.

There was more variance in AUC with trough-based monitoring than anticipated by the original guideline authors. Neely et al. evaluated three data sets through modeling and simulation to compare obtained trough values to AUC estimations. The simulation results suggest that an AUC/MIC ≥ 400 mg·h/L can be achieved with a trough <15 mg/L in 60% of patients [53]. A retrospective study by Ghosh et al. reported that 61% of patients achieving an AUC/MIC ≥ 400 mg·h/L had a vancomycin trough <15 mg/L [54]. A prospective trial of 252 patients found that 31% of patients with an AUC/MICs ≥ 400 mg·h/L had a trough concentration <10 mg/L and 68% had a trough concentration <15 mg/L [55]. Therefore, multiple studies have shown that AUC provides a better estimate of vancomycin exposure than a single trough concentration.

A recent meta-analysis of eight observational studies ($n = 2491$) suggested a cutpoint of 650 mg·h/L for the risk of vancomycin-associated nephrotoxicity. Patients with an AUC/MIC < 650 mg·h/L were less likely to develop nephrotoxicity whether the AUC was calculated in the first 24 h period (OR 0.36; 95% CI 0.23–0.56) or second 24 h period (OR 0.45; 95% CI 0.27–0.75) [56]. Using an AUC monitoring strategy was associated with significantly lower rates of nephrotoxicity than trough-guided monitoring

(OR 0.68; 95% CI 0.46–0.99). However, this finding is based on only two studies, with one retrospective study representing 90% of the total sample in the analysis.

The primary issue with all of these analyses is that they all fail to identify if increased vancomycin concentrations are the cause of nephrotoxicity or if they are increased as a result of nephrotoxicity. In addition, the reliance upon retrospective analyses and computer-generated cutpoints brings the stability of the values generated into question. The lack of randomized, controlled trials targeting different trough or AUC values is particularly concerning in that we may be continuously creating risk factors for nephrotoxicity that are never validated prospectively in a randomized trial.

5.2. Fluid Status

The European Society of Intensive Care Medicine issued strong recommendations (lower-level evidence) regarding the use of controlled fluid resuscitation with crystalloids and avoiding fluid overload to prevent the development of nephrotoxicity [57]. To our knowledge, no data exist assessing the association between hypovolemia and nephrotoxicity specifically related to vancomycin therapy. However, we believe continuous reassessment of volume status should take place throughout the course of treatment as part of the patient and drug monitoring process, as the detrimental effects of either hypovolemia or fluid overload have been reviewed elsewhere [58].

5.3. Reassessment of Nephrotoxicity Risk

We are unaware of literature that documents the clinical benefit of re-assessing the patient's risk of nephrotoxicity. However, we feel that this should be a routine part of clinical care, as it makes common sense that assessing for the risk of adverse events should be a continual process.

6. Diagnosis of AKI

More than 35 definitions of acute renal dysfunction have previously been identified in the literature [59]. The most commonly utilized definitions of vancomycin-associated nephrotoxicity are consistent with the Acute Kidney Injury Network (AKIN), Kidney Disease Improving Global Outcomes (KDIGO), and Risk, Injury, Failure, Loss, End stage renal disease (RIFLE) criteria but vary between studies [60–62]. The 2009 version of the vancomycin consensus guidelines defines vancomycin-induced nephrotoxicity based on an increase in serum creatinine of 0.5 mg/dL or a ≥50% increase from baseline [4]. Most of these definitions allow for classification based on serum creatinine or urine output as a surrogate for the diagnosis of kidney injury. The vast majority of studies evaluating vancomycin and nephrotoxicity have focused on serum creatinine changes due to their retrospective nature. Data regarding urine output has typically not been evaluated in these retrospective evaluations due to the lack of information regarding the urine volume and/or the accuracy of the data for timing and volume charted.

Clinicians have used serum creatinine as a diagnostic criterion for AKI for decades. This surrogate measure is plagued by several issues. The accuracy of serum creatinine in estimating renal function in patients with extremes of weight (e.g., anorexics, weight lifters) or decreased muscle mass (e.g., elderly, long-term spinal cord injury patients) may be less accurate, since creatinine is a product of muscle catabolism [63–65]. Additionally, the kinetics of creatinine often result in a delay between kidney injury and the subsequent rise in serum creatinine. This may lead to delays in recognition and diagnosis of nephrotoxicity [66].

Various medications have also been associated with increases in serum creatinine without changes to renal function. Similar to piperacillin-tazobactam, there are several agents including trimethoprim, cimetidine, pyrimethamine, and various antiretroviral agents that have been found to increase serum creatinine through inhibition of creatinine tubular secretion without decreasing glomerular filtration rate [67–71].

More sensitive urinary biomarkers have been evaluated recently as potential replacement(s) to serum creatine, given its issues in estimating glomerular filtration rate and/or diagnosing

AKI. These candidates to serve as next-generation biomarkers include urinary KIM-1, neutrophil gelatinase-associated lipocalin (NGAL), interleukin-18 (IL-18), cystatin C, clusterin, fatty acid binding protein-liver type (L-FABP), and osteopontin [72]. Animal studies have suggested that KIM-1 and/or clusterin monitoring may identify nephrotoxicity in the setting of vancomycin exposure more quickly [73,74]. Continuous monitoring of renal function is also being explored as an alternative to conventional methods. The optimal molecule to facilitate the continuous monitoring has not been identified in the last ten years [75]. Additional research is needed to assess the feasibility and utility of these monitoring methods in clinical practice.

7. Prognosis of AKI

In general, patient outcomes after AKI are poorly described in current literature. The rate of in-hospital death associated with AKI ranges from 15–60% depending upon the patient population studied and the degree of renal impairment reached [76,77]. The presence of any KDIGO stage of AKI has been associated with death up to 10 years (OR 1.30; 95% CI 1.1–1.6) from being admitted to an intensive care unit (ICU) [78]. This effect was not observed when only patients who survived the first 28 days were evaluated (OR 1.26; 95% CI 1.0–1.6).

Nephrotoxicity in the setting of vancomycin therapy appears to be reversible in most cases. Jeffres and colleagues observed that 73% of patients with nephrotoxicity had reductions in serum creatinine levels to near baseline by hospital discharge [6]. A larger study found that 81% of cases of nephrotoxicity resolved [11]. A meta-analysis found that short-term dialysis was only required in 3% (6/192) of all patients who developed nephrotoxicity [20]. None of these patients required long-term dialysis. A retrospective study evaluating the timing of serum creatinine lowering in patients with AKI observed that serum creatinine remained 50% above baseline for a median duration of seven days (interquartile range (IQR0 3, 20 days) [10]. While vancomycin had higher rates of nephrotoxicity (18.2% vs. 8.4%) compared to linezolid in a randomized, controlled trial of patients with MRSA nosocomial pneumonia, its use was not associated with 60-day mortality (26.6% vs. 28.1%) [79].

8. Conclusions

Vancomycin remains a first-line agent for the treatment of MRSA infections despite different generations questioning its nephrotoxic potential. The lack of prospective randomized, controlled trials evaluating various vancomycin dosing strategies and/or combination empiric therapy regimens has left clinicians to depend on data from cohorts (primarily retrospective) to evaluate vancomycin's nephrotoxic potential. These gold standard trials could have a dramatic impact by informing which dosing strategies and vancomycin-based combinations are safest to use, particularly in patients at risk of nephrotoxicity.

Clinicians should not fear using vancomycin in the absence of these data. Patients who develop AKI while receiving vancomycin infrequently require acute renal replacement therapy and even fewer chronic therapy The short-term mortality increase associated with AKI may be an indicator of more acute illness, or it could even be a result of more aggressive/risky interventions being used in these patients. We would advise to evaluate the patient in addition to the serum creatinine instead of basing treatment decisions solely on laboratory values.

We are hopeful that the novel biomarkers for kidney injury will help clear the issues regarding the timing of renal injury and better elucidate the potential causes. Several medications can compete with creatinine via tubular secretion. This competition creates uncertainty regarding whether serum creatinine increases represent damage to the kidneys or not. The most frequent instance is piperacillin-tazobactam being prescribed along with vancomycin to provide empiric gram-negative and anaerobic coverage. Having a more accurate marker of kidney function could potentially help clinicians from unnecessarily avoiding this combination. In addition, some clinicians are choosing alternatives that may result in other safety issues in select patients (e.g., cefepime and neurotoxicity) [80].

Antimicrobial stewardship efforts can be conducted in the meantime to decrease the duration of combination empiric therapy. This approach has additional benefits outside of the AKI prevention.

We recognize that some clinicians may seek to avoid vancomycin in patients with multiple risk factors for nephrotoxicity. This makes common sense even though there are no data to validate this approach. One study that sought to evaluate the random assignment of other anti-MRSA agents versus vancomycin in patients at risk of nephrotoxicity failed to observe a difference between these approaches [81]. However, another study has shown improvements in clinical outcomes by avoiding nephrotoxins [82]. This is why we advocate using a patient-specific approach that evaluates the patient, severity of illness, and concomitant medications in order to make an informed decision that takes the specific patient's baseline (and ongoing) risk into account.

Author Contributions: Conceptualization, methodology, resources, writing—original draft preparation, and writing—review and editing, A.R.S. and R.G.H.

References

1. Hazlewood, K.A.; Brouse, S.D.; Pitcher, W.D.; Hall, R.G. Vancomycin-associated nephrotoxicity: Grave concern or death by character assassination? *Am. J. Med.* **2010**, *123*, 182. [CrossRef]
2. Farber, B.F.; Moellering, R.C., Jr. Retrospective study of the toxicity of preparations of vancomycin from 1974 to 1981. *Antimicrob. Agents Chemother.* **1983**, *23*, 138–141. [CrossRef]
3. Downs, N.J.; Neihart, R.E.; Dolezal, J.M.; Hodges, G.R. Mild nephrotoxicity associated with vancomycin use. *Arch. Intern. Med.* **1989**, *149*, 1777–1781. [CrossRef]
4. Rybak, M.J.; Lomaestro, B.M.; Rotschafer, J.C.; Moellering, R.C.; Craig, W.A.; Billeter, M.; Dalovisio, J.R.; Levine, D.P. Vancomycin therapeutic guidelines: A summary of consensus recommendations from the Infectious Diseases Society of America, the American Society of Health-System Pharmacists, and the Society of Infectious Diseases Pharmacists. *Clin. Infect. Dis.* **2009**, *49*, 325–327. [CrossRef]
5. Baggs, J.; Fridkin, S.K.; Pollack, L.A.; Srinivasan, A.; Jernigan, J.A. Estimating national trends in inpatient antibiotic use among us hospitals from 2006 to 2012. *JAMA Intern. Med.* **2016**, *176*, 1639–1648. [CrossRef]
6. Jeffres, M.N.; Isakow, W.; Doherty, J.A.; Micek, S.T.; Kollef, M.H. A retrospective analysis of possible renal toxicity associated with vancomycin in patients with health care-associated methicillin-resistant Staphylococcus aureus pneumonia. *Clin. Ther.* **2007**, *29*, 1107–1115. [CrossRef]
7. Davies, S.W.; Guidry, C.A.; Petroze, R.T.; Hranjec, T.; Sawyer, R.G. Vancomycin and nephrotoxicity; just another myth? *J. Trauma Acute Care Surg.* **2013**, *75*, 830–835. [CrossRef]
8. Hall, R.G., II; Hazlewood, K.A.; Brouse, S.D.; Giuliano, C.A.; Haase, K.K.; Frei, C.R.; Forcade, N.A.; Bell, T.; Bedimo, R.J.; Alvarez, C.A. Empiric guideline-recommended weight-based vancomycin dosing and nephrotoxicity rates in patients with methicillin-resistant Staphylococcus aureus bacteremia: A retrospective cohort study. *BMC Pharmacol. Toxicol.* **2013**, *14*, 1–6. [CrossRef]
9. Lodise, T.P.; Lomaestro, B.; Graves, L.; Drusano, G.L. Larger vancomycin doses (at least four grams per day) are associated with an increased incidence of nephrotoxicity. *Antimicrob. Agents Chemother.* **2008**, *52*, 1330–1336. [CrossRef]
10. Lodise, T.P.; Patel, N.; Lomaestro, B.M.; Rodvold, K.A.; Drusano, G.L. Relationship between initial vancomycin concentration-time profile and nephrotoxicity among hospitalized patients. *Clin. Infect. Dis.* **2009**, *49*, 507–514. [CrossRef]
11. Pritchard, L.; Baker, C.; Leggett, J.; Sehdev, P.; Brown, A.; Bayley, K.B. Increasing vancomycin serum trough concentrations and incidence of nephrotoxicity. *Am. J. Med.* **2010**, *123*, 1143–1149. [CrossRef] [PubMed]
12. Hall, R.G., II; Yoo, E.; Faust, A.; Smith, T.; Goodman, E.; Mortensen, E.M.; Felder, V.; Alvarez, C.A. Impact of total body weight on acute kidney injury in patients with gram-negative bacteremia. *Expert Rev. Clin. Pharmacol.* **2018**, *11*, 651–654. [CrossRef]
13. Hall, R.G., II; Yoo, E.; Faust, A.; Smith, T.; Goodman, E.; Mortensen, E.M.; Raza, J.; Dehmami, F.; Alvarez, C.A. Impact of piperacillin/tazobactam on nephrotoxicity in patients with Gram-negative bacteraemia. *Int. J. Antimicrob. Agents* **2019**, *53*, 343–346. [CrossRef] [PubMed]

14. Rutter, W.C.; Burgess, D.R.; Talbert, J.C.; Burgess, D.S. Acute kidney injury in patients treated with vancomycin and piperacillin-tazobactam: A retrospective cohort analysis. *J. Hosp. Med.* **2017**, *12*, 77–82. [CrossRef]

15. Minejima, E.; Choi, J.; Beringer, P.; Lou, M.; Tse, E.; Wong-Beringer, A. Applying new diagnostic criteria for acute kidney injury to facilitate early identification of nephrotoxicity in vancomycin-treated patients. *Antimicrob. Agents Chemother.* **2011**, *55*, 3278–3283. [CrossRef]

16. Mullins, B.P.; Kramer, C.J.; Bartel, B.J.; Catlin, J.S.; Gilder, R.E. Comparison of the nephrotoxicity of vancomycin in combination with cefepime, meropenem, or piperacillin/tazobactam: A prospective, multicenter study. *Ann. Pharmacother.* **2018**, *52*, 639–644. [CrossRef] [PubMed]

17. Bosso, J.A.; Nappi, J.; Rudisill, C.; Wellein, M.; Bookstaver, P.B.; Swindler, J.; Mauldin, P.D. Relationship between vancomycin trough concentrations and nephrotoxicity: A prospective multicenter trial. *Antimicrob. Agents Chemother.* **2011**, *55*, 5475–5479. [CrossRef] [PubMed]

18. Horey, A.; Mergenhagen, K.A.; Mattappallil, A. The relationship of nephrotoxicity to vancomycin trough serum concentrations in a veteran's population: A retrospective analysis. *Ann. Pharmacother.* **2012**, *46*, 1477–1483. [CrossRef]

19. Meaney, C.J.; Hynicka, L.M.; Tsoukleris, M.G. Vancomycin-associated nephrotoxicity in adult medicine patients: Incidence, outcomes, and risk factors. *Pharmacotherapy* **2014**, *34*, 653–661. [CrossRef]

20. van Hal, S.J.; Paterson, D.L.; Lodise, T.P. Systematic review and meta-analysis of vancomycin-induced nephrotoxicity associated with dosing schedules that maintain troughs between 15 and 20 milligrams per liter. *Antimicrob. Agents Chemother.* **2013**, *57*, 734–744. [CrossRef] [PubMed]

21. Mingeot-Leclercq, M.P.; Tulkens, P.M. Aminoglycosides: Nephrotoxicity. *Antimicrob. Agents Chemother.* **1999**, *43*, 1003–1012. [CrossRef]

22. Fanos, V.; Cataldi, L. Amphotericin B-induced nephrotoxicity: A review. *J. Chemother.* **2000**, *12*, 463–470. [CrossRef] [PubMed]

23. Hidayat, L.K.; Hsu, D.I.; Quist, R.; Shriner, K.A.; Wong-Beringer, A. High-dose vancomycin therapy for methicillin-resistant Staphylococcus aureus infections: Efficacy and toxicity. *Arch. Intern. Med.* **2006**, *166*, 2138–2144. [CrossRef] [PubMed]

24. Hanrahan, T.P.; Kotapati, C.; Roberts, M.J.; Rowland, J.; Lipman, J.; Roberts, J.A.; Udy, A. Factors associated with vancomycin nephrotoxicity in the critically ill. *Anaesth. Intensive Care* **2015**, *43*, 594–599. [CrossRef]

25. Rutter, W.C.; Cox, J.N.; Martin, C.A.; Burgess, D.R.; Burgess, D.S. Nephrotoxicity during vancomycin therapy in combination with piperacillin-tazobactam or cefepime. *Antimicrob. Agents Chemother.* **2017**, *62*, e02089-16. [CrossRef] [PubMed]

26. Hammond, D.A.; Smith, M.N.; Li, C.; Hayes, S.M.; Lusardi, K.; Bookstaver, P.B. Systematic review and meta-analysis of acute kidney injury associated with concomitant vancomycin and piperacillin/tazobactam. *Clin. Infect. Dis.* **2017**, *64*, 666–674. [CrossRef]

27. Luther, M.K.; Timbrook, T.T.; Caffrey, A.R.; Dosa, D.; Lodise, T.P.; LePlant, K.L. Vancomycin plus piperacillin-tazobactam and acute kidney injury in adults: A systematic review and meta-analysis. *Crit. Care Med.* **2018**, *46*, 12–20. [CrossRef] [PubMed]

28. Carreno, J.; Smiraglia, T.; Hunter, C.; Tobin, E.; Lomaestro, B. Comparative incidence and excess risk of acute kidney injury in hospitalised patients receiving vancomycin and piperacillin/tazobactam in combination or as monotherapy. *Int. J. Antimicrob. Agents* **2018**, *52*, 643–650. [CrossRef]

29. Hammond, D.A.; Smith, M.N.; Painter, J.T.; Meena, N.K.; Lusardi, K. Comparative incidence of acute kidney injury in critically ill patients receiving vancomycin with concomitant piperacillin-tazobactam or cefepime: A retrospective cohort study. *Pharmacotherapy* **2016**, *36*, 463–571. [CrossRef]

30. Buckley, M.S.; Hartsock, N.C.; Berry, A.J.; Bikin, D.S.; Richards, E.C.; Yerondopoulos, M.J.; Kobic, E.; Wicks, L.M.; Hammond, D.A. Comparison of acute kidney injury risk associated with vancomycin and concomitant piperacillin/tazobactam or cefepime in the intensive care unit. *J. Crit. Care* **2018**, *48*, 32–38. [CrossRef]

31. Schreier, D.J.; Kashani, K.B.; Sakhuja, A.; Mara, K.C.; Toottooni, M.S.; Personett, M.S.; Nelson, S.; Rule, A.D.; Steckelberg, J.M.; Tande, A.J.; et al. Incidence of acute kidney injury among critically ill patients with brief empiric use of antipseudomonal β-lactams with vancomycin. *Clin. Infect. Dis.* **2018**. Epub ahead of print. [CrossRef] [PubMed]

32. Rutter, W.C.; Burgess, D.S. Acute kidney injury in patients treated with iv beta-lactam/beta-lactamase inhibitor combinations. *Pharmacotherapy* **2017**, *37*, 593–598. [CrossRef] [PubMed]

33. Choudhury, D.; Ahmed, Z. Drug-associated renal dysfunction and injury. *Nat. Clin. Pract. Nephrol.* **2006**, *2*, 80–91. [CrossRef] [PubMed]

34. Pais, G.M.; Liu, J.; Avedissian, S.N.; Xanthos, T.; Chalkias, A.; d'Aloja, E.; Locci, E.; Gilchrist, A.; Prozialeck, W.C.; Rhodes, N.J.; et al. Urinary Biomarker and Histopathological Evaluation of Vancomycin and Piperacillin Tazobactam Nephrotoxicity in Comparison with Vancomycin in a Rat Model and a Confirmatory Cellular Model. *bioRxiv* **2019**. Epub ahead of print. [CrossRef]

35. Dellit, T.H.; Owens, R.C.; McGowan, J.E., Jr.; Gerding, D.N.; Weinstein, R.A.; Burke, J.P.; Huskins, W.C.; Paterson, D.L.; Fishman, N.O.; Carpenter, C.F.; et al. Infectious Diseases Society of America and the Society for Healthcare Epidemiology of America guidelines for developing an institutional program to enhance antimicrobial stewardship. *Clin. Infect. Dis.* **2007**, *44*, 159–177. [CrossRef]

36. Stevens, D.L.; Bisno, A.L.; Chambers, H.F.; Dellinger, E.P.; Goldstein, E.J.; Gorbach, S.L.; Hirschmann, J.V.; Kaplan, S.L.; Montoya, J.G.; Wade, J.C. Practice guidelines for the diagnosis and management of skin and soft tissue infections: 2014 update by the Infectious Diseases Society of America. *Clin. Infect. Dis.* **2014**, *59*, e10–e52. [CrossRef] [PubMed]

37. Lipsky, B.A.; Berendt, A.R.; Cornia, P.B.; Pile, J.C.; Peters, E.J.; Armstrong, D.G.; Deery, H.G.; Embil, J.M.; Joseph, W.S.; Karchmer, A.W.; et al. 2012 infectious diseases society of america clinical practice guideline for the diagnosis and treatment of diabetic foot infections. *J. Am. Podiatr. Med. Assoc.* **2013**, *103*, 2–7. [CrossRef]

38. Baddour, L.M.; Wilson, W.R.; Bayer, A.S.; Fowler, V.G., Jr.; Tleyjeh, I.M.; Rybak, M.J.; Barsic, B.; Lockhart, P.B.; Gewitz, M.H.; Levison, M.E.; et al. Infective endocarditis in adults: Diagnosis, antimicrobial therapy, and management of complications: A scientific statement for healthcare professionals from the American Heart Association. *Circulation* **2015**, *132*, 1435–1486. [CrossRef] [PubMed]

39. Freifeld, A.G.; Bow, E.J.; Sepkowitz, K.A.; Boeckh, M.J.; Ito, J.I.; Mullen, C.A.; Raad, I.I.; Rolston, K.V.; Young, J.A.; Wingard, J.R. Clinical practice guideline for the use of antimicrobial agents in neutropenic patients with cancer: 2010 update by the Infectious Diseases Society of America. *Clin. Infect. Dis.* **2011**, *52*, 56–93. [CrossRef] [PubMed]

40. Tunkel, A.R.; Hartman, B.J.; Kaplan, S.L.; Kaufman, B.A.; Roos, K.L.; Scheld, W.M.; Whitley, R.J. Practice guidelines for the management of bacterial meningitis. *Clin. Infect. Dis.* **2004**, *39*, 1267–1284. [CrossRef]

41. Mandell, L.A.; Wunderink, R.G.; Anzueto, A.; Bartlett, J.G.; Campbell, G.D.; Dean, N.C.; Dowell, S.F.; File, T.M., Jr.; Musher, D.M.; Niederman, M.S.; et al. Infectious Diseases Society of America/American Thoracic Society consensus guidelines on the management of community-acquired pneumonia in adults. *Clin. Infect. Dis.* **2007**, *44* (Suppl. 2), 27–72. [CrossRef] [PubMed]

42. Kalil, A.C.; Metersky, M.L.; Klompas, M.; Muscedere, J.; Sweeney, D.A.; Palmer, L.B.; Napolitano, L.M.; O'Grady, N.P.; Bartlett, J.G.; Carratalà, J.; et al. Management of adults with hospital-acquired and ventilator-associated pneumonia: 2016 Clinical practice guidelines by the Infectious Diseases Society of America and the American Thoracic Society. *Clin. Infect. Dis.* **2016**, *63*, 61–111. [CrossRef] [PubMed]

43. Bratzler, D.W.; Dellinger, E.P.; Olsen, K.M.; Perl, T.M.; Auwaerter, P.G.; Bolon, M.K.; Fish, D.N.; Napolitano, L.M.; Sawyer, R.G.; Slain, D.; et al. Clinical practice guidelines for antimicrobial prophylaxis in surgery. *Surg. Infect. (Larchmt)* **2013**, *14*, 73–156. [CrossRef] [PubMed]

44. Iversen, K.; Ihlemann, N.; Gill, S.U.; Madsen, T.; Elming, H.; Jensen, K.T.; Bruun, N.E.; Høfsten, D.E.; Fursted, K.; Christensen, J.J.; et al. Partial oral versus intravenous antibiotic treatment of endocarditis. *N. Engl. J. Med.* **2019**, *380*, 415–424. [CrossRef] [PubMed]

45. Li, H.K.; Rombach, I.; Zambellas, R.; Walker, A.S.; McNally, M.A.; Atkins, B.L.; Lipsky, B.A.; Hughes, H.C.; Bose, D.; Kümin, M.; et al. Oral versus intravenous antibiotics for bone and joint infection. *N. Engl. J. Med.* **2019**, *380*, 425–436. [CrossRef] [PubMed]

46. Cowley, M.C.; Ritchie, D.J.; Hampton, N.; Kollef, M.H.; Micek, S.T. Outcomes associated with de-escalating therapy for methicillin-resistant Staphylococcus aureus in culture-negative nosocomial pneumonia. *Chest* **2019**, *155*, 53–59. [CrossRef]

47. Dangerfield, B.; Chung, A.; Webb, B.; Seville, M.T. Predictive value of methicillin-resistant Staphylococcus aureus (MRSA) nasal swab PCR assay for MRSA pneumonia. *Antimicrob. Agents Chemother.* **2014**, *58*, 859–864. [CrossRef]

48. Parente, D.M.; Cunha, C.B.; Mylonakis, E.; Timbrook, T.T. The clinical utility of methicillin-resistant Staphylococcus aureus (MRSA) nasal screening to rule out MRSA pneumonia: A diagnostic meta-analysis with antimicrobial stewardship implications. *Clin. Infect. Dis.* **2018**, *67*, 1–7. [CrossRef] [PubMed]

49. Baby, N.; Faust, A.C.; Smith, T.; Sheperd, L.A.; Knoll, L.; Goodman, E.L. Nasal methicillin-resistant Staphylococcus aureus (MRSA) PCR testing reduces the duration of MRSA-targeted therapy in patients with suspected MRSA pneumonia. *Antimicrob. Agents Chemother.* **2017**, *61*, e02432-16. [CrossRef]

50. Barlam, T.F.; Cosgrove, S.E.; Abbo, L.M.; MacDougall, C.; Schuetz, A.N.; Septimus, E.J.; Srinivasan, A.; Dellit, T.H.; Falck-Ytter, Y.T.; Fishman, N.O.; et al. Implementing an antibiotic stewardship program: Guidelines by the Infectious Diseases Society of America and the Society for Healthcare Epidemiology of America. *Clin. Infect. Dis.* **2016**, *62*, 51–77. [CrossRef]

51. Fernández de Gatta, M.D.; Calvo, M.V.; Hernández, J.M.; Caballero, D.; San Miguel, J.F.; Domínguez-Gil, A. Cost-effectiveness analysis of serum vancomycin concentration monitoring in patients with hematologic malignancies. *Clin. Pharmacol. Ther.* **1996**, *60*, 332–340. [PubMed]

52. Luque, Y.; Louis, K.; Jouanneau, C.; Placier, S.; Esteve, E.; Bazin, D.; Rondeau, E.; Letavernier, E.; Wolfromm, A.; Gosset, C.; et al. Vancomycin-Associated Cast Nephropathy. *J. Am. Soc. Nephrol.* **2017**, *28*, 1723–1728. [CrossRef]

53. Neely, M.N.; Youn, G.; Jones, B.; Jelliffe, R.W.; Drusano, G.L.; Rodvold, K.A.; Lodise, T.P. Are vancomycin trough concentrations adequate for optimal dosing? *Antimicrob. Agents. Chemother.* **2014**, *58*, 309–316. [CrossRef]

54. Ghosh, N.; Chavada, R.; Maley, M.; van Hal, S.J. Impact of source of infection and vancomycin AUC_{0-24}/MIC_{BMD} targets on treatment failure in patients with methicillin-resistant Staphylococcus aureus bacteraemia. *Clin. Microbiol. Infect.* **2014**, *20*, 1098–1105. [CrossRef] [PubMed]

55. Neely, M.N.; Kato, L.; Youn, G.; Kraler, L.; Bayard, D.; van Guilder, M.; Schumitzky, A.; Yamada, W.; Jones, B.; Minejima, E. Prospective trial on the use of trough concentration versus area under the curve to determine therapeutic vancomycin dosing. *Antimicrob. Agents Chemother.* **2018**, *62*, e02042-17. [CrossRef] [PubMed]

56. Aljefri, D.M.; Avedissian, S.N.; Rhodes, N.J.; Postelnick, M.J.; Nguyen, K.; Scheetz, M.H. Vancomycin Area under the Curve and Acute Kidney Injury: A Meta-analysis. *Clin. Infect. Dis.* **2019**. Epub ahead of print. [CrossRef] [PubMed]

57. Joannidis, M.; Druml, W.; Forni, L.G.; Groeneveld, A.B.J.; Honore, P.M.; Hoste, E.; Ostermann, M.; Oudemans-van Straaten, H.M.; Schetz, M. Prevention of acute kidney injury and protection of renal function in the intensive care unit: Update 2017: Expert opinion of the Working Group on Prevention, AKI section, European Society of Intensive Care Medicine. *Intensive Care Med.* **2017**, *43*, 730–749. [CrossRef]

58. Ostermann, M.; Straaten, H.M.; Forni, L.G. Fluid overload and acute kidney injury: Cause or consequence? *Crit. Care* **2015**, *19*, 443. [CrossRef]

59. Kellum, J.A.; Levin, N.; Bouman, C.; Lameire, N. Developing a consensus classification system for acute renal failure. *Curr. Opin. Crit. Care* **2002**, *8*, 509–514. [CrossRef]

60. Bellomo, R.; Ronco, C.; Kellum, J.A.; Mehta, R.L.; Palevsky, P.; Acute Dialysis Quality Initiative workgroup. Acute renal failure—Definition, outcome measures, animal models, fluid therapy and information technology needs: The Second International Consensus Conference of the Acute Dialysis Quality Initiative (ADQI) Group. *Crit. Care* **2004**, *8*, 204–212. [CrossRef]

61. Mehta, R.L.; Kellum, J.A.; Shah, S.V.; Molitoris, B.A.; Ronco, C.; Warnock, D.G.; Levin, A. Acute Kidney Injury Network. cute Kidney Injury Network: Report of an initiative to improve outcomes in acute kidney injury. *Crit. Care* **2007**, *11*, R31. [CrossRef]

62. Kidney Disease: Improving Global Outcomes (KDIGO); Acute Kidney Injury Work Group. KDIGO clinical practice guidelines for acute kidney injury. *Kidney Int. Suppl.* **2012**, *2*. [CrossRef]

63. Perrone, R.D.; Madias, N.E.; Levey, A.S. Serum creatinine as an index of renal function: New insights into old concepts. *Clin. Chem.* **1992**, *38*, 1933–1953.

64. Spencer, K. Analytical reviews in clinical biochemistry: The estimation of creatinine. *Ann. Clin. Biochem.* **1986**, *23*, 1–25. [CrossRef]

65. Heymsfield, S.B.; Arteaga, C.; McManus, C.; Smith, J.; Moffitt, S. Measurement of muscle mass in humans: Validity of the 24-hour urinary creatinine method. *Am. J. Clin. Nutr.* **1983**, *37*, 478–494. [CrossRef] [PubMed]

66. Waikar, S.S.; Bonventre, J.V. Creatinine kinetics and the definition of acute kidney injury. *Am. Soc. Nephrol.* **2009**, *20*, 672–679. [CrossRef]

67. Delanaye, P.; Mariat, C.; Cavalier, E.; Maillard, N.; Krzesinski, J.M.; White, C.A. Trimethoprim, creatinine and creatinine-based equations. *Nephron Clin. Pract.* **2011**, *119*, 187–194. [CrossRef]

68. van Acker, B.A.; Koomen, G.C.; Koopman, M.G.; de Waart, D.R.; Arisz, L. Creatinine clearance during cimetidine administration for measurement of glomerular filtration rate. *Lancet* **1992**, *340*, 1326–1329. [CrossRef]

69. Opravil, M.; Keusch, G.; Luthy, R. Pyrimethamine inhibits renal secretion of creatinine. *Antimicrob. Agents Chemother.* **1993**, *37*, 1056–1060. [CrossRef]

70. German, P.; Liu, H.C.; Szwarcberg, J.; Hepner, M.; Andrews, J.; Kearney, B.P.; Mathias, A. Effect of cobicistat on glomerular filtration rate in subjects with normal and impaired renal function. *J. Acquir. Immune Defic. Syndr.* **2012**, *61*, 32–40. [CrossRef]

71. Maggi, P.; Montinaro, V.; Mussini, C.; Di Biagio, A.; Bellagamba, R.; Bonfanti, P.; Calza, L.; Cherubini, C.; Corsi, P.; Gargiulo, M.; et al. Novel antiretroviral drugs and renal function monitoring of HIV patients. *AIDS Rev.* **2014**, *16*, 144–151.

72. Bonventre, J.V.; Vaidya, V.S.; Schmouder, R.; Feig, P.; Dieterie, F. Next-generation biomarkers for detecting kidney toxicity. *Nat. Biotechnol.* **2010**, *28*, 436–440. [CrossRef]

73. O'Donnell, J.N.; Rhodes, N.J.; Lodise, T.P.; Prozialeck, W.C.; Miglis, C.M.; Joshi, M.D.; Venkatesan, N.; Pais, G.; Cluff, C.; Lamar, P.C.; et al. 24-Hour pharmacokinetic relationships for vancomycin and novel urinary biomarkers of acute kidney injury. *Antimicrob. Agents Chemother.* **2017**, *61*, e00416-17. [CrossRef]

74. Pais, G.M.; Avedissian, S.N.; O'Donnell, J.N.; Rhodes, N.J.; Lodise, T.P.; Prozialeck, W.C.; Lamar, P.C.; Cluff, C.; Gulati, A.; Fitzgerald, J.C.; et al. Comparative performance of urinary biomarkers for vancomycin induced kidney injury according to timeline of injury. *Antimicrob. Agents Chemother.* **2019**. Epub ahead of print. [CrossRef] [PubMed]

75. Dorshow, R.B.; Asmelash, B.; Chinen, L.K.; Debreczeny, M.P.; Fitch, R.M.; Freskos, J.K.; Galen, K.P.; Gaston, K.R.; Marzan, T.A.; Poreddy, A.R.; et al. *New Optical Probes for the Continuous Monitoring of Renal Function*; Proceedings of SPIE; SPIE: Bellingham, WA, USA, 2008; Volume 6867, pp. 1–11.

76. Uchino, S.; Kellum, J.A.; Bellomo, R.; Doig, G.S.; Morimatsu, H.; Morgera, S.; Schetz, M.; Tan, I.; Bouman, C.; Macedo, E.; et al. Acute renal failure in critically ill patients: A multinational, multicenter study. *JAMA* **2005**, *294*, 813–818. [CrossRef]

77. Xue, J.L.; Daniels, F.; Star, R.A.; Kimmel, P.L.; Eggers, P.W.; Molitoris, B.A.; Himmelfarb., J.; Collins, A.J. Incidence and mortality of acute renal failure in Medicare beneficiaries, 1992 to 2001. *J. Am. Soc. Nephrol.* **2006**, *17*, 1135–1142. [CrossRef] [PubMed]

78. Linder, A.; Fjell, C.; Levin, A.; Walley, K.R.; Russell, J.A.; Boyd, J.H. Small acute increases in serum creatinine are associated with decreased long-term survival in the critically ill. *Am. J. Respir. Crit. Care Med.* **2014**, *189*, 1075–1081. [CrossRef]

79. Chavanet, P. The ZEPHyR study: A randomized comparison of linezolid and vancomycin for MRSA pneumonia. *Med. Mal. Infect.* **2013**, *43*, 451–455. [CrossRef]

80. Payne, L.E.; Gagnon, D.J.; Riker, R.R.; Seder, D.B.; Glisic, E.K.; Morris, J.G.; Fraser, G.L. Cefepime-induced neurotoxicity: A systematic review. *Crit. Care* **2017**, *21*, 276. [CrossRef]

81. Carreno, J.J.; Kenney, R.M.; Divine, G.; Vazquez, J.A.; Davis, S. Randomized controlled trial to determine the efficacy of early switch from vancomycin to vancomycin alternatives as a strategy to prevent nephrotoxicity in patients with multiple risk factors for adverse renal outcomes (STOP-NT). *Ann. Pharmacother.* **2017**, *51*, 185–193. [CrossRef]

82. Meersch, M.; Schmidt, C.; Hoffmeier, A.; Van Aken, H.; Wempe, C.; Gerss, J.; Zarbock, A. Prevention of cardiac surgery-associated AKI by implementing the KDIGO guidelines in high risk patients identified by biomarkers: The PrevAKI randomized controlled trial. *Intensive Care Med.* **2017**, *43*, 1551–1561. [CrossRef] [PubMed]

12

A New Vision of IgA Nephropathy: The Missing Link

Fabio Sallustio [1,2,*], **Claudia Curci** [2,3,*], **Vincenzo Di Leo** [3], **Anna Gallone** [2], **Francesco Pesce** [3] and **Loreto Gesualdo** [3]

[1] Interdisciplinary Department of Medicine (DIM), University of Bari "Aldo Moro", 70124 Bari, Italy
[2] Department of Basic Medical Sciences, Neuroscience and Sense Organs, University of Bari "Aldo Moro", 70124 Bari, Italy; anna.gallone@uniba.it
[3] Nephrology, Dialysis and Transplantation Unit, DETO, University "Aldo Moro", 70124 Bari, Italy; vincenzodileo88@yahoo.it (V.D.L.); f.pesce81@gmail.com (F.P.); loreto.gesualdo@uniba.it (L.G.)
[*] Correspondence: fabio.sallustio@uniba.it (F.S.); claudiacurci@gmail.com (C.C.)

Abstract: IgA Nephropathy (IgAN) is a primary glomerulonephritis problem worldwide that develops mainly in the 2nd and 3rd decade of life and reaches end-stage kidney disease after 20 years from the biopsy-proven diagnosis, implying a great socio-economic burden. IgAN may occur in a sporadic or familial form. Studies on familial IgAN have shown that 66% of asymptomatic relatives carry immunological defects such as high IgA serum levels, abnormal spontaneous in vitro production of IgA from peripheral blood mononuclear cells (PBMCs), high serum levels of aberrantly glycosylated IgA1, and an altered PBMC cytokine production profile. Recent findings led us to focus our attention on a new perspective to study the pathogenesis of this disease, and new studies showed the involvement of factors driven by environment, lifestyle or diet that could affect the disease. In this review, we describe the results of studies carried out in IgAN patients derived from genomic and epigenomic studies. Moreover, we discuss the role of the microbiome in the disease. Finally, we suggest a new vision to consider IgA Nephropathy as a disease that is not disconnected from the environment in which we live but influenced, in addition to the genetic background, also by other environmental and behavioral factors that could be useful for developing precision nephrology and personalized therapy.

Keywords: IgA Nephropathy; microbiome; virome; environment

1. Introduction

IgA-Nephropathy (IgA-N) is the most common form of primary glomerulonephritis worldwide. It is characterized by the manifestation of mesangial IgA deposits in the glomeruli leading to frequent episodes of intra-infectious macroscopic hematuria or continuous microscopic hematuria and/or proteinuria. The aberrant synthesis of deglycosylated IgA1, selective mesangial IgA1 deposition with ensuing mesangial cell proliferation and extracellular matrix expansion lead to renal fibrosis, with molecular mechanisms still poorly understood. Approximately 40% of patients older than 20 years develop end-stage renal disease within 20 years after the renal biopsy-proven diagnosis [1,2]. The prevalence of IgA-N ranges widely worldwide, from 16.7% in the USA to 48.7% in Australia of all patients with biopsy-proven primary glomerulonephritis as reported in regional biopsy registries. The frequency of the disease increases from the Western (USA 16.7%) to the Eastern regions of the world (Japan 47.4%) [2,3]. IgAN is the most common glomerulonephritis in Asia, where it accounts for 40% of glomerulonephritis; it is also very common among the native Americans in Manitoba, the Zuni and the Australian aborigines; it is rare in African native populations and in the Indian [2–7]. The family aggregation has been widely described in the world, in sibling pairs, in families and in extensive pedigrees belonging to geographically-isolated populations [8–10]. The difference in percentages in all countries may be only partially attributed to late referral to nephrologists, routine screening of urine in some countries, and disparities in the indication to perform a kidney biopsy in individuals with permanent urinary abnormalities.

Several studies describe immunological abnormalities involving B and T lymphocytes throughout the clinical course of the disease [11]. Naive B cells express surface IgM/IgD and have to go through a process of clonal expansion, isotype switching, affinity maturation, and differentiation before IgA plasma cells develop. During the process of class switching, recombination occurs by looping out and deletions of segments of DNA. In IgA-N patients, B cells not only seem to be increased in number in both bone marrow and tonsils [12–14], but also show reduced susceptibility to Fas-mediated apoptosis with a marked expression of BCL-2 [12]. In addition, B cells produce polymeric IgA1 abnormally glycosylated in response to a variety of antigens that initiate the formation of IgA immune complexes [15,16].

The regulation of IgA production by B cells is regulated in both a T cell-dependent and a T cell-independent manner, through molecular signals involving the TNF-Receptor superfamily, which is expressed on the surface of dendritic cells. In both cases, dendritic cells are thought to play a critical role in this process. A functional defect of these cells has been observed in the nasal mucosa of IgA-N patients, thus inducing dysregulation of the immune response [16].

Mucosal immunity is largely involved in the pathogenesis of the disease, as the exposure of the upper respiratory tract to bacteria or virus is often associated with recurrent episodes of macroscopic hematuria. There is increasing support for the hypothesis of altered cell homing in IgAN patients, in which there is a displacement of mucosal derived plasma cells and a secretion of mucosal-type antibodies in the systemic compartment [17,18]. In particular, $CD4^+$ T cells represent a key component of the mucosal immune defense against pathogens, altered homing from mucosal to systemic sites, and excessive activation of this leukocyte subset has been demonstrated by Batra et al. [19].

Numerous observations point towards an important role for alterations in IgA biology in the pathogenesis of the disease. Deposited IgA is predominantly polymeric IgA (pIgA) of the IgA1 subclass [20] and has been shown to be differently glycosylated [21], since there is a reduced galactosylation of the O-linked glycans in the hinge region of serum IgA1 and in IgA1 located in the mesangial deposits. Levels of plasma IgA1 are elevated in about half of the IgA-N patients [21]. This is the result of a higher production of deglycosylated IgA1 by plasma cells in the bone marrow and by tonsillar lymphocytes [22,23]. IgA1 glycosylation takes place in the Golgi apparatus of the B cells. These IgA1 proteins with altered glycans represent an autologous antigen recognized by ubiquitous, naturally occurring antibodies, mostly of the IgG isotype with anti-glycan or anti-glycopeptide specificities [24]. Thus, the presence of glycan-specific anti-IgA1 antibodies promotes the formation of circulating immune-complexes which are relatively large [25]. Because of their size, they are not efficiently cleared from the circulation, and thus tend to deposit in the renal mesangium. Deposited immune-complexes and/or polymeric IgA1 aggregated for their de-glycosylation stimulate mesangial cell proliferation and production of cytokines (IL-6 or TGFβ) [26]. Continuous deposition of circulating IgA1-IgG immune complexes induces activation of mesangial cells and of the innate immune system with the attraction of macrophages that produce inflammatory mediators leading to renal damage. Interstitial infiltration by T cells at the renal level causes tubular injury and sets in motion irreversible interstitial fibrosis leading to end-stage renal failure. Hence, a dynamic constellation of B and T lymphocytes and their soluble mediators participate at all levels in disease pathogenesis: Initiation, perpetuation, amplification, regulation, disease relapse, and tissue and organ destruction.

2. Genetics Involvement in IgAN

IgA-N may occur in a sporadic or a familial form according to the clinical evidence that one or more subjects belonging to the same family are affected by biopsy-proven IgA-N. The routine urinalysis carried out in first-degree relatives frequently evidences the occurrence of urinary abnormalities. Such abnormalities have been detected in 25% of first-degree relatives of IgA-N patients as compared to 4% of unrelated subjects [27]. Moreover, first-degree relatives have a higher risk of developing the disease, with an odds ratio (OR) of 16.4 (95% CI 5.7–47.8), than second-degree relatives (OR = 2.4; 95% CI 0.7–7.9) [10]. Three loci linked for familial IgA-N have been found by our group [8,9] (7,8), and some genetic variants which may predispose individuals to sporadic IgA-N have been identified [28]. The IGAN 1 locus is located on chromosome 6q22-23, with a LOD score of 5.6 [9]. IGAN 2 and 3 loci are located on chromosome 4q26-31 and 17q12-22, respectively [8]. These chromosomal traits may contain causative and/or susceptibility genes for familial IgAN which may be involved in the development of, or susceptibility to, overt IgA-N.

Advancements in the field of knowledge on the genetics of IgAN have recently been achieved by the application of genome-wide association studies (GWAS) on large cohorts of IgAN cases and controls. GWAS is an approach aimed at providing comprehensive coverage of the entire genome in order to find variants associated with susceptibility to developing the disease. The major limitation of GWAS is that they only identify common variants of susceptibility, and these obviously have only a modest effect. However, a well-conducted GWAS can offer additional bias-free knowledge on the biology of a human disease that could be clinically relevant, allowing for the identification of new unknown pathways and of potential targets of innovative drug therapies. What is needed for an informative GWAS is the collection of very large numbers of sporadic patients affected by IgAN and healthy controls, comparable in age, sex and geographical origin. The recent GWAS have allowed the discovery of common susceptibility variants to IgAN development. To date, several GWAS related to IgAN have been published and, overall, have led to the identification of 15 disability susceptibilities due to illness.

Regarding classical genetics, several hypotheses have been made on the type of inheritance in the course of family IgAN. The autosomal recessive transmission would seem to be the most unlikely. Many families have affected members in different generations of the pedigree; moreover, a high incidence of the disease in children of consanguineous parents has not been found. An X-linked transmission was considered, given that IgAN is more frequent in males; however, this hypothesis can be excluded as the male-male transmission has also been observed. An autosomal dominant transmission with complete penetrance has been excluded because, in the pedigrees there are numerous examples of subjects that should be obligated carriers but that are healthy. Autosomal dominant transmission with incomplete penetrance would seem to be the most plausible hypothesis as it would be a suitable model to explain most pedigrees. This model would explain the presence of cases in many arms of the pedigree and the recurrence of the disease in subsequent generations. Incomplete penetrance may justify the presence of another genetic factor or environmental exposure. The other model that would explain this type of family aggregation is the hypothesis of a multifactorial etiology in which the combined effect of more genes and/or environmental factors is necessary for the development of the disease in each individual [29].

The three major GWAS on IgAN, performed between 2010 and 2012, had shown a strong contribution of the MHC locus in determining the risk of developing the disease; in addition to this locus, the studies had identified 4 additional non-HLA susceptibility loci (chromosome 1q32, containing the CFH cluster; chromosomal 8p23, comprising the DEFA gene cluster, coding α-defensin; chromosome 17p13, including TNFSF13; chromosome 22, including HORMAD2) [8,9,30]. Cumulatively, these 9 loci are responsible for around 5% of the risk of developing IgAN. In addition, the variation in the frequency of risk alleles is able to explain a substantial proportion of the variation observed in the various ethnic groups with regard to the prevalence of the disease, with the risk alleles showing a higher frequency in Asians compared to Europeans.

The 3 loci in the MHC region (with the strongest signal at the HLA DQB1/DQA1/DRB1 locus) suggested pathways involved in antigen processing and presentation [31]; a locus on chromosome 1q32 containing the Complement Factor H (CFH) gene cluster, suggested a metabolic pathway involved in regulating the activation of the complement pathway. However, the locus on chromosome 22 (HORMAD2) is active in the regulation of mucosal immunity, through the regulation of IgA levels. Moreover, the two regions on chromosome 17p13 and 8q23, containing respectively the TNFSF13 genes (Tumor Necrosis Factor ligand superfamily member 13, encoding a protein which plays an important role in the development of B cells) and DEFA (coding a protein, defensin, which has natural antimicrobial properties, having a role in innate immunity) were also involved in the regulation of mucosal immunity [31,32]. TNFSF13 codifies for APRIL, a potent B-cell stimulating cytokine that is stimulated by intestinal bacteria and leads to CD40-independent IgA class switching [33]. APRIL concentrations are high in patients with IgAN [34] and may upregulate intestinal IgA production [32] (Table 1).

Table 1. Evidence of Potential Relationship with Environmental and Alimentary Hit in IgAN.

References	Loci	Chormosomes	Year	Notes on Potential Relationship with Environmental and Alimentary Hit
Sallustio [35]	TRIM27 DUSP3 VTRNA2-1	6p22 17q21.31 5q31.1	2016	TRIM27 and DUSP3 and the hyper-methylation of VTRNA2-1 lead to the overexpression of TGFβ and to a reduced TCR signal strength of the CD4$^+$ T-cells, with a consequent T helper cell imbalance
AI [36]	DEFA	8p23	2016	The DEFA locus may probably regulate intestinal microbial pathogens and inflammation.
Sallustio [37]	GALNT13 COL11A2 TLR9	2q24 6p21 3p21	2015	The TLR9 loss in IgAN may result in impaired elimination of mucosal antigens, prolonged antigen exposure to B cells and an increase in immunologic memory leading to deal with a continuous antigenic challenge that triggers the production of nephritogenic IgA1
Kiryluk [38]	VAV3 HLA-DR HLA-DQ DEFA CARD9 ITGAM-ITGAX	1p13 6p21 8p23 9q34 16p11	2014	MHC class II molecules are critical for antigen presentation and adaptive immunity. MHC class II molecules participate in the regulation of intestinal inflammation and IgA production. VAV3 may modulate the intestinal inflammation, IgA secretion, the glomerular inflammation, the phagocytosis, and the clearance of immune complexes. CARD9 may intervene in the regulation of bacterial infection after intestinal epithelial injury. Integrins codified by ITGAM and ITGAX are expressed in intestinal dendritic cells and bring to T-cell independent IgA class-switch.
Kiryluk [39]	HLA-DR– HLA-DQ	6p21	2012	There are four independent classical HLA alleles associated with IgAN at this locus; two risk alleles (DQA1*0101, DQB1*0301) and two protective alleles (DQA1*0102, DQB1*0201). Some class II alleles have a permissive role in autoimmunity, and thus may be associated with a greater risk of antiglycan response
Yu [32]	DEFA TNFSF13	8p23 17p13	2012	TNFSF13 codify for APRIL, a potent B-cell stimulating cytokine which is stimulated by intestinal bacteria and lead to CD40-independent IgA class switching
Gharavi [31]	HLA-DR– HLA-DQ HLA-DPA1-DPB1-DPB2 TAP1-PSMB9 CFHR3-CFHR1 del HORMAD2	6p21 6p21 6p21 1p32 22q12	2011	HLA-DP are MHC class II molecules, less well studied compared with HLA-DQ and HLA-DR. Some class II alleles have a permissive role in autoimmunity, and thus may be associated with a greater risk of antiglycan response. Elevated expression of TAP2, PSMB8, and PSMB9, may lead to a proinflammatory intestinal state. HORMAD2 regulates mucosal immunity, through the control of IgA levels.
Feehally [40]	HLA-DR– HLA-DQ	6p21	2010	

These data, however, suggested the possible existence of additional loci of susceptibility to developing the disease. For this reason, new GWAS larger than the previous ones were performed [38]. In addition to replicating the 9 loci described in the previous GWAS, including the loci on chromosome 6p21 (HLA-DQ–HLA-DR, TAP1-PSMB8 and HLA-DP), on chromosome 1q32 (CFHR3-CFHR1), on chromosome 8p23 (DEFA), on chromosome 17p13 (TNFSF13) and on chromosome 22q12 (HORMAD2), new signals were identified, 4 of which in three new loci [38]: Integrin alpha M- Integrin alpha X (ITGAM-ITGAX) on the 16p11 chromosome, implicated in the adhesion and migration of leukocytes and in phagocytosis complement-mediated by monocytes and macrophages and associated with the development of erythematous systemic lupus; CARD9, on chromosome 9q34, implicated in the activation of nuclear factor NF-κB in macrophages, which gives an increased risk of ulcerative colitis and Crohn's disease; and VAV3, on chromosome 1p13, implicated in the development of B and T lymphocytes and in the antigen presentation process. PSMB8 and PSMB9 constitute interferon-inducible immunoproteasome mediating intestinal NF-κB activation in inflammatory bowel diseases (IBD) [41,42]. The TAP gene encodes a protein involved in the transport of antigens from the cytoplasm to the endoplasmic reticulum for association with MHC class I molecules. Elevated expression of TAP2, PSMB8, and PSMB9 may lead to a proinflammatory intestinal state [42]. Moreover, two new independent signals (HLA-DQB1 and DEFA, respectively) were identified in previously known regions (Table 1).

Some case-control association studies identified the C1GALT1 as an important gene for the pathogenesis of IgAN and highlighted some C1GALT1 genetic variants associated with the IgAN pathogenesis in the Italian and Chinese populations [43,44]. C1GALT1 codifies for the enzyme core 1,b1,3-galactosyltransferase 1 that adds a galactose to the IgA1 heavy-chain hinge region. In IgAN, IgA1are aberrantly glycosylated, since the hinge-region O-linked glycans of the IgA1 heavy-chain lack galactose. This contributes to the kidney mesangial deposition of IgA1.

In particular, these studies associated the disease to a C1GALT1 SNP (rs1047763) in the gene promoter region. This variant was also correlated with a decreased C1GALT1 expression in homozygous people [43]. Interestingly, the SNP is contained within the gene region binding the microRNA miR-148b that was found regulating the *C1GALT1* expression and the IgA1 O-glycosylation [45–47]. We do not know whether this SNP effectively influences the disease pathogenesis, but probably it can affect the miR-148b binding to C1GALT1.

Overall, the identified loci seem to be implicated in critical mechanisms for the development of IgAN: The maintenance of the intestinal mucosal barrier, the synthesis of IgA at the mucosal level, the modulation of the signal by NF-kB, the defense against intracellular pathogens and complement activation. The innovative finding is that most of these loci are directly associated with the risk of developing inflammatory bowel disease (HLA-DQ, HLA-DR, CARD9, and HORMAD2), or maintenance of intestinal epithelial barrier integrity and response to various pathogenic pathogens (DEFA, TNFSF13, VAV3, ITGAM-ITGAX, and PSMB8) (Table 1). In fact, abnormal glycosylation mainly consists of polymeric IgA1, which is generated by mucosal IgA1-secreting cells. Also, 107 Immunocompetent B cells can migrate to the gut mucosal lamina propria, where they mature into IgA-secreting plasma cells. These plasma cells can release dimeric IgA1, which can form dimeric IgA or polymeric IgA proteins. The risen levels of polymeric IgA1 in the circulation may be the result of 'spillover' from mucosal sites to the vascular space. Instead, the preponderance of the IgA that achieves the circulation from the bone marrow is predominantly in a monomeric form [48,49].

VAV proteins are guanine nucleotide exchange proteins crucial for adaptive immune function and NF-κB triggering in B cells, stimulating IgA production [50]. They are necessary for appropriate differentiation of colonic enterocytes and avoiding natural ulcerations of intestinal mucosa [50]. Moreover, VAV3 may modulate the intestinal inflammation, IgA secretion, the glomerular inflammation, the phagocytosis, and the clearance of immune complexes. DEFA genes codify for α-defensins that are antimicrobial peptides keeping innate immunity against microbial pathogens. α-defensin 1 and 3 are synthesized in neutrophils, whereas α-defensin 5 and 6 (DEFA5 and DEFA6) are synthesized by the intestinal Paneth cells. Whether DEFA IgAN risk alleles constitute a risk haplotype per se or are associated with close variants of DEFA5 or DEFA6 genes is not clear. Anyway, the DEFA locus may probably regulate intestinal microbial pathogens and inflammation. CARD9 codifies for a protein necessary for the assemblage of a BCL10 signaling complex. It triggers NF-κB, which is involved in both innate and adaptive immunity [51]. CARD9 intervenes in intestinal repair, T-helper 17 responses, and regulation of bacterial infection after intestinal epithelial injury in mice [52].

ITGAM and ITGAX codify for integrins αM and αX that, together with the integrin β2 chain, constitute leukocyte-specific complement receptors 3 and 4 (CR3 and CR4, respectively). High quantity of these integrins, expressed in intestinal dendritic cells bringing to T-cell independent IgA class-switch [53,54]. In addition, ITGAM and ITGAX are also present in macrophages and contribute to the phagocytosis process (Table 1).

Indications on the involvement of genes correlated with environmental factors or eating habits have also come from studies on copy number variations (CNV) in IgAN patients. Ai Z. et al. identified CNV of DEFA locus, including DEFA1A3, DEFA3 [36], and Sallustio et al. identified GALNT13, COL11A2, and TLR9 loci that are associated with susceptibility to and progression of IgAN [37] (Table 1). In particular, a TLR9 loss has been found associated with IgAN progression and renal dysfunction. TLR9 is expressed in immune system cells such as B cells, dendritic cells, macrophages, natural killer cells, and other antigen-presenting cells [55]. TLR9 preferentially binds unmethylated CpG dinucleotides (CpG DNA) released by bacteria and viruses and triggers signaling cascades that lead to a pro-inflammatory cytokine response [56,57]. In IgAN, the TLR9 CNV loss may lead to the failure of CpG to induce the proliferation of memory B cells because of the lower expression levels of TLR9, thus exacerbating IgA class switching in naive B cells via BCR. This may result in impaired elimination of mucosal antigens, prolonged antigen exposure to B cells, and an increase in immunologic memory leading to deal with a continuous antigenic challenge that triggers the production of nephritogenic IgA1 [58–61].

Taken together, these data seem to suggest that IgAN is an inflammatory disease with an autoimmune genesis that involves or perhaps even originates in the intestine. GWAS study of the Gharavi group also showed that the frequency of the 15 identified genetic risk factors reflects the different distribution of IgAN frequency in the various areas of the world. It was confirmed that the loci of susceptibility to develop IgAN were, in fact, more frequent in Asian populations, which have the highest incidence of disease, and less frequent in African populations, which have the lowest incidence [38]. This data strongly suggested that the distinctive geographic pattern of IgAN risk alleles could have been modeled by an adaptation to the local environment.

The environmental influence on IgAN is supported also from DNA methylation studies showing that aberrant DNA methylation in IgAN patients influences the expression of some genes involved in the T-cell receptor signaling, the pathway that transfers the signal of the presence of antigens and that activates the T-cells [35]. In particular, the hypo-methylation of TRIM27 and DUSP3 and the hyper-methylation of VTRNA2-1 lead to the overexpression of TGFβ and to a reduced TCR signal strength of the CD4$^+$ T-cells, with a consequent T helper cell imbalance. DNA methylation studies are important because the structural modifications of the DNA can be established through environmental programming. Moreover, the DNA methylation can be dynamic and potentially reversible [62]. For these reasons, further studies about the DNA methylation in IgAN will be needed to better understand environmental influences on this disease.

The last GWAS study of the Gharavi group suggested that the distinctive geographical pattern of IgAN risk alleles could have been modeled by adaptation to the local environment [38]. It was also able to better define potential environmental factors able to explain such an adaptation process. The authors carried out an association analysis of the genetic risk score to develop IgAN with some ecological variables present in the populations enrolled in the study, reflecting the local climate, pathogenic load, and dietary factors. A strong positive association emerged between the score of genetic risk for IgAN and the diversity of local pathogens such as viruses, bacteria, protozoa, helminths. The strongest correlation was the diversity of parasitic worms (helminths), which often infest the intestine. The increased incidence of IgAN in some geographical areas, therefore, could be the accidental consequence of a protective adaptation from intestinal worm mucosal invasion. Helminth infection has been an important source of morbidity and mortality in human history, and still occurs in 25% of the world's population, with the highest global burden of soil-transmitted helminth infections (geo-helminthiasis) in Asia, where it contributes significantly to pediatric mortality. Schistosomiasis, a common helminthic infection that is a long-known cause of secondary IgAN, further supports this hypothesis.

On the other hand, it is known that host-pathogen interactions have exerted a critical influence on the genetic architecture of IBD. According to these data, IgAN susceptibility loci appear to be either directly associated with the risk of IBD or encode proteins involved in maintaining the intestinal mucosal barrier or in regulating the mucosal immune response. Thanks to these latest studies it is possible to link inflammatory diseases of the intestinal mucosa, including IBD, with the risk of IgAN, and to explain why these two diseases occur simultaneously more often than expected. These data are also consistent with the clinical observations that mucosal infections often trigger episodes of acute nephritis during IgAN, with the key role of IgA in defense at the mucosal surface level.

3. Microbiota and IgA Nephropathy: The "Chicken or Egg" Question

The ensemble of bacteria, bacteriophages, fungi, protozoa, and viruses that live in the digestive tract of humans, called microbiota, is in contact with the gut epithelium and plays a role in the development of the mucosal-associated lymphoid tissue (MALT) and, reciprocally, the composition of the commensal microbiota depends on MALT function [63,64]. In humans, the MALT is the primary source of IgA [65], and numerous studies indicate that IgA Nephropathy (IgAN) is closely associated with alterations in the gut microbiota [34,66,67]. To date, it is unclear whether dysbiosis precedes the disease or if the IgAN can lead to gut dysbiosis.

A transgenic mouse model of IgA nephropathy that overexpresses the B cell activation factor of the TNF family (BAFF) fails to develop glomerular IgA deposits when raised in germ-free conditions until gut microbiota are introduced [34].

In a cross-sectional study, Gesualdo et al. [66] identified reduced fecal microbial diversity in patients with progressive IgAN compared to those with non-progressive IgAN and healthy subjects. IgAN patients have been found to have microbial dysbiosis with an increased Firmicutes/Bacteroidetes ratio. Specifically, in the fecal samples of IgAN patients, a high level of Firmicutes has been found. They are characterized by high percentages of some genera/species of Ruminococcaceae, Lachnospiraceae, Eubacteriaceae, and Streptococcaeae. Instead, healthy controls presented a higher level of Clostridium, Enterococcus and Lactobacillus genera.

4. Microbiome Modulation in IgAN: "State of the Art"

In the context of detection of microbiota dysbiosis in IgAN patients, restoring some microbial gaps could lead to new supportive therapeutic strategies, such as the use of antibiotics or dietary implementation with prebiotics and/or probiotics, or through fecal microbiota transplantation (FMT).

In this scenario, the first therapeutic approach was conducted by Monteiro et al. [67]. The authors have demonstrated that antibiotic treatment (ampicillin, vancomycin, neomycin, and metronidazole) of a double transgenic mice model of IgAN reverses the phenotype of the disease; but this antibiotic cocktail may have other collateral effects on the gut and weight. Moreover, it is not feasible to give to patients a broad-spectrum antibiotic mix, and it could generate resistant strains of bacteria.

The use of probiotics, prebiotics or symbiotics may prove to be a viable and low-risk therapeutic strategy in the future. Probiotics have anti-inflammatory, anti-oxidative, and other favorable gut-modulating properties [68]. Especially species from the Lactobacilli and Bifidobacteria genera were shown to support the humoral immune responses against environmental toxins and antigens [69]. The use of probiotics or symbiotics in patients with chronic kidney disease has been shown to have some beneficial effects on the uremic toxins, blood urea nitrogen, oxidative stress, and markers of inflammation also by enhancing barrier function [70–73]. In that regard, the study of Soylu et al. [74] showed that the administration of Saccharomyces boulardii, which is able to decrease intestinal inflammation through modulation of the T-cell [75], reduced systemic IgA response and protected induced IgAN mice from the disease.

Another future weapon against the IgAN could be the FMT. This approach consists of stool transfer from a selected healthy donor to the gastrointestinal tract of a recipient patient suffering from microbial dysbiosis [76]. Currently, FMT is recommended as the most effective therapy for the recurrent Clostridium difficile infection [77]. Although there is no strong evidence that supports the use of the FMT in IgAN, promising studies are focusing on revealing whether this therapeutic option may play a role in the management of this disease. Indeed, an interesting interventional ongoing study (clinical trial NCT03633864) aims to determine the safety and efficacy of FMT in IgAN patients not responding to the standard treatment or not responding to immunosuppressive treatments.

5. The Interplay between the Microbiome and Virome: A New Vision of Human Metagenome

The human gut microbiome is a complex ecosystem that begins with colonization at birth and continues to alter and adapt throughout the life of an individual [78]. The bacterial and archaeal communities of the microbiome provide their host with an array of functions, including immune system development, synthesis of vitamins, and energy generation [79]. The bacterial components are characterized by high temporal stability in a healthy subject but can be transiently affected by events such as travel, sickness, and antibiotic usage [80].

Recently, the scientific community focused attention also on the human virome. The human virome consists of both the viral component of the microbiome, dominated by bacteriophages [80], and a variety of DNA viruses that directly infect eukaryotic cells [81]. Viruses access the human body through mucosal surfaces, where they interact with the host immune defense, commensal bacteria included. Bacteria of microbiota interact with viruses to eliminate or reduce their infectivity, ensuring the homeostasis of the mucosal sites, but viruses had mechanisms to take advantage of the microbiota, and thereby evade the immune system [82]. The concept of the virome as a stable part of the human metagenome has been raised from studies on chronic viral infections. During a chronic viral infection, a dynamic relationship between the host and viral agents occurs, creating a continuous state of immune surveillance. This immune system dynamism is neutral for the host, but it has a critically important role in shaping the "normal" human immune system [83]. The virome is one of the most variable components of the human gut microbiome, changing from childhood to adult life [84] in response to different environments, lifestyles or infections. A number of cross-sectional population studies reported disease-specific alterations of the gut virome in a number of gastrointestinal and systemic disorders, such as inflammatory bowel disease [85,86], AIDS [87], diabetes [88], and malnutrition [89]. However, to date, interpretation of these data is inconsistent, due to the very high variability in the virome composition and the lack of exact taxonomic classification and biological properties of several viral groups [80].

Recent studies have shed light on how resident enteric viruses may affect host physiology beyond causing disease [90]. Despite the partial picture of the taxonomic composition of the mammalian virome, recent investigations showed that the preponderance of viruses residing in the intestine are bacteriophages, which infect bacteria and can be released from them in response to stress signals [91]. As a consequence of the lysis of bacteria by phages, bacterial cell wall components and bacterial and phage DNA can trigger pattern recognition receptors in intestinal or immune cells, influencing intestinal homeostasis and immunity [92,93]. This hypothesis has been investigated in several studies with discordant results. In fact, some in vitro studies showed that phages were internalized by phagocytosis or endocytosis in lysosomes of lymphocytes and degraded without inflammation [94]. A different study performed on mice showed activation of myeloid differentiation primary response 88 (MyD88)-dependent pathway, with consequent involvement of TLRs [95]. Despite controversial results, it is clear that enteric phages have a key role in the modulation of the bacterial microbiome on the intestinal mucosal surface [90].

It is known that IgAN and other glomerulonephritides are clinically associated with viral infections, such as hepatitis B virus [96], respiratory syncytial virus [97] or HIV [98]. Most viral pathogens for mammals produce double-stranded RNA (dsRNA) incidental to viral replication. dsRNAs are recognized by TLR3, which is expressed on the cellular membrane surface of many immune cells [99]. TLR3 binds primarily to dsRNA and induce antiviral and inflammatory responses, mediated by the TNFs system and NFkB [100,101].

Yamashita et al. investigated the cellular podocyte response to dsRNA [102]. Cell cultures of human or murine podocytes were cultured and stimulated with Polyinosinic-polycytidylic acid (Poly(I:C)), a synthetic double-stranded (ds) RNA. RT-PCR, immunoblotting, phenotype characterization and functional assays were then performed to study alterations in podocyte marker expression or cellular functions. They found that human and murine podocytes expressed TLR3 and other proteins of its correlated activation pathway. Stimulation with synthetic dsRNA led to the activation of the TLR3 signaling, and exposed podocytes showed alteration in migration processes and defective expression of proteins podocyte-specific such as nephrin, podocin or CD2AP, and increased transepithelial albumin flux [102]. Although these results need to be validated by in vivo experiments, they support the hypothesis that dsRNA exposure can contribute to glomerular injury associated with immune complex deposition and could be associated with the progression of IgAN.

The group of He L. et al. [103] offered more direct evidence of the involvement of dsRNA in IgAN. In this paper, human leukocytes, isolated from tonsil tissue and whole blood, were cultured with or without poly(I:C) for 1–7 days. They also analyzed lymphomonocyte, urine, kidney and spleen samples from rats administered with or without poly(I:C) in the presence or absence of IgAN. In both in vivo and in vitro experiments, theTLR3-dependent BAFF expression was upregulated after a viral infection, especially in IgAN patients or animals. The TLR3 crosstalk with BAFF plays a vital role in the over-production of IgA and in the Recombinant Class Switch to IgA in IgAN. Thus, the inhibition of TLR3/BAFF axis activation could be an interesting option for preventing IgAN progression [103].

These studies demonstrated that exposure to viral products can directly influence the IgAN progression. However, to date, there are no data available about a direct role of the virome in the modulation of IgAN pathogenesis and/or progression. Specific studies aimed to study the influence of virome in healthy and pathological processes are in very early stages, and efforts must be made to improve our knowledge in this challenging field.

6. Conclusions

The GWAS and the other whole-genome genomic studies, thanks to technological developments in the field of genetics, have allowed researchers to identify multiple susceptibility loci for the IgAN and, consequently, they have shed new light on the pathogenesis of this disease, revealing the close connections with multiple environmental, alimentary and behavioral factors. Nevertheless, these studies have made possible the correlation of the genetic risk to develop IgAN with the geo-epidemiological aspects of the disease. These findings focalize attention on a new perspective to study the IgAN pathogenesis and show the involvement of factors driven by environment, lifestyle, or diet affecting the disease (Table 1). These factors may represent the missing link in IgAN pathogenesis. Many steps forward have been taken in the characterization of IgAN, and new studies through an integrated genomic approach will be needed to deepen the etiopathogenetic mechanisms and to suggest new potential therapeutic targets. Nevertheless, recent data suggest a new vision to consider the IgA Nephropathy as a disease which is not disconnected from the environment in which we live but influenced by, in addition to the genetic background, other environmental and behavioral factors that could be useful for developing precision nephrology and personalized therapy.

Author Contributions: Conceptualization, F.S. and L.G.; investigation, C.C., F.S., F.P.; resources, V.D.L., F.P.; data curation, C.C., V.D.L.; writing—original draft preparation, C.C., F.S., F.P., V.D.L.; writing—review and editing, F.S., A.G., F.P., L.G.; supervision, F.S., F.P., L.G.; funding acquisition, L.G. All authors have read and agreed to the published version of the manuscript.

Abbreviations

IgAN	IgA Nephropathy
PBMC	Peripheral blood mononuclear cells
OR	Odds ratio
GWAS	Genome-wide association studies
IBD	Inflammatory bowel diseases

References

1. D'Amico, G. The commonest glomerulonephritis in the world: IgA nephropathy. *Q. J. Med.* **1987**, *64*, 709–727. [PubMed]
2. Suzuki, H.; Kiryluk, K.; Novak, J.; Moldoveanu, Z.; Herr, A.B.; Renfrow, M.B.; Wyatt, R.J.; Scolari, F.; Mestecky, J.; Gharavi, A.G.; et al. The Pathophysiology of IgA Nephropathy. *J. Am. Soc. Nephrol.* **2011**, *22*, 1795–1803. [CrossRef] [PubMed]
3. Paolo Schena, F. A retrospective analysis of the natural history of primary IgA nephropathy worldwide. *Am. J. Med.* **1990**, *89*, 209–215. [CrossRef]
4. Julian, B.A.; Waldo, F.B.; Rifai, A.; Mestecky, J. IgA nephropathy, the most common glomerulonephritis worldwide. *Am. J. Med.* **1988**, *84*, 129–132. [CrossRef]
5. Smith, S.M.; Harford, A.M. IgA Nephropathy in Renal Allografts: Increased Frequency in Native American Patients. *Ren. Fail.* **1995**, *17*, 449–456. [CrossRef]
6. Hughson, M.D.; Megill, D.M.; Smith, S.M.; Tung, K.S.; Miller, G.; Hoy, W.E. Mesangiopathic glomerulonephritis in Zuni (New Mexico) Indians. *Arch. Pathol. Lab. Med.* **1989**, *113*, 148–157.
7. O'connell, P.J.; Ibels, L.S.; Thomas, M.A.; Harris, M.; Eckstein, R.P. Familial IgA nephropathy: A Study of renal disease in an australian aboriginal family. *Aust. N. Z. J. Med.* **1987**, *17*, 27–33. [CrossRef]
8. Bisceglia, L.; Cerullo, G.; Forabosco, P.; Torres, D.D.; Scolari, F.; Di Perna, M.; Foramitti, M.; Amoroso, A.; Bertok, S.; Floege, J.; et al. Genetic heterogeneity in Italian families with IgA nephropathy: Suggestive linkage for two novel IgA nephropathy loci. *Am. J. Hum. Genet.* **2006**, *79*, 1130–1134. [CrossRef]
9. Gharavi, A.G.; Yan, Y.; Scolari, F.; Schena, F.P.; Frasca, G.M.; Ghiggeri, G.M.; Cooper, K.; Amoroso, A.; Viola, B.F.; Battini, G.; et al. IgA nephropathy, the most common cause of glomerulonephritis, is linked to 6q22–23. *Nat. Genet.* **2000**, *26*, 354–357. [CrossRef]
10. Schena, F.P.; Cerullo, G.; Rossini, M.; Lanzilotta, S.G.; D'Altri, C.; Manno, C. Increased risk of end-stage renal disease in familial IgA nephropathy. *J. Am. Soc. Nephrol.* **2002**, *13*, 453–460.
11. Emancipator, P. Discussant: S.N. Immunoregulatory factors in the pathogenesis of IgA nephropathy. *Kidney Int.* **1990**, *38*, 1216–1229. [CrossRef] [PubMed]
12. Kodama, S.; Suzuki, M.; Arita, M.; Mogi, G. Increase in tonsillar germinal centre B-1 cell numbers in IgA nephropathy (IgAN) patients and reduced susceptibility to Fas-mediated apoptosis. *Clin. Exp. Immunol.* **2001**, *123*, 301–308. [CrossRef] [PubMed]
13. Harper, S.J.; Allen, A.C.; Pringle, J.H.; Feehally, J. Increased dimeric IgA producing B cells in the bone marrow in IgA nephropathy determined by in situ hybridisation for J chain mRNA. *J. Clin. Pathol.* **1996**, *49*, 38–42. [CrossRef] [PubMed]
14. Harper, S.J.; Allen, A.C.; Béné, M.C.; Pringle, J.H.; Faure, G.; Lauder, I.; Feehally, J. Increased dimeric IgA-producing B cells in tonsils in IgA nephropathy determined by in situ hybridization for J chain mRNA. *Clin. Exp. Immunol.* **2008**, *101*, 442–448. [CrossRef]
15. Suzuki, H.; Moldoveanu, Z.; Hall, S.; Brown, R.; Vu, H.L.; Novak, L.; Julian, B.A.; Tomana, M.; Wyatt, R.J.; Edberg, J.C.; et al. IgA1-secreting cell lines from patients with IgA nephropathy produce aberrantly glycosylated IgA1. *J. Clin. Investig.* **2008**, *118*, 629–639. [CrossRef]
16. Eijgenraam, J.W.; Woltman, A.M.; Kamerling, S.W.A.; Briere, F.; De Fijter, J.W.; Daha, M.R.; Van Kooten, C. Dendritic cells of IgA nephropathy patients have an impaired capacity to induce IgA production in naïve B cells. *Kidney Int.* **2005**, *68*, 1604–1612. [CrossRef]
17. Kennel-de March, A.; Bene, M.C.; Renoult, E.; Kessler, M.; Faure, G.C.; Kolopp-Sarda, M.N. Enhanced expression of L-selectin on peripheral blood lymphocytes from patients with IgA nephropathy. *Clin. Exp. Immunol.* **1999**, *115*, 542–546. [CrossRef]

18. Barratt, J.; Bailey, E.M.; Buck, K.S.; Mailley, J.; Moayyedi, P.; Feehally, J.; Turney, J.H.; Crabtree, J.E.; Allen, A.C. Exaggerated systemic antibody response to mucosal Helicobacter pylori infection in IgA nephropathy. *Am. J. Kidney Dis.* **1999**, *33*, 1049–1057. [CrossRef]

19. Batra, A.; Smith, A.C.; Feehally, J.; Barratt, J. T-cell homing receptor expression in IgA nephropathy. *Nephrol. Dial. Transplant.* **2007**, *22*, 2540–2548. [CrossRef]

20. Allen, A.C.; Bailey, E.M.; Barratt, J.; Buck, K.S.; Feehally, J. Analysis of IgA1 O-glycans in IgA nephropathy by fluorophore-assisted carbohydrate electrophoresis. *J. Am. Soc. Nephrol.* **1999**, *10*, 1763–1771.

21. Allen, A.C.; Bailey, E.M.; Brenchley, P.E.C.; Buck, K.S.; Barratt, J.; Feehally, J. Mesangial IgA1 in IgA nephropathy exhibits aberrant O-glycosylation: Observations in three patients. *Kidney Int.* **2001**, *60*, 969–973. [CrossRef] [PubMed]

22. Horie, A.; Hiki, Y.; Odani, H.; Yasuda, Y.; Takahashi, M.; Kato, M.; Iwase, H.; Kobayashi, Y.; Nakashima, I.; Maeda, K. IgA1 molecules produced by tonsillar lymphocytes are under-O-glycosylated in IgA nephropathy. *Am. J. Kidney Dis.* **2003**, *42*, 486–496. [CrossRef]

23. Van den Wall Bake, A.W.; Daha, M.R.; Valentijn, R.M.; van Es, L.A. The bone marrow as a possible origin of the IgA1 deposited in the mesangium in IgA nephropathy. *Semin. Nephrol.* **1987**, *7*, 329–331. [PubMed]

24. Kokubo, T.; Hashizume, K.; Iwase, H.; Arai, K.; Tanaka, A.; Toma, K.; Hotta, K.; Kobayashi, Y. Humoral immunity against the proline-rich peptide epitope of the IgA1 hinge region in IgA nephropathy. *Nephrol. Dial. Transplant.* **2000**, *15*, 28–33. [CrossRef]

25. Tomana, M.; Novak, J.; Julian, B.A.; Matousovic, K.; Konecny, K.; Mestecky, J. Circulating immune complexes in IgA nephropathy consist of IgA1 with galactose-deficient hinge region and antiglycan antibodies. *J. Clin. Investig.* **1999**, *104*, 73–81. [CrossRef]

26. Gómez-Guerrero, C.; López-Armada, M.J.; González, E.; Egido, J. Soluble IgA and IgG aggregates are catabolized by cultured rat mesangial cells and induce production of TNF-alpha and IL-6, and proliferation. *J. Immunol.* **1994**, *153*, 5247–5255.

27. Schena, F.P. Immunogenetic aspects of primary IgA nephropathy. *Kidney Int.* **1995**, *48*, 1998–2013. [CrossRef]

28. Schena, F.P.; D'Altri, C.; Cerullo, G.; Manno, C.; Gesualdo, L. ACE gene polymorphism and IgA nephropathy: An ethnically homogeneous study and a meta-analysis. *Kidney Int.* **2001**, *60*, 732–740. [CrossRef]

29. Hsu, S.I.-H.; Ramirez, S.B.; Winn, M.P.; Bonventre, J.V.; Owen, W.F. Evidence for genetic factors in the development and progression of IgA nephropathy. *Kidney Int.* **2000**, *57*, 1818–1835. [CrossRef]

30. Paterson, A.D.; Liu, X.Q.; Wang, K.; Magistroni, R.; Song, X.; Kappel, J.; Klassen, J.; Cattran, D.; St George-Hyslop, P.; Pei, Y. Genome-wide linkage scan of a large family with IgA nephropathy localizes a novel susceptibility locus to chromosome 2q36. *J. Am. Soc. Nephrol.* **2007**, *18*, 2408–2415. [CrossRef]

31. Gharavi, A.G.; Kiryluk, K.; Choi, M.; Li, Y.; Hou, P.; Xie, J.; Sanna-Cherchi, S.; Men, C.J.; Julian, B.A.; Wyatt, R.J.; et al. Genome-wide association study identifies susceptibility loci for IgA nephropathy. *Nat. Genet.* **2011**, *43*, 321–327. [CrossRef] [PubMed]

32. Yu, X.Q.; Li, M.; Zhang, H.; Low, H.Q.; Wei, X.; Wang, J.Q.; Sun, L.D.; Sim, K.S.; Li, Y.; Foo, J.N.; et al. A genome-wide association study in Han Chinese identifies multiple susceptibility loci for IgA nephropathy. *Nat. Genet.* **2011**, *44*, 178–182. [CrossRef] [PubMed]

33. Litinskiy, M.B.; Nardelli, B.; Hilbert, D.M.; He, B.; Schaffer, A.; Casali, P.; Cerutti, A. DCs induce CD40-independent immunoglobulin class switching through BLyS and APRIL. *Nat. Immunol.* **2002**, *3*, 822–829. [CrossRef] [PubMed]

34. McCarthy, D.D.; Kujawa, J.; Wilson, C.; Papandile, A.; Poreci, U.; Porfilio, E.A.; Ward, L.; Lawson, M.A.E.; Macpherson, A.J.; McCoy, K.D.; et al. Mice overexpressing BAFF develop a commensal flora–dependent, IgA-associated nephropathy. *J. Clin. Investig.* **2011**, *121*, 3991–4002. [CrossRef]

35. Sallustio, F.; Serino, G.; Cox, S.N.; Gassa, A.D.; Curci, C.; De Palma, G.; Banelli, B.; Zaza, G.; Romani, M.; Schena, F.P. Aberrantly methylated DNA regions lead to low activation of CD4$^+$ T-cells in IgA nephropathy. *Clin. Sci.* **2016**, *130*, 733–746. [CrossRef]

36. Ai, Z.; Li, M.; Liu, W.; Foo, J.N.; Mansouri, O.; Yin, P.; Zhou, Q.; Tang, X.; Dong, X.; Feng, S.; et al. Low alpha-defensin gene copy number increases the risk for IgA nephropathy and renal dysfunction. *Sci. Transl. Med.* **2016**, *8*, 345ra88. [CrossRef]

37. Sallustio, F.; Cox, S.N.; Serino, G.; Curci, C.; Pesce, F.; De Palma, G.; Papagianni, A.; Kirmizis, D.; Falchi, M.; Schena, F.P. Genome-wide scan identifies a copy number variable region at 3p21.1 that influences the TLR9 expression levels in IgA nephropathy patients. *Eur. J. Hum. Genet.* **2015**, *23*, 940–948. [CrossRef]

38. Kiryluk, K.; Li, Y.; Scolari, F.; Sanna-Cherchi, S.; Choi, M.; Verbitsky, M.; Fasel, D.; Lata, S.; Prakash, S.; Shapiro, S.; et al. Discovery of new risk loci for IgA nephropathy implicates genes involved in immunity against intestinal pathogens. *Nat. Genet.* **2014**, *46*, 1187–1196. [CrossRef]

39. Kiryluk, K.; Li, Y.; Sanna-Cherchi, S.; Rohanizadegan, M.; Suzuki, H.; Eitner, F.; Snyder, H.J.; Choi, M.; Hou, P.; Scolari, F.; et al. Geographic differences in genetic susceptibility to IgA nephropathy: GWAS replication study and geospatial risk analysis. *PLoS Genet.* **2012**, *8*, e1002765. [CrossRef]

40. Feehally, J.; Farrall, M.; Boland, A.; Gale, D.P.; Gut, I.; Heath, S.; Kumar, A.; Peden, J.F.; Maxwell, P.H.; Morris, D.L.; et al. HLA has strongest association with IgA nephropathy in genome-wide analysis. *J. Am. Soc. Nephrol.* **2010**, *21*, 1791–1797. [CrossRef]

41. Wu, F.; Dassopoulos, T.; Cope, L.; Maitra, A.; Brant, S.R.; Harris, M.L.; Bayless, T.M.; Parmigiani, G.; Chakravarti, S. Genome-wide gene expression differences in Crohn's disease and ulcerative colitis from endoscopic pinch biopsies: Insights into distinctive pathogenesis. *Inflamm. Bowel. Dis.* **2007**, *13*, 807–821. [CrossRef] [PubMed]

42. Visekruna, A.; Joeris, T.; Seidel, D.; Kroesen, A.; Loddenkemper, C.; Zeitz, M.; Kaufmann, S.H.E.; Schmidt-Ullrich, R.; Steinhoff, U. Proteasome-mediated degradation of IκBα and processing of p105 in Crohn disease and ulcerative colitis. *J. Clin. Investig.* **2006**, *116*, 3195–3203. [CrossRef] [PubMed]

43. Li, G.S.; Zhang, H.; Lv, J.C.; Shen, Y.; Wang, H.Y. Variants of C1GALT1 gene are associated with the genetic susceptibility to IgA nephropathy. *Kidney Int.* **2007**, *71*, 448–453. [CrossRef] [PubMed]

44. Pirulli, D.; Crovella, S.; Ulivi, S.; Zadro, C.; Bertok, S.; Rendine, S.; Scolari, F.; Foramitti, M.; Ravani, P.; Roccatello, D.; et al. Genetic variant of C1GalT1 contributes to the susceptibility to IgA nephropathy. *J. Nephrol.* **2009**, *22*, 152–159.

45. Serino, G.; Sallustio, F.; Cox, S.N.; Pesce, F.; Schena, F.P. Abnormal miR-148b expression promotes aberrant glycosylation of IgA1 in IgA nephropathy. *J. Am. Soc. Nephrol.* **2012**, *23*, 814–824. [CrossRef]

46. Serino, G.; Pesce, F.; Sallustio, F.; De Palma, G.; Cox, S.N.; Curci, C.; Zaza, G.; Lai, K.N.; Leung, J.C.K.; Tang, S.C.W.; et al. In a retrospective international study, circulating miR-148b and let-7b were found to be serum markers for detecting primary IgA nephropathy. *Kidney Int.* **2016**, *89*, 683–692. [CrossRef]

47. Serino, G.; Sallustio, F.; Curci, C.; Cox, S.N.; Pesce, F.; De Palma, G.; Schena, F.P. Role of let-7b in the regulation of N-acetylgalactosaminyltransferase 2 in IgA nephropathy. *Nephrol. Dial. Transplant.* **2015**, *30*, 1132–1139. [CrossRef]

48. Floege, J.; Feehally, J. The mucosa-kidney axis in IgA nephropathy. *Nat. Rev. Nephrol.* **2016**, *12*, 147–156. [CrossRef]

49. Magistroni, R.; D'Agati, V.D.; Appel, G.B.; Kiryluk, K. New developments in the genetics, pathogenesis, and therapy of IgA nephropathy. *Kidney Int.* **2015**, *88*, 974–989. [CrossRef]

50. Vigorito, E.; Gambardella, L.; Colucci, F.; McAdam, S.; Turner, M. Vav proteins regulate peripheral B-cell survival. *Blood* **2005**, *106*, 2391–2398. [CrossRef]

51. Bertin, J.; Guo, Y.; Wang, L.; Srinivasula, S.M.; Jacobson, M.D.; Poyet, J.-L.; Merriam, S.; Du, M.-Q.; Dyer, M.J.S.; Robison, K.E.; et al. CARD9 Is a Novel Caspase Recruitment Domain-containing Protein That Interacts with BCL10/CLAP and Activates NF-κB. *J. Biol. Chem.* **2000**, *275*, 41082–41086. [CrossRef] [PubMed]

52. Sokol, H.; Conway, K.L.; Zhang, M.; Choi, M.; Morin, B.; Cao, Z.; Villablanca, E.J.; Li, C.; Wijmenga, C.; Yun, S.H.; et al. Card9 Mediates Intestinal Epithelial Cell Restitution, T-Helper 17 Responses, and Control of Bacterial Infection in Mice. *Gastroenterology* **2013**, *145*, 591–601.e3. [CrossRef] [PubMed]

53. Uematsu, S.; Fujimoto, K.; Jang, M.H.; Yang, B.-G.; Jung, Y.J.; Nishiyama, M.; Sato, S.; Tsujimura, T.; Yamamoto, M.; Yokota, Y.; et al. Regulation of humoral and cellular gut immunity by lamina propria dendritic cells expressing Toll-like receptor 5. *Nat. Immunol.* **2008**, *9*, 769–776. [CrossRef] [PubMed]

54. Fujimoto, K.; Karuppuchamy, T.; Takemura, N.; Shimohigoshi, M.; Machida, T.; Haseda, Y.; Aoshi, T.; Ishii, K.J.; Akira, S.; Uematsu, S. A New Subset of CD103⁺ CD8α⁺ Dendritic Cells in the Small Intestine Expresses TLR3, TLR7, and TLR9 and Induces Th1 Response and CTL Activity. *J. Immunol.* **2011**, *186*, 6287–6295. [CrossRef] [PubMed]

55. Du, X.; Poltorak, A.; Wei, Y.; Beutler, B. Three novel mammalian toll-like receptors: Gene structure, expression, and evolution. *Eur. Cytokine Netw.* **2000**, *11*, 362–371. [PubMed]

56. Notley, C.A.; Jordan, C.K.; McGovern, J.L.; Brown, M.A.; Ehrenstein, M.R. DNA methylation governs the dynamic regulation of inflammation by apoptotic cells during efferocytosis. *Sci. Rep.* **2017**, *7*, 42204. [CrossRef]

57. Martínez-Campos, C.; Burguete-García, A.I.; Madrid-Marina, V. Role of TLR9 in Oncogenic Virus-Produced Cancer. *Viral Immunol.* **2017**, *30*, 98–105. [CrossRef]

58. Bernasconi, N.L.; Onai, N.; Lanzavecchia, A. A role for Toll-like receptors in acquired immunity: Up-regulation of TLR9 by BCR triggering in naive B cells and constitutive expression in memory B cells. *Blood* **2003**, *101*, 4500–4504. [CrossRef]

59. Gesualdo, L.; Lamm, M.E.; Emancipator, S.N. Defective oral tolerance promotes nephritogenesis in experimental IgA nephropathy induced by oral immunization. *J. Immunol.* **1990**, *145*, 3684–3691.

60. Bernasconi, N.L. Maintenance of Serological Memory by Polyclonal Activation of Human Memory B Cells. *Science* **2002**, *298*, 2199–2202. [CrossRef]

61. Blaas, S.H.; Stieber-Gunckel, M.; Falk, W.; Obermeier, F.; Rogler, G. CpG-oligodeoxynucleotides stimulate immunoglobulin A secretion in intestinal mucosal B cells. *Clin. Exp. Immunol.* **2009**, *155*, 534–540. [CrossRef] [PubMed]

62. Nagy, C.; Turecki, G. Sensitive periods in epigenetics: Bringing us closer to complex behavioral phenotypes. *Epigenomics* **2012**, *4*, 445–457. [CrossRef] [PubMed]

63. Nakajima, A.; Vogelzang, A.; Maruya, M.; Miyajima, M.; Murata, M.; Son, A.; Kuwahara, T.; Tsuruyama, T.; Yamada, S.; Matsuura, M.; et al. IgA regulates the composition and metabolic function of gut microbiota by promoting symbiosis between bacteria. *J. Exp. Med.* **2018**, *215*, 2019–2034. [CrossRef] [PubMed]

64. Bunker, J.J.; Erickson, S.A.; Flynn, T.M.; Henry, C.; Koval, J.C.; Meisel, M.; Jabri, B.; Antonopoulos, D.A.; Wilson, P.C.; Bendelac, A. Natural polyreactive IgA antibodies coat the intestinal microbiota. *Science* **2017**, *358*. [CrossRef]

65. Coppo, R. The Gut-Renal Connection in IgA Nephropathy. *Semin. Nephrol.* **2018**, *38*, 504–512. [CrossRef]

66. De Angelis, M.; Montemurno, E.; Piccolo, M.; Vannini, L.; Lauriero, G.; Maranzano, V.; Gozzi, G.; Serrazanetti, D.; Dalfino, G.; Gobbetti, M.; et al. Microbiota and metabolome associated with Immunoglobulin a Nephropathy (IgAN). *PLoS ONE* **2014**. [CrossRef]

67. Chemouny, J.M.; Gleeson, P.J.; Abbad, L.; Lauriero, G.; Boedec, E.; Le Roux, K.; Monot, C.; Bredel, M.; Bex-Coudrat, J.; Sannier, A.; et al. Modulation of the microbiota by oral antibiotics treats immunoglobulin A nephropathy in humanized mice. *Nephrol. Dial. Transpl.* **2018**, *34*, 1135–1144. [CrossRef]

68. Cavalcanti Neto, M.P.; Aquino, J.S.; da Romao Silva, L.F.; de Oliveira Silva, R.; Guimaraes, K.S.L.; de Oliveira, Y.; de Souza, E.L.; Magnani, M.; Vidal, H.; de Brito Alves, J.L. Gut microbiota and probiotics intervention: A potential therapeutic target for management of cardiometabolic disorders and chronic kidney disease? *Pharmacol. Res.* **2018**, *130*, 152–163. [CrossRef]

69. Vitetta, L.; Vitetta, G.; Hall, S. Immunological Tolerance and Function: Associations between Intestinal Bacteria, Probiotics, Prebiotics, and Phages. *Front. Immunol.* **2018**, *9*, 2240. [CrossRef]

70. Rao, R.K.; Samak, G. Protection and Restitution of Gut Barrier by Probiotics: Nutritional and Clinical Implications. *Curr. Nutr. Food Sci.* **2013**, *9*, 99–107.

71. Ranganathan, N.; Friedman, E.A.; Tam, P.; Rao, V.; Ranganathan, P.; Dheer, R. Probiotic dietary supplementation in patients with stage 3 and 4 chronic kidney disease: A 6-month pilot scale trial in Canada. *Curr. Med. Res. Opin.* **2009**, *25*, 1919–1930. [CrossRef] [PubMed]

72. Ranganathan, N.; Ranganathan, P.; Friedman, E.A.; Joseph, A.; Delano, B.; Goldfarb, D.S.; Tam, P.; Rao, A.V.; Anteyi, E.; Musso, C.G. Pilot study of probiotic dietary supplementation for promoting healthy kidney function in patients with chronic kidney disease. *Adv. Ther.* **2010**, *27*, 634–647. [CrossRef] [PubMed]

73. Guida, B.; Germano, R.; Trio, R.; Russo, D.; Memoli, B.; Grumetto, L.; Barbato, F.; Cataldi, M. Effect of short-term synbiotic treatment on plasma p-cresol levels in patients with chronic renal failure: A randomized clinical trial. *Nutr. Metab. Cardiovasc. Dis.* **2014**, *24*, 1043–1049. [CrossRef] [PubMed]

74. Soylu, A.; Berktas, S.; Sarioglu, S.; Erbil, G.; Yilmaz, O.; Demir, B.K.; Tufan, Y.; Yesilirmak, D.; Turkmen, M.; Kavukcu, S. Saccharomyces boulardii prevents oral-poliovirus vaccine-induced IgA nephropathy in mice. *Pediatr. Nephrol.* **2008**, *23*, 1287–1291. [CrossRef] [PubMed]

75. Dalmasso, G.; Cottrez, F.; Imbert, V.; Lagadec, P.; Peyron, J.F.; Rampal, P.; Czerucka, D.; Groux, H.; Foussat, A.; Brun, V. Saccharomyces boulardii inhibits inflammatory bowel disease by trapping T cells in mesenteric lymph nodes. *Gastroenterology* **2006**, *131*, 1812–1825. [CrossRef] [PubMed]

76. Zipursky, J.S.; Sidorsky, T.I.; Freedman, C.A.; Sidorsky, M.N.; Kirkland, K.B. Patient attitudes toward the use of fecal microbiota transplantation in the treatment of recurrent Clostridium difficile infection. *Clin. Infect. Dis.* **2012**, *55*, 1652–1658. [CrossRef]

77. Wortelboer, K.; Nieuwdorp, M.; Herrema, H. Fecal microbiota transplantation beyond Clostridioides difficile infections. *EBioMedicine* **2019**, *44*, 716–729. [CrossRef]

78. Rodríguez, J.M.; Murphy, K.; Stanton, C.; Ross, R.P.; Kober, O.I.; Juge, N.; Avershina, E.; Rudi, K.; Narbad, A.; Jenmalm, M.C.; et al. The composition of the gut microbiota throughout life, with an emphasis on early life. *Microb. Ecol. Health Dis.* **2015**, *26*, 1–17. [CrossRef]

79. Qin, J.; Li, R.; Raes, J.; Arumugam, M.; Burgdorf, S.; Manichanh, C.; Nielsen, T.; Pons, N.; Yamada, T.; Mende, D.R.; et al. Europe PMC Funders Group Europe PMC Funders Author Manuscripts A human gut microbial gene catalog established by metagenomic sequencing. *Nature* **2010**, *464*, 59–65. [CrossRef]

80. Shkoporov, A.N.; Clooney, A.G.; Sutton, T.D.S.; Ryan, F.J.; Daly, K.M.; Nolan, J.A.; McDonnell, S.A.; Khokhlova, E.V.; Draper, L.A.; Forde, A.; et al. The Human Gut Virome Is Highly Diverse, Stable, and Individual Specific. *Cell Host Microbe* **2019**, *26*, 527–541.e5. [CrossRef]

81. Wylie, K.M.; Mihindukulasuriya, K.A.; Zhou, Y.; Sodergren, E.; Storch, G.A.; Weinstock, G.M. Metagenomic analysis of double-stranded DNA viruses in healthy adults. *BMC Med.* **2014**, *12*, 71. [CrossRef] [PubMed]

82. Domínguez-Díaz, C.; García-Orozco, A.; Riera-Leal, A.; Padilla-Arellano, J.R.; Fafutis-Morris, M. Microbiota and Its Role on Viral Evasion: Is It with Us or Against Us? *Front. Cell. Infect. Microbiol.* **2019**, *9*, 1–7. [CrossRef] [PubMed]

83. Virgin, H.W.; Wherry, E.J.; Ahmed, R. Redefining Chronic Viral Infection. *Cell* **2009**, *138*, 30–50. [CrossRef] [PubMed]

84. Moreno-Gallego, J.L.; Chou, S.P.; Di Rienzi, S.C.; Goodrich, J.K.; Spector, T.D.; Bell, J.T.; Youngblut, N.D.; Hewson, I.; Reyes, A.; Ley, R.E. Virome Diversity Correlates with Intestinal Microbiome Diversity in Adult Monozygotic Twins. *Cell Host Microbe* **2019**, *25*, 261–272.e5. [CrossRef]

85. Norman, J.M.; Handley, S.A.; Baldridge, M.T.; Droit, L.; Liu, C.Y.; Keller, B.C.; Kambal, A.; Monaco, C.L.; Zhao, G.; Fleshner, P.; et al. Disease-specific alterations in the enteric virome in inflammatory bowel disease. *Cell* **2015**, *160*, 447–460. [CrossRef]

86. Zuo, T.; Lu, X.J.; Zhang, Y.; Cheung, C.P.; Lam, S.; Zhang, F.; Tang, W.; Ching, J.Y.L.; Zhao, R.; Chan, P.K.S.; et al. Gut mucosal virome alterations in ulcerative colitis. *Gut* **2019**, *68*, 1169–1179. [CrossRef]

87. Monaco, C.L.; Gootenberg, D.B.; Zhao, G.; Handley, S.A.; Musie, S.; Lim, E.S.; Lankowski, A.; Baldridge, M.T.; Wilen, C.B.; Flagg, M.; et al. Altered Virome and Bacterial Microbiome in Human Immuni. *Cell Host Microbe* **2017**, *19*, 311–322. [CrossRef]

88. Ma, Y.; You, X.; Mai, G.; Tokuyasu, T.; Liu, C. A human gut phage catalog correlates the gut phageome with type 2 diabetes. *Microbiome* **2018**, *6*, 1–12. [CrossRef]

89. Reyes, A.; Blanton, L.V.; Cao, S.; Zhao, G.; Manary, M.; Trehan, I.; Smith, M.I.; Wang, D.; Virgin, H.W.; Rohwer, F.; et al. Gut DNA viromes of Malawian twins discordant for severe acute malnutrition. *Proc. Natl. Acad. Sci. USA* **2015**, *112*, 11941–11946. [CrossRef]

90. Metzger, R.N.; Krug, A.B.; Eisenächer, K. Enteric virome sensing—Its role in intestinal homeostasis and immunity. *Viruses* **2018**, *10*, 146. [CrossRef]

91. Duerkop, B.A.; Hooper, L.V. Resident viruses and their interactions with the immune system. *Nat. Immunol.* **2013**, *14*, 654–659. [CrossRef] [PubMed]

92. Duerkop, B.A.; Clements, C.V.; Rollins, D.; Rodrigues, J.L.M.; Hooper, L.V. A composite bacteriophage alters colonization by an intestinal commensal bacterium. *Proc. Natl. Acad. Sci. USA* **2012**, *109*, 17621–17626. [CrossRef] [PubMed]

93. Reyes, A.; Wu, M.; McNulty, N.P.; Rohwer, F.L.; Gordon, J.I. Gnotobiotic mouse model of phage-bacterial host dynamics in the human gut. *Proc. Natl. Acad. Sci. USA* **2013**, *110*, 20236–20241. [CrossRef] [PubMed]

94. Jończyk-Matysiak, E.; Weber-Dąbrowska, B.; Owczarek, B.; Międzybrodzki, R.; Łusiak-Szelchowska, M.; Łodej, N.; Górski, A. Phage-phagocyte interactions and their implications for phage application as therapeutics. *Viruses* **2017**, *9*, 150. [CrossRef] [PubMed]

95. Eriksson, F.; Tsagozis, P.; Lundberg, K.; Parsa, R.; Mangsbo, S.M.; Persson, M.A.A.; Harris, R.A.; Pisa, P. Tumor-Specific Bacteriophages Induce Tumor Destruction through Activation of Tumor-Associated Macrophages. *J. Immunol.* **2009**, *182*, 3105–3111. [CrossRef] [PubMed]

96. Ozdamar, S.O.; Gucer, S.; Tinaztepe, K. Hepatitis-B virus associated nephropathies: A clinicopathological study in 14 children. *Pediatr. Nephrol.* **2003**, *18*, 23–28. [CrossRef] [PubMed]

97. Hu, X.; Feng, J.; Zhou, Q.; Luo, L.; Meng, T.; Zhong, Y.; Tang, W.; Deng, S.; Li, X. Respiratory syncytial virus exacerbates kidney damages in IgA nephropathy mice via the C5a-C5AR1 axis orchestrating Th17 cell responses. *Front. Cell Infect. Microbiol.* **2019**, *9*, 151. [CrossRef]

98. Kupin, W.L. Viral-associated GN hepatitis B and other viral infections. *Clin. J. Am. Soc. Nephrol.* **2017**, *12*, 1529–1533. [CrossRef]

99. Sallustio, F.; Curci, C.; Stasi, A.; De Palma, G.; Divella, C.; Gramignoli, R.; Castellano, G.; Gallone, A.; Gesualdo, L. Role of Toll-Like Receptors in Actuating Stem/Progenitor Cell Repair Mechanisms: Different Functions in Different Cells. *Stem Cells Int.* **2019**, *2019*, 1–12. [CrossRef]

100. Ozato, K.; Tailor, P.; Kubota, T. The interferon regulatory factor family in host defense: Mechanism of action. *J. Biol. Chem.* **2007**, *282*, 20065–20069. [CrossRef]

101. Sarkar, S.N.; Elco, C.P.; Peters, K.L.; Chattopadhyay, S.; Sen, G.C. Two tyrosine residues of toll-like receptor 3 trigger different steps of NF-κB activation. *J. Biol. Chem.* **2007**, *282*, 3423–3427. [CrossRef] [PubMed]

102. Yamashita, M.; Millward, C.A.; Inoshita, H.; Saikia, P.; Chattopadhyay, S.; Sen, G.C.; Emancipator, S.N. Antiviral innate immunity disturbs podocyte cell function. *J. Innate Immun.* **2013**, *5*, 231–241. [CrossRef] [PubMed]

103. He, L.; Peng, X.; Wang, J.; Tang, C.; Zhou, X.; Liu, H.; Liu, F.; Sun, L.; Peng, Y. Synthetic double-stranded RNA Poly(I:C) aggravates IgA nephropathy by triggering IgA class switching recombination through the TLR3-BAFF axis. *Am. J. Nephrol.* **2015**, *42*, 185–197. [CrossRef] [PubMed]

13

Incidence and Impact of Acute Kidney Injury after Liver Transplantation

Charat Thongprayoon [1], Wisit Kaewput [2], Natanong Thamcharoen [3], Tarun Bathini [4], Kanramon Watthanasuntorn [5], Ploypin Lertjitbanjong [5], Konika Sharma [5], Sohail Abdul Salim [6], Patompong Ungprasert [7], Karn Wijarnpreecha [8], Paul T. Kröner [8], Narothama Reddy Aeddula [9], Michael A Mao [10] and Wisit Cheungpasitporn [6,*]

[1] Division of Nephrology and Hypertension, Mayo Clinic, Rochester, MN 55905, USA; charat.thongprayoon@gmail.com

[2] Department of Military and Community Medicine, Phramongkutklao College of Medicine, Bangkok 10400, Thailand; wisitnephro@gmail.com

[3] Division of Nephrology, Beth Israel Deaconess Medical Center, Harvard Medical School, Boston, MA 02215, USA; natthamcharoen@gmail.com

[4] Department of Internal Medicine, University of Arizona, Tucson, AZ 85721, USA; tarunjacobb@gmail.com

[5] Department of Internal Medicine, Bassett Medical Center, Cooperstown, NY 13326, USA; kanramon@gmail.com (K.W.); ploypinlert@gmail.com (P.L.); drkonika@gmail.com (K.S.)

[6] Division of Nephrology, Department of Medicine, University of Mississippi Medical Center, MS 39216, USA; sohail3553@gmail.com

[7] Clinical Epidemiology Unit, Department of Research and Development, Faculty of Medicine, Siriraj Hospital, Mahidol University, Bangkok 10700, Thailand; p.ungprasert@gmail.com

[8] Department of Medicine, Division of Gastroenterology and Hepatology, Mayo Clinic, Jacksonville, FL 32224, USA; karnjuve10@gmail.com (K.W.); thomaskroner@gmail.com (P.T.K.)

[9] Division of Nephrology, Department of Medicine, Deaconess Health System, Evansville, IN 47747, USA; dr.anreddy@gmail.com

[10] Department of Medicine, Division of Nephrology and Hypertension, Mayo Clinic, Jacksonville, FL 32224, USA; mao.michael@mayo.edu

* Correspondence: wcheungpasitporn@gmail.com

Abstract: Background: The study's aim was to summarize the incidence and impacts of post-liver transplant (LTx) acute kidney injury (AKI) on outcomes after LTx. Methods: A literature search was performed using the MEDLINE, EMBASE and Cochrane Databases from inception until December 2018 to identify studies assessing the incidence of AKI (using a standard AKI definition) in adult patients undergoing LTx. Effect estimates from the individual studies were derived and consolidated utilizing random-effect, the generic inverse variance approach of DerSimonian and Laird. The protocol for this systematic review is registered with PROSPERO (no. CRD42018100664). Results: Thirty-eight cohort studies, with a total of 13,422 LTx patients, were enrolled. Overall, the pooled estimated incidence rates of post-LTx AKI and severe AKI requiring renal replacement therapy (RRT) were 40.7% (95% CI: 35.4%–46.2%) and 7.7% (95% CI: 5.1%–11.4%), respectively. Meta-regression showed that the year of study did not significantly affect the incidence of post-LTx AKI ($p = 0.81$). The pooled estimated in-hospital or 30-day mortality, and 1-year mortality rates of patients with post-LTx AKI were 16.5% (95% CI: 10.8%–24.3%) and 31.1% (95% CI: 22.4%–41.5%), respectively. Post-LTx AKI and severe AKI requiring RRT were associated with significantly higher mortality with pooled ORs of 2.96 (95% CI: 2.32–3.77) and 8.15 (95%CI: 4.52–14.69), respectively. Compared to those without post-LTx AKI, recipients with post-LTx AKI had significantly increased risk of liver graft failure and chronic kidney disease with pooled ORs of 3.76 (95% CI: 1.56–9.03) and 2.35 (95% CI: 1.53–3.61), respectively. Conclusion: The overall estimated incidence rates of post-LTx AKI and severe AKI requiring RRT are 40.8% and 7.0%, respectively. There are significant associations of post-LTx AKI with increased mortality and graft failure after transplantation. Furthermore, the incidence of post-LTx AKI has remained stable over the ten years of the study.

Keywords: Acute renal failure; Acute kidney injury; Epidemiology; Incidence; Meta-analysis; Liver Transplantation; Transplantation; Systematic reviews

1. Introduction

Acute kidney injury (AKI) is associated with high mortality worldwide (1.7 million deaths per year) [1–4]. Patients who survive AKI are at increased risk for significant morbidities such as hypertension and progressive chronic kidney disease (CKD) [5]. The incidence of AKI has steadily increased in recent years [2]. It has been suggested that AKI's global burden is 13.3 million cases a year [6]. In the United States, hospitalizations for AKI have been steeply rising, and data from national inpatient sample shows that the number of hospitalizations due to AKI increased from 953,926 in 2000 to 1,823,054 in 2006 and 3,959,560 in 2014, which accounts for one hospitalization associated with AKI every 7.5 minutes [7,8].

AKI is a common and significant complication after liver transplantation (LTx), and is associated with increased mortality, hospital length of stay, utilization of resources, and health care costs [9–27]. Although the survival of LTx recipients has improved substantially over the past five decades, mortality rates related to post-LTx AKI and subsequent progressive CKD remain high and are of increasing concern [14,15,28–31]. The underlying mechanisms for post-LTx AKI appear to be complex and differ from other medical or surgery-associated AKI [11,23–25,32–35]. Recent studies have suggested several important factors that influence post-LTx AKI, including hepatic ischemia-reperfusion injury (HIRI) [36–38], increased use of high-risk or marginal grafts, and transplantation of liver grafts to sicker patients with higher Model For End-Stage Liver Disease (MELD) score or with more comorbidities [23,39–51]. In our literature review, the reported incidences are a farrago, having a range between 5% to 94% [10,11,14–25,28–35,39–49,52–80]. These wide variabilities are possibly due to non-uniform definitions of AKI [10,11,14–25,28–35,39–49,52–80]. In addition, despite progress in transplant medicine, the incidence, risk factors, and mortality associated with AKI in post-LTx patients and their trends remain unclear [10,11,14–25,28–35,39–49,52–83].

Thus, we performed a systematic review to summarize the incidence (using standard AKI definitions of Risk, Injury, Failure, Loss of kidney function, and End-stage kidney disease (RIFLE), Acute Kidney Injury Network (AKIN), and Kidney Disease: Improving Global Outcomes (KDIGO) classifications), risk factors, and mortality and their trends for AKI in patients undergoing LTx.

2. Methods

2.1. Search Strategy and Literature Review

The protocol for this systematic review was registered with PROSPERO (International Prospective Register of Systematic Reviews; no. CRD42018100664). A systematic literature search of MEDLINE (1946 to December 2018), EMBASE (1988 to December 2018) and the Cochrane Database of Systematic Reviews (database inception to December 2018) was performed to evaluate the incidence of AKI in adult patients undergoing LTx. The systematic literature review was conducted independently by two investigators (C.T. and W.C.) using the search strategy that consolidated the terms "acute kidney injury" OR "renal failure" AND "liver transplantation," which is provided in online supplementary data 1. No language limitation was implemented. A manual search for conceivably related studies using references of the included articles was also performed. This study was conducted by the Preferred Reporting Items for Systematic Reviews and Meta-Analysis (PRISMA) statement [84] and the Strengthening the Reporting of Observational Studies in Epidemiology (STROBE) [85].

2.2. Selection Criteria

Eligible studies must be clinical trials or observational studies (cohort, case-control, or cross-sectional studies) that reported the incidence of post-LTx AKI in adult patients (age >/= 18 years old). Included studies must provide data to estimate the incidence of post-LTx AKI with 95% confidence intervals (CI). Retrieved articles were individually reviewed for eligibility by the two investigators (C.T. and W.C.). Discrepancies were addressed and solved by mutual consensus. Inclusion was not limited by the size of study.

2.3. Data Abstraction

A structured data collecting form was used to obtain the following information from each study, including title, name of the first author, year of the study, publication year, country where the study was conducted, post-LTx AKI definition, incidence of AKI post-LTx, risk factors for post-LTx AKI, and impact of post-LTx AKI on patient outcomes.

2.4. Statistical Analysis

Analyses were performed utilizing the Comprehensive Meta-Analysis 3.3 software (Biostat Inc, Englewood, NJ, USA). Adjusted point estimates from each study were consolidated by the generic inverse variance approach of DerSimonian and Laird, which designated the weight of each study based on its variance [86]. Given the possibility of between-study variance, we used a random-effect model rather than a fixed-effect model. Cochran's Q test and I^2 statistic were applied to determine the between-study heterogeneity. A value of I^2 of 0%–25% represents insignificant heterogeneity, 26%–50% low heterogeneity, 51%–75% moderate heterogeneity and 76–100% high heterogeneity [87]. The presence of publication bias was assessed by the Egger test [88].

3. Results

A total of 2525 potentially eligible articles were identified using our search strategy. After the exclusion of 1994 articles based on title and abstract for clearly not fulfilling inclusion criteria on the basis of type of article, patient population, study design, or outcome of interest, and 417 due to being duplicates, 114 articles were left for full-length review. Thirty-six of them were excluded from the full-length review as they did not report the outcome of interest, while 17 were excluded because they were not observational studies or clinical trials. Twenty-three studies were subsequently excluded because they did not use a standard AKI definition. Thus, we included 38 cohort studies [14,18,19,21,28–32,39,41–44,48,49,55–60,62–66,69,70,72–80] in the meta-analysis of post-LTx AKI incidence with 13,422 patients enrolled. The literature retrieval, review, and selection process are demonstrated in Figure 1. The characteristics of the included studies are presented in Table 1.

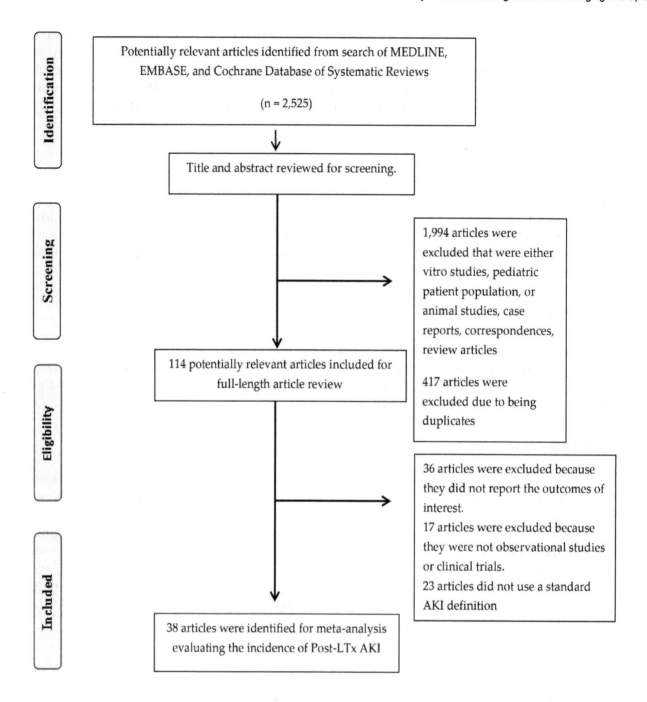

Figure 1. Outline of our search methodology.

Table 1. Main characteristics of studies included in meta-analysis of AKI in patients undergoing LTx [14,18,19,21,28–32,39,41–44,48,49,55–60,62–66,69,70,72–80].

Study	Year	Country	Procedure/Patients	Number	Deceased Donor	AKI Definition	Incidence	Mortality in AKI
O'riordan et al. [32]	2007	Ireland	Deceased donor orthotopic liver transplant	350	350 (100%)	ARI/ARF; RIFLE Injury and Failure stage within 2 weeks after transplant	ARI/ARF 129/350 (36.9%) Dialysis 68/350 (19.4%)	1-year mortality 56/129 (43%)
Kundakci et al. [41]	2010	Turkey	Orthotopic liver transplant	112	75 (67%)	AKI; RIFLE criteria	AKI 64/112 (57.1%)	1-year mortality 23/64 (36%)
Portal et al. [55]	2010	UK	Liver transplant	80	N/A	AKI; AKIN criteria within 48 hours after transplants	AKI 30/80 (37.5%)	N/A
Zhu et al. [42]	2010	China	Deceased donor orthotopic liver transplant	193	193 (100%)	AKI; AKIN criteria within 28 days after transplants	AKI 116/193 (60.1%) Dialysis 10/193 (5.2%)	1-year mortality 30/116 (26%)
Lee et al. [56]	2010	Korea	Liver transplant	431	99 (23%)	AKI; RIFLE criteria	AKI 118/431 (27.4%) Dialysis 14/431 (3.2%)	N/A
Ferreira et al. [57]	2010	Portugal	Orthotopic liver transplant	708	N/A	AKI; RIFLE criteria within 21 days after transplant	AKI 235/708 (33.2%) Dialysis 73/708 (10.3%)	Mortality 43/235 (18%)
Tinti et al. [58]	2010	Italy	Deceased donor orthotopic liver transplant	24	24 (100%)	AKI; RIFLE criteria within 15 days after transplant	AKI 9/24 (37.5%)	N/A
Chen et al. (1) [18]	2011	USA	Liver transplant	334	N/A	ARI/ARF; RIFLE Injury and Failure stage within 2 weeks after transplant within 7 days after transplant	ARI/ARF 118/334 (38.3%)	Mortality 13/118 (11%)
Umbro et al. [59]	2011	Italy	Deceased donor liver transplant	46	46 (100%)	AKI; RIFLE criteria within 7 days after transplant	AKI 26/46 (56.5%)	N/A
Karapanagiotou et al. (1) [43]	2012	Greece	Orthotopic liver transplant	75	N/A	AKI; an increase in SCr 1.5 times above baseline or value > 2.0 mg/dL within 7 days after transplant	AKI 22/75 (29.3%) Dialysis 7/75 (9.3%)	1-year mortality 11/22 (50%)
Utsumi et al. [44]	2013	Japan	Living donor liver transplant	200	0 (0%)	AKI; RIFLE criteria within 28 days after transplants	AKI 121/200 (60.5%) ARI/ARF 74/200 (37%)	Hospital mortality AKI 14/121 (12%) ARI/ARF 12/74 (16%) 1-year mortality AKI 24/121 (20%) ARI/ARF 22/74 (30%)

Table 1. *Cont.*

Study	Year	Country	Procedure/Patients	Number	Deceased Donor	AKI Definition	Incidence	Mortality in AKI
Narciso et al. [60]	2013	Brazil	Liver transplant	315	181 (57%)	AKI; AKIN criteria within 48 hours after transplants	AKI 48 hours: 101/315 (32.1%) 1 week: 255/315 (81%) Hospitalization: 293/315 (93%) Dialysis Any: 48/315 (15.2%) 1 week: 31/315 (9.8%)	Dialysis 28/48 (58%)
Leithead et al. [39]	2014	UK	Liver transplant	1152	1152 (100%) DCD 112 (10%)	AKI; KDIGO criteria within 7 days after transplants	AKI 381/1152 (33.1%) Dialysis 238/1152 (20.7%)	AKI 152/381 (40%)
Karapanagiotou et al. (2) [48]	2014	Greece	Liver transplant	71	N/A	AKI; RIFLE within 7 days or AKIN criteria within 48 hours	RIFLE AKI 28/71 (39.4%) AKIN AKI 37/71 (52.1%)	6-month mortality RIFLE AKI 15/28 (54%) AKIN AKI 17/37 (46%)
Nadeem et al. [49]	2014	Saudi Arabia	Liver transplant	158	N/A	AKI; RIFLE criteria within 72 hours after transplants	AKI 57/158 (36.1%)	N/A
Lewandowska et al. [62]	2014	Poland	Orthotopic liver transplant	63	N/A	AKI; RIFLE criteria within 72 hours after transplant	AKI 35/63 (55.6%)	N/A
Barreto et al. [63]	2015	Brazil	Orthotopic liver transplant	134	N/A	AKI; AKIN criteria 2 or 3 within 72 hours after transplants	AKIN stage 2 or 3 64/134 (47.8%) Dialysis 33/134 (24.6%)	N/A
Hilmi et al. [19]	2015	USA	Deceased donor liver transplant	424	424 (100%) ECD 257 (61%)	AKI; KDIGO criteria within 72 hours after transplant	AKI 221/424 (52.1%)	30-day mortality 3/221 (1%)
Park et al. [64]	2015	Korea	Living donor liver transplant	538	0 (0%)	AKI; RIFLE criteria within 30 days after transplant	AKI 147/538 (27.3%) Dialysis 34/538 (6.3%)	Hospital mortality 26/147 (18%) 1-year mortality 29/147 (20%)
Mukhtar et al. [65]	2015	Egypt	Living donor liver transplant	303	0 (0%)	AKI; AKIN criteria within 96 hours after transplant	AKI 115/303 (38%) Dialysis 28/303 (9.2%)	N/A

Table 1. *Cont.*

Study	Year	Country	Procedure/Patients	Number	Deceased Donor	AKI Definition	Incidence	Mortality in AKI
Sang et al. [66]	2015	Korea	Living donor liver transplant	998	0 (0%)	AKI; RIFLE or AKIN criteria within 7 days after transplant	RIFLE AKI 709/998 (71.0%) AKIN AKI 593/998 (59.4%)	RIFLE AKI 79/709 (11%) AKIN AKI 66/593 (11%)
Biancofiore et al. [69]	2015	Italy	Deceased donor liver transplant	295	295 (100%)	AKI; AKIN criteria within 7 days after transplant	AKIN stage 2 AKI 51/295 (17.3%)	N/A
Jun et al. [70]	2016	Korea	Living donor liver transplant	1617	0 (0%)	AKI; KDIGO criteria within 7 days after transplant	AKI 999/1617 (61.8%) Dialysis 9/448 (2%)	N/A
Erdost et al. [72]	2016	Turkey	Liver transplant	440	194 (44%)	AKI; RIFLE, AKIN, KDIGO criteria within 7 days after transplant	RIFLE AKI 35/440 (8.0%) AKIN AKI 63/440 (14.3%) KDIGO AKI 64/440 (14.5%)	30-day mortality RIFLE AKI 8/35 (23%) AKIN AKI 34/63 (54%) KDIGO AKI 35/64 (55%)
Kamei et al. [73]	2016	Japan	Liver transplant	62	DBD 4 (6%)	AKI; RIFLE injury or failure stage within 4 weeks after transplant	AKI 13/62 (21%) Dialysis 4/62 (6.5%)	N/A
Mizota et al. (1) [74]	2016	Japan	Living donor liver transplant	320	0 (0%)	AKI; KDIGO criteria within 7 days after transplant	AKI 199/320 (62.2%)	Hospital mortality 39/199 (20%)
Sun et al. [21]	2017	USA	Liver transplant	1037	N/A	AKI; AKIN criteria within 48 hours after transplant	AKI 549/1037 (54.9%)	N/A
Chae et al. [75]	2017	Korea	Living donor liver transplant	334	0 (0%)	AKI; AKIN criteria within 48 hours after transplant	AKI 76/334 (22.7%)	Hospital mortality 10/76 (13.2%)
Mizota et al. (2) [76]	2017	Japan	Living donor liver transplant	231	0 (0%)	Severe AKI; KDIGO stage 2 or 3 criteria within 7 days after transplant	Severe AKI 71/231 (30.7%)	Hospital mortality 23/71 (32.4%)
Trinh et al. [77]	2017	Canada	Deceased donor liver transplant	491	491 (100%)	AKI; KDIGO criteria within 7 days after transplant	AKI 278/491 (56.6%)	N/A
Kalisvaart et al. [78]	2017	Netherlands	Donation after brain death liver transplant	155	155 (100%) DBD 155 (100%)	AKI; AKIN criteria within 7 days after transplant	AKI 61/155 (39.4%) Dialysis 5/155 (3.2%)	Hospital mortality 9/61 (15%)
Chen et al. (2) [79]	2017	China	Liver transplant in hepatocellular carcinoma	566	N/A	AKI; AKIN criteria within 48 hours after transplant	AKI 109/566 (19.3%) Dialysis 13/566 (2.3%)	30-day mortality 9/109 (8%)

Table 1. *Cont.*

Study	Year	Country	Procedure/Patients	Number	Deceased Donor	AKI Definition	Incidence	Mortality in AKI
Baron-Stefaniak et al. [80]	2017	Austria	Orthotopic liver transplant	45	N/A	AKI; KDIGO criteria within 48 hours after transplant	AKI 34/45 (75.6)	N/A
Zhou et al. [30]	2017	China	Donation after circulatory death orthotopic liver transplant	103	103 (100%) DCD 103 (100%)	AKI; KDIGO criteria within 7 days after transplant	AKI 42/103 (40.8%) CRRT 7/103 (6.8%)	N/A
Yoo et al. [31]	2017	Korea	Liver transplant	304	84 (28%)	AKI; RIFLE criteria within 7 days after transplant	AKI 132/304 (43.4%)	N/A
Jochmans [29]	2017	Belgium	Orthotopic liver transplant	80	80 (100%) DCD 13 (16%) DBD 67 (84%)	AKI; RIFLE criteria within 5 days after reperfusion	AKI 21/80 (26.3%) Dialysis 4/80 (5%)	1-year mortality 2/21 (10%)
Kandil et al. [28]	2017	Egypt	Living donor liver transplant	50	0 (0%)	AKI; AKIN criteria within 48 hours	AKI 23/50 (46%)	N/A
Kim et al. [14]	2018	Korea	Living donor liver transplant	583	0 (0%)	AKI; KDIGO criteria within 7 days after transplant	AKI 205/583 (35.2%)	N/A

Abbreviations: AKIN, Acute Kidney Injury Network; DCD, donation after circulatory death; EDC, extended donor criteria liver allografts; KDIGO, Kidney Disease Improving Global Outcomes; RIFLE, Risk, Injury, Failure, Loss of kidney function, and End-stage kidney disease; UK, United Kingdom; USA, United States of America.

3.1. Incidence of Post-LTx AKI

Overall, the pooled estimated incidence rates of post-LTx AKI and severe AKI requiring RRT following LTx were 40.7% (95% CI: 35.4%–46.2%, I^2 = 97%, Figure 2) and 7.7% (95% CI: 5.1%–11.4%, I^2 = 95%, Figure 3), respectively.

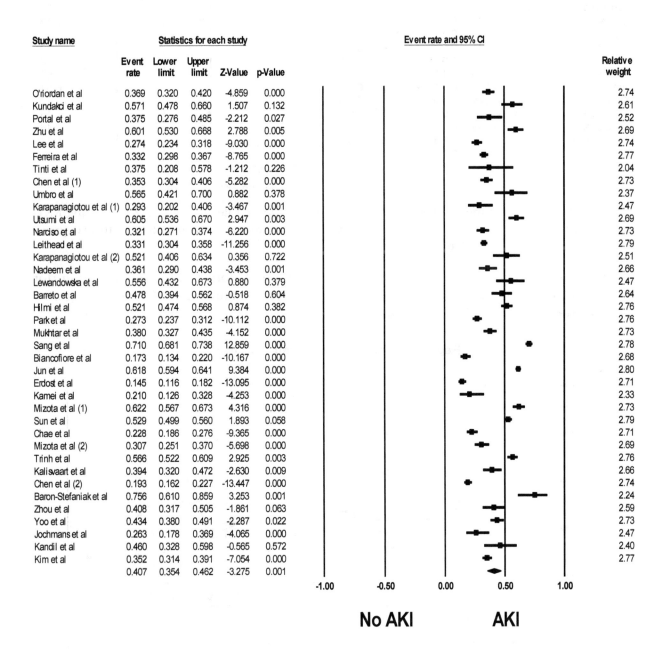

Study name	Event rate	Lower limit	Upper limit	Z-Value	p-Value		Relative weight
O'riordan et al	0.369	0.320	0.420	-4.859	0.000		2.74
Kundakci et al	0.571	0.478	0.660	1.507	0.132		2.61
Portal et al	0.375	0.276	0.485	-2.212	0.027		2.52
Zhu et al	0.601	0.530	0.668	2.788	0.005		2.69
Lee et al	0.274	0.234	0.318	-9.030	0.000		2.74
Ferreira et al	0.332	0.298	0.367	-8.765	0.000		2.77
Tinti et al	0.375	0.208	0.578	-1.212	0.226		2.04
Chen et al (1)	0.353	0.304	0.406	-5.282	0.000		2.73
Umbro et al	0.565	0.421	0.700	0.882	0.378		2.37
Karapanagiotou et al (1)	0.293	0.202	0.406	-3.467	0.001		2.47
Utsumi et al	0.605	0.536	0.670	2.947	0.003		2.69
Narciso et al	0.321	0.271	0.374	-6.220	0.000		2.73
Leithead et al	0.331	0.304	0.358	-11.256	0.000		2.79
Karapanagiotou et al (2)	0.521	0.406	0.634	0.356	0.722		2.51
Nadeem et al	0.361	0.290	0.438	-3.453	0.001		2.66
Lewandowska et al	0.556	0.432	0.673	0.880	0.379		2.47
Barreto et al	0.478	0.394	0.562	-0.518	0.604		2.64
Hilmi et al	0.521	0.474	0.568	0.874	0.382		2.76
Park et al	0.273	0.237	0.312	-10.112	0.000		2.76
Mukhtar et al	0.380	0.327	0.435	-4.152	0.000		2.73
Sang et al	0.710	0.681	0.738	12.859	0.000		2.78
Biancofiore et al	0.173	0.134	0.220	-10.167	0.000		2.68
Jun et al	0.618	0.594	0.641	9.384	0.000		2.80
Erdost et al	0.145	0.116	0.182	-13.095	0.000		2.71
Kamei et al	0.210	0.126	0.328	-4.253	0.000		2.33
Mizota et al (1)	0.622	0.567	0.673	4.316	0.000		2.73
Sun et al	0.529	0.499	0.560	1.893	0.058		2.79
Chae et al	0.228	0.186	0.276	-9.365	0.000		2.71
Mizota et al (2)	0.307	0.251	0.370	-5.698	0.000		2.69
Trinh et al	0.566	0.522	0.609	2.925	0.003		2.76
Kalisvaart et al	0.394	0.320	0.472	-2.630	0.009		2.66
Chen et al (2)	0.193	0.162	0.227	-13.447	0.000		2.74
Baron-Stefaniak et al	0.756	0.610	0.859	3.253	0.001		2.24
Zhou et al	0.408	0.317	0.505	-1.861	0.063		2.59
Yoo et al	0.434	0.380	0.491	-2.287	0.022		2.73
Jochmans et al	0.263	0.178	0.369	-4.065	0.000		2.47
Kandil et al	0.460	0.328	0.598	-0.565	0.572		2.40
Kim et al	0.352	0.314	0.391	-7.054	0.000		2.77
	0.407	0.354	0.462	-3.275	0.001		

Figure 2. Forest plots of the included studies assessing incidence rates of post-LTx AKI. A diamond data marker represents the overall rate from each included study (square data marker) and 95% confidence interval.

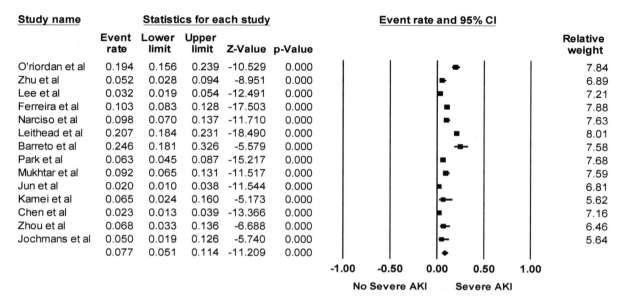

Figure 3. Forest plots of the included studies assessing incidence rates of severe AKI requiring RRT following LTx. A diamond data marker represents the overall rate from each included study (square data marker) and 95% confidence interval.

Meta-regression showed no significant impact of type of donor (deceased vs living donors) ($p = 0.33$) on the incidence of post-LTx AKI. In addition, the year of study ($p = 0.81$) did not significantly affect the incidence of post-LTx AKI (Figure 4).

Regression of Logit event rate on Year

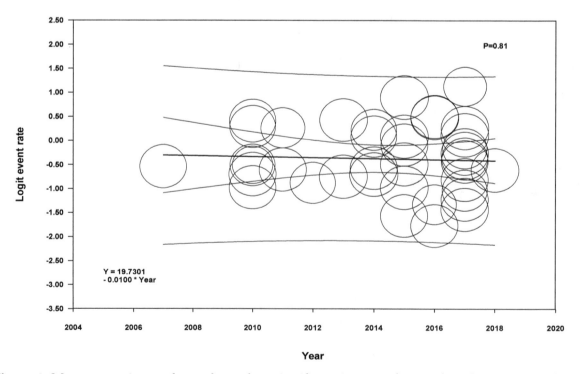

Figure 4. Meta-regression analyses showed no significant impact of year of study on the incidence of post-LTx AKI ($p = 0.81$). The solid black line represents the weighted regression line based on variance-weighted least squares. The inner and outer lines show the 95% confidence interval and prediction interval around the regression line. The circles indicate log event rates in each study.

3.2. *Risk Factors for Post-LTx AKI*

Reported risk factors for post-LTx AKI are demonstrated in Table 2. Higher pretransplant SCr [11,23–25,32–35], high body mass index (BMI) [39,64,66,67], high MELD/MELD-Na score [23,39–49], intraoperative blood loss and perioperative blood transfusion [18,25,39,48,54,65], high APACHE II score [25,43,48,55], hypotension and vasopressor requirement [18,24,48,54], cold and warm ischemia time [14,35,78], graft dysfunction [11,40,53], post-reperfusion syndrome [20,64,66,75,78], infection prior to transplant [25,45,48], and hypoalbuminemia [18,64,66] were consistently identified as important risk factors for Post-LTx AKI.

3.3. *Impacts of Post-LTx AKI on Patient Outcomes*

The impacts of post-LTx AKI on patient outcomes are demonstrated in Table 3. Overall, the pooled estimated in-hospital or 30-day mortality, and 1-year mortality rates of patients with post-LTx AKI were 16.5% (95% CI: 10.8%–24.3%, $I^2 = 94\%$) and 31.1% (95% CI: 22.4%–41.5%, $I^2 = 78\%$), respectively. Post-LTx AKI was associated with significantly higher mortality with a pooled OR of 2.96 (95% CI: 2.32–3.77, $I^2 = 59\%$). In addition, severe post-LTx AKI requiring RRT was associated with significantly higher mortality with a pooled OR of 8.15 (95% CI: 4.52–14.69, $I^2 = 90\%$). Compared to those without post-LTx AKI, recipients with post-LTx AKI had significantly increased risks of liver graft failure and CKD with pooled ORs of 3.76 (95% CI: 1.56–9.03, $I^2 = 91\%$, Figure 5) and 2.35 (95% CI: 1.53–3.61, $I^2 = 75\%$, Figure 6), respectively. AKI was associated with prolonged intensive care (ICU) and hospital stay [17,18,23,24,29,32,35,40,42,44,48,49,53,61,64,75,78] (Table 3).

Study name	Odds ratio	Lower limit	Upper limit	Z-Value	p-Value	Relative weight
Bilbao et al	4.110	1.811	9.326	3.381	0.001	19.65
Barri et al	2.560	1.732	3.784	4.714	0.000	22.65
Chen et al	1.910	0.891	4.094	1.663	0.096	20.11
Jochmans et al	2.540	0.611	10.563	1.282	0.200	14.58
Zongyi et al	11.730	8.569	16.058	15.367	0.000	23.02
	3.756	1.563	9.025	2.958	0.003	

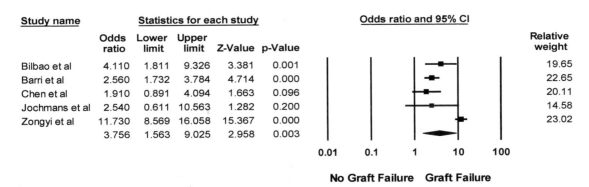

Figure 5. Forest plots of the included studies assessing liver graft failure among patients with post-LTx AKI. A diamond data marker represents the overall rate from each included study (square data marker) and 95% confidence interval.

Study name	Odds ratio	Lower limit	Upper limit	Z-Value	p-Value	Relative weight
Ferreira et al	4.840	3.447	6.795	9.110	0.000	17.89
Lee et al	1.540	1.017	2.333	2.038	0.042	16.95
Hilmi et al	1.690	1.109	2.577	2.439	0.015	16.86
Inoue et al	2.330	0.657	8.258	1.310	0.190	7.33
Mizota et al	2.460	1.508	4.014	3.604	0.000	15.96
Trinh et al	2.390	1.274	4.484	2.714	0.007	14.06
Jochmans et al	1.170	0.399	3.431	0.286	0.775	8.89
Utsumi et al	25.973	1.529	441.132	2.254	0.024	2.06
	2.347	1.528	3.605	3.894	0.000	

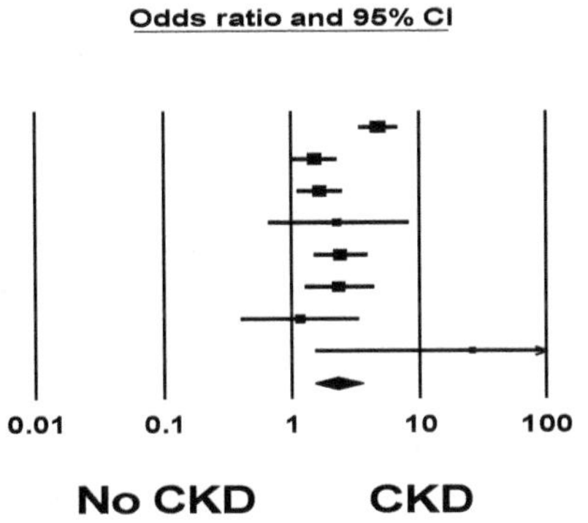

Figure 6. Forest plots of the included studies assessing CKD risk among patients with post-LTx AKI. A diamond data marker represents the overall rate from each included study (square data marker) and 95% confidence interval.

Table 2. Reported Potential Predictors/Associated-Risk Factors of Post-LTx AKI.

Donor and Graft Factors	Recipient Factors	Surgical and Postoperative Factors
Cold ischemia time [14,35,78], warm ischemic time [35,39,63,64,66], Small-for-size graft/Graft-recipient body weight ratio [40,44,65,66], Deceased donor [20,47], Graft dysfunction [11,53], DCD [39], ABO incompatibility [70], Lower donor BMI [39], Older donor age [39]	Higher MELD score/MELD-Na [23,39-49,64,67,89], APACHE II25 [43,48,55], Preoperative SCr11 [23-25,32-35], Preoperative BUN [23,24], Preoperative renal dysfunction/ARF [40,43,53], Child-Pugh score [19], SOFA [48], Male sex [42], female sex [19,31], Preoperative hepatic encephalopathy [47], Infection [25,48,71], Hypoalbuminemia [18,53,64,66], Preoperative low hemoglobin [14,72], High body weight, BMI [14,19,39,44,64,66,67,75], Pretransplant hypertension [32,54], Preoperative DM [19,44], Alcoholic liver disease [32], Pretransplant hepatitis B and/or C [54,63], Tumor as indication for transplant [47], Elevated lactate [54,63], Elevated plasma NGAL [55], Hyponatremia [39], Pulmonary hypertension [31]	Intra-operative hypotension, low MAP [24,33,34,54,66,79], Inotrope/vasopressor requirement [18,30,32,48,65], dopamine [35], intra-operative need of noradrenaline [33,67], Duration of treatment with dopamine [53], Blood loss [35,44,47,64,70,71], RBC transfusion [14,18,25,33,39,48,54,65,66,72,89], Need of cryoprecipitate [64], Anesthetic/Operation time [30,64,66,70], Post-reperfusion syndrome [20,64,66,78], SvO2 reduction with oliguria [14], Oxygen content 5 min after graft reperfusion [75], Terlipressin (protective) [65], Venovenous bypass (protective) [21], Postoperative ICU days [23,48], Duration of ventilator support [48], Aminoglycoside use [32], Duration of anhepatic phase [41,79], Intra-operative acidosis [41], Intra-operative urine output [14,24,30,33], Overexposure to calcineurin inhibitor [35,44,64], Need of diuretics [46,75], Chloride-liberal fluid received within the 24 h posttransplant [49], Crystalloid administration [14], Use of 6% HES [89], Mean blood glucose during the day of surgery [64], glucose variability [31], Peak AST occurring at 6 h [29]

Abbreviations:: ABO incompatibility, incompatibility of the ABO blood group; AKI, acute kidney injury; AKIN, Acute Kidney Injury Network; ALP, alkaline phosphatase; APACHE, Acute Physiology and Chronic Health Evaluation; ARI, acute renal injury; ARF, acute renal failure; AST, aspartate aminotransferase; ATG, Anti-thymocyte globulin; BMI, body mass index; BUN, blood urea nitrogen; CMV, cytomegalovirus; DBD, graft donated after brain death; DCD, donation after circulatory death; DM, diabetes mellitus; eGFR, estimated glomerular filtration rate; FFP, fresh frozen plasma; HCV, hepatitis C virus; HES, hydroxyethyl starch; ICU, intensive care unit; KDIGO, Kidney Disease Improving Global Outcomes; SCr, serum creatinine; MAP, mean arterial pressure; MELD, Model For End-Stage Liver Disease; MME, mycophenolate mofetil; N/A, not available; NGAL, neutrophil gelatinase-associated lipocalin; PBC, primary biliary cirrhosis; RBC, red blood cell; RRT, renal replacement therapy; RIFLE, Risk, Injury, Failure, Loss of kidney function, and End-stage kidney disease; SOFA, Sequential Organ Failure Assessment; SvO2, mixed venous oxygen saturation.

Table 3. Reported Outcomes of Post-LTx AKI.

Study	Outcomes	Confounder Adjustment
Bilbao et al. [11]	Mortality Dialysis: 6.47 (2.73–15.35) Graft failure Dialysis: 4.11 (1.81–9.32)	None
Contreras et al. [24]	Hospital mortality Dialysis: 9.91 (3.45–28.51) ICU LOS Dialysis: 15 ± 13 vs. 7 ± 11 days Hospital LOS Dialysis: 34 ± 27 vs. 19 ± 20 days	None
Lebrón Gallardo et al. [25]	Mortality Early renal dysfunction: 2.47 (1.29–4.72) Dialysis: 8.80 (3.65–21.23)	None
Sanchez et al. [23]	1-year mortality Dialysis: 9.07 (5.49–14.97) ICU LOS 2.1 ± 3.0 in no dialysis vs. 8.6 ± 11.6 in hemodialysis vs. 10.5 ± 12.8 days in CRRT	None
Wyatt et al. [22]	Mortality ARF without RRT: 8.69 (3.25–23.19) ARF with RRT: 12.07 (3.90–37.32)	Age, sex, race, DM, transplant centers
Cabezuelo et al. [53]	ICU LOS ARF: 12.9 ± 7.4 vs. 7.2 ± 4.0 days	N/A
O'Riordan et al. [32]	1-year mortality ARF: 2.6 (1.5–4.5) Hospital LOS 39.3 ± 79.5 in no ARI/ARF vs. 53.3 ± 72.8 in ARI vs. 73.0 ± 129.8 days in ARF	DM, pretransplant, SCr, PBC, inotrope use, CMV infection/disease, rejection
Lee et al. [40]	Hospital LOS Renal dysfunction: 75 ± 144 vs. 45.2 ± 34.5 days	N/A
Rueggeberg et al. [54]	1-year mortality AKI: 10.93 (3.64–32.83)	None
Barri et al. [17]	2-year mortality AKI: 2.33 (1.53–3.53) 2-year graft failure AKI: 2.56 (1.73–3.78) ICU LOS AKI: 8 ± 19 vs. 3 ± 5 days Hospital LOS AKI: 20 ± 24 vs. 11 ± 10 days	None
Kundakci et al. [41]	1-year mortality AKI: 6.73 (2.15–21.06)	None

Table 3. *Cont.*

Study	Outcomes	Confounder Adjustment
Zhu et al. [42]	1-year mortality AKI: 12.1 (1.57–93.54) ICU LOS AKI: 6 (4–9) vs. 4 (3–5) days Hospital LOS AKI: 29 (16–47) vs. 29 (20–48) days	Hypertension, infection and APACHE II
Ferreira et al. [57]	Mortality AKI: 0.73 (0.59–1.08) CKD AKI: 4.84 (3.45–6.80)	None
Lee et al. [56]	CKD AKI: 1.54 (1.02–2.34)	Age, sex, period of transplant, BMI, pretransplant DM, pretransplant hypertension, history of cardiovascular disease, donor type, underlying liver disease, HBV-related liver disease, hepatocellular carcinoma, use of adefovir, calcineurin inhibitors, purine metabolism inhibitors, acute rejection, pretransplant hemoglobin, pretransplant GFR, pretransplant proteinuria, hepatorenal syndrome, Child-Pugh score, MELD score
Chen et al. [18]	1-year mortality ARI/ARF: 2.79 (0.96–8.12) 1-year graft failure ARI/ARF: 1.91 (0.89–4.09) Hospital LOS 21.8 ± 22.1 in no ARI/ARF vs. 24 ± 25 in ARI and 37 ± 49 days in ARF	None
Karapanagiotou et al. [43]	1-year mortality 9.61 (1.48–62.55)	Infection, hemorrhage, MELD, APACHE score
Utsumi et al. [44]	Hospital mortality AKI: 5.04 (1.11–22.81) ARI/ARF: 5.90 (1.83–19.06) 1-year mortality AKI: 9.53 (2.18–41.56) ARI/ARF: 12.90 (4.24–39.30) CKD AKI: 15/107 (14%) vs. 0/77 (0%) ARI/ARF: 35.29 (4.51–275.82) Hospital LOS ARI/ARF: 101.5 ± 68.8 vs. 69.7 ± 48.5 days	None
Narciso et al. [60]	Mortality Dialysis: 6.7 (3.49–12.96)	None
Romano et al. [45]	Hospital mortality AKI: 1.88 (0.76–4.65)	None

Table 3. *Cont.*

Study	Outcomes	Confounder Adjustment
Leithead et al. [39]	Mortality 1.71 (1.35–2.17)	Age, sex, MELD score, eGFR, DM
Klaus et al. [46]	Mortality AKI: 5.11 (1.39–18.71) Dialysis:14.4 (4.60–45.09)	None
Kim et al. [47]	1-year mortality Dialysis: 56.5 (12.32–259.20)	None
Karapanagiotou et al. [48]	6-month mortality RIFLE: 3.08 (1.09–1.95) AKIN: 9.34 (1.20–15.69) ICU LOS RIFLE: 15.44 ± 15.41 vs. 8.65 ± 12.59 days AKIN: 13.75 ± 14.53 vs. 9.1 ± 13.08 days	Vasopressor use, RBC transfusion
Nadeem et al. [49]	ICU LOS AKI: 13.4 ± 19 vs. 5.5 ± 4.7 days	N/A
Kirnap et al. [61]	Mortality AKI: 1.85 (0.65–5.23) ICU LOS AKI: 10 ± 8 vs. 3 ± 2 days Hospital LOS AKI: 26 ± 70 vs. 16 ± 7 days	None
Barreto et al. [63]	Hospital mortality AKIN stage 2 or 3: 4.3 (1.3–14.6)	None
Hilmi et al. [19]	30-day mortality AKI: 3/221(1.4%) vs. 0/203 (0%) CKD AKI: 1.69 (1.11–2.58)	None
Park et al. [64]	Hospital mortality 3.44 (1.89–6.25) 1-year mortality AKI: 1.57 (0.95–2.58) ICU LOS 6 (6–7) in no AKI vs. 6 (6–9) in Risk vs. 7 (6–18) in Injury vs. 11 (10–85) in Failure group Hospital LOS 29 (23–42) in no AKI vs. 31 (21–43) in Risk vs. 33 (26–47) in Injury vs. 46 (16–108) in Failure group	None
Mukhtar et al. [65]	Mortality AKI: 2.1 (1.18–4.0)	Graft weight to recipient body weight ratio, baseline creatinine, MELD score, DM, Terlipressin use, massive transfusion, vasopressor use

Table 3. *Cont.*

Study	Outcomes	Confounder Adjustment
Sang et al. [66]	Mortality RIFLE AKI: 2.29 (1.29–4.05) AKIN AKI: 1.69 (1.06–2.67)	None
Wyssusek et al. [67]	Mortality AKI: 3.23 (0.43–24.27)	None
Jun et al. [70]	Mortality AKI: 0.36 (0.09–1.43)	ABO incompatibility, MELD score, hypertension, coronary artery disease, age, post-reperfusion syndrome, vasopressor, crystalloid, RBC transfusion, FFP transfusion, operation time, cold ischemic time
Inoue et al. [71]	1-year mortality AKI: 4.54 (1.27–16.32) CKD AKI: 2.33 (0.66–8.29)	None
Mizota et al. [74]	Hospital mortality AKI: 2.53 (1.23–5.22) CKD AKI: 2.46 (1.51–4.02)	Age, MELD score, blood type incompatibility, re-transplantation
Erdost et al. [72]	30-day mortality RIFLE AKI: 4.15 (1.72–10.00) AKIN AKI: 440.83 (58.24–3336.87) KDIGO AKI: 35/64 (55%) vs. 0/376	None
Chae et al. [75]	Hospital mortality AKI: 1.63 (0.73–3.60) ICU LOS AKI: 7 (6–8) vs. 7 (5–7) days Hospital LOS AKI: 28 (22–39) vs. 23 (21–31) days	None
Mizota et al. [76]	Hospital mortality Severe AKI: 3.56 (1.78–7.09)	None
Trinh et al. [77]	Mortality AKI: 1.41 (1.03–1.92) CKD stage 4–5 AKI: 2.39 (1.27–4.47)	Age, sex, MELD score, baseline eGFR, ATG induction, pretransplant hypertension and DM
Kalisvaart et al. [78]	Hospital mortality AKI: 7.96 (1.66–38.25) ICU LOS AKI: 3 (2–5) vs. 2 (2–3) days Hospital LOS AKI: 24 (19–35) vs. 17 (14–27) days	None

Table 3. *Cont.*

Study	Outcomes	Confounder Adjustment
Nadkarni et al. [16]	Hospital mortality Dialysis: 2.00 (1.55–2.59)	Not specified
Chen et al. [79]	30-day mortality AKI: 4.05 (1.02–16.18)	ALP, MELD score, operation time, blood transfusion
Zongyi et al. [35]	1-year mortality RIFLE failure stage AKI: 12.25 (8.99–16.70) 1-year graft failure RIFLE failure stage AKI: 11.73 (8.57–16.06) Hospital LOS RIFLE failure stage AKI: 16 (6–34.5) vs. 25 (18–35) days	None
Zhou et al. [30]	14-day mortality AKI: 3.35 (0.94–11.98) Hospital LOS AKI: 28.13 ± 20.04 vs. 26.16 ± 11.91 days	None
Jochmans et al. [29]	1-year mortality AKI: 6.11 (0.52–71.16) 1-year graft failure AKI: 2.54 (0.61–10.55) CKD AKI:1.17 (0.40–3.44) ICU LOS AKI: 4 (3–9) vs. 2 (2–4) Hospital LOS AKI: 23 (17–46) vs. 16 (13–26)	None

Abbreviations:: ABO incompatibility, incompatibility of the ABO blood group; AKI, acute kidney injury; AKIN, Acute Kidney Injury Network; ALP, alkaline phosphatase; APACHE, Acute Physiology and Chronic Health Evaluation; ARI, acute renal injury; ARF, acute renal failure; AST, aspartate aminotransferase; ATG, Anti-thymocyte globulin; BMI, body mass index; BUN, blood urea nitrogen; CMV, cytomegalovirus; DCD, donation after circulatory death; DM, diabetes mellitus; eGFR, estimated glomerular filtration rate; FFP, fresh frozen plasma; HCV, hepatitis C virus; HES, hydroxyethyl starch; ICU, intensive care unit; KDIGO, Kidney Disease Improving Global Outcomes; SCr, serum creatinine; MAP, mean arterial pressure; MELD, Model For End-Stage Liver Disease; MMF, mycophenolate mofetil; N/A, not available; NGAL, neutrophil gelatinase-associated lipocalin; PBC, primary biliary cirrhosis; RBC, red blood cell; RRT, renal replacement therapy; RIFLE, Risk, Injury, Failure, Loss of kidney function, and End-stage kidney disease; SOFA, Sequential Organ Failure Assessment; SvO2, mixed venous oxygen saturation.

3.4. Evaluation for Publication Bias

Funnel plot (Supplementary Figure S1) and Egger's regression asymmetry test were performed to evaluate for publication bias in the analysis evaluating incidence of post-LTx AKI and mortality risk of post-LTx AKI. There was no significant publication bias in meta-analysis assessing the incidence of post-LTx AKI, p-value = 0.12.

4. Discussion

In this meta-analysis, we found that AKI and severe AKI requiring RRT after LTx are common, with an incidence of 40.8% and 7.0%, respectively. In addition, our findings showed no significant correlation between the incidence of post-LTx AKI and study year for the ten years of the study. Furthermore, compared to patients without post-LTx AKI, those with post-LTx AKI carry a 2.96-fold increased risk of mortality and a 3.76-fold higher risk of liver graft failure.

The development of post-LTx AKI appears to be multifactorial with a number of preoperative, intraoperative and postoperative factors involved [90]. Pre-LTx factors include high MELD/MELD-Na score, high APACHE II score, hypoalbuminemia, and reduced eGFR [11,23–25,32–35]. Preexisting renal impairment is common among patients with end-stage liver disease [91]. Although cirrhotic patients with significant CKD are eligible to receive a combined liver-kidney transplantation [92], a lower baseline GFR among those who received LTx alone remained an important risk factor for post-operative AKI [11,23–25,32–35]. Studies have demonstrated that hepatorenal syndrome before LTx can also lead to renal insufficiency and render LTx recipients more susceptible to post-LTx AKI [22,90,93]. In addition, sepsis, graft dysfunction, thrombotic microangiopathy, and calcineurin inhibitor nephrotoxicity may all contribute to AKI [22,37,94–96].

Studies have shown that higher MELD scores were associated with post-LTx AKI [23,39–49]. In patients with high MELD scores >30, the majority required RRT post LTx [44,97]. Although SCr is an important determinant of the MELD score, other components of MELD such as pre-LTx INR has also been demonstrated to be strongly associated with post-LT AKI, suggesting that the severity of the liver disease itself, as reflected by the MELD score, is associated with post-LT AKI [45]. Identified perioperative factors for post-LTx AKI include cardiopulmonary failure, vasopressor requirement, hemodynamic effects of prolonged surgery, and blood loss/RBC transfusion [18,24,25,39,48,54,65]. Moreover, it has been hypothesized that HIRI is an important cause of post-LTx AKI [37,38]. Aspartate aminotransferase (AST), as a surrogate marker for HIRI, has been shown to be correlated with post-LTx AKI. [38,78] HIRI has a close relationship with the systemic inflammatory response, which in turn is related to AKI and multiorgan dysfunction in similar settings such as sepsis [37]. Early hepatic graft dysfunction has also been shown to be associated to post-LTx AKI [98]. In addition, recipients of donation after circulatory death (DCD) grafts are reported to have a higher incidence of post-LTx AKI compared to donation after brain death (DBD grafts). After DCD LTx, peak AST levels were an independent predictor of post-LTx AKI [99]. Other known factors that influence HIRI such as donor age, cold and warm ischemia times and graft steatosis have also been associated with post-LTx AKI [37].

As demonstrated in our study, post-LTx AKI is associated with an increased risk of death and liver graft failure. Several pharmacological and non-pharmacological interventions have been studied, but so far these have failed to demonstrate any significant benefit in the prevention of post-LTx AKI [37,100,101]. To continue efforts to mitigate post-LTx AKI, it is important to identify those who are at high-risk for post-LTx AKI in order to develop earlier protective strategies [37]. There have been many attempts to develop predictive models for post-LTx AKI [37]. Seven published predictive models addressing a diverse range of AKI definitions for post-LT AKI have been developed [19,23,24,33,47,54,55]. However, the numbers of patients in these studies were limited [19,23,24,33,47,54,55], and future prospective external validation, ideally with multi-center studies with large number of patients, is required.

Several limitations in our meta-analysis are worth mentioning. First, there were statistical heterogeneities present in our study. Possible sources for heterogeneities were the differences in the patient characteristics in the individual studies. However, we performed a meta-regression analysis which demonstrated that the type of donor (deceased vs. living donors); the year of study did not significantly affect the incidence of post-LTx AKI. Second, there is a lack of data from included studies on novel AKI biomarkers. Novel biomarkers for AKI are emerging and could be useful for the early identification and characterization of AKI. Thus, future studies evaluating predictive models with novel biomarkers are needed. Lastly, this is a systematic review and meta-analysis of cohort studies. Thus, it can demonstrate associations of post-LTx AKI with increased risk of mortality and liver graft failure, but not a causal relationship.

5. Conclusions

In conclusion, there are overall high incidence rates of post-LTx AKI and severe AKI requiring RRT of 40.8% and 7.0%. Post-LTx AKI is significantly associated with increased mortality and liver graft failure. In addition, the incidence of post-LTx AKI has remained stable over time. This study provides an epidemiological perspective to support the need for future large-scale multi-center studies to identify preventive strategies for post-LTx AKI.

Author Contributions: Conceptualization, M.A.M. and W.C.; Data curation, C.T., N.T., and K.W. Formal analysis, C.T. and W.C.; Investigation, C.T., N.T., T.B., P.L., K.S., S.A.S., P.U. and W.C.; Methodology, C.T., W.K., T.B., P.U., K.W., P.T.K., N.R.A. and W.C.; Project administration, W.K., T.B., K.W., P.L., K.S. and S.A.S.; Resources, T.B., K.W., P.L., K.S. and S.A.S. and P.U.; Software, K.W.; Supervision, W.K., M.A.M. and W.C.; Validation, P.U., M.A.M. and W.C.; Visualization, W.C.; Writing—original draft, C.T.; Writing—review & editing, C.T., W.K., N.T., T.B., K.W., P.L., K.S. and S.A.S., P.U., K.W., P.T.K., N.R.A., M.A.M. and W.C.

Acknowledgments: None. All authors had access to the data and played essential roles in writing of the manuscript.

References

1. Gameiro, J.; Agapito Fonseca, J.; Jorge, S.; Lopes, J.A. Acute Kidney Injury Definition and Diagnosis: A Narrative Review. *J. Clin. Med.* **2018**, *7*, 307. [CrossRef] [PubMed]
2. Hoste, E.A.J.; Kellum, J.A.; Selby, N.M.; Zarbock, A.; Palevsky, P.M.; Bagshaw, S.M.; Goldstein, S.L.; Cerdá, J.; Chawla, L.S. Global epidemiology and outcomes of acute kidney injury. *Nat. Rev. Nephrol.* **2018**, *14*, 607–625. [CrossRef] [PubMed]
3. Mehta, R.L.; Burdmann, E.A.; Cerdá, J.; Feehally, J.; Finkelstein, F.; García-García, G.; Godin, M.; Jha, V.; Lameire, N.H.; Levin, N.W.; et al. Recognition and management of acute kidney injury in the International Society of Nephrology 0by25 Global Snapshot: A multinational cross-sectional study. *Lancet* **2016**, *387*, 2017–2025. [CrossRef]
4. Mehta, R.L.; Burdmann, E.A.; Cerdá, J.; Feehally, J.; Finkelstein, F.; García-García, G.; Godin, M.; Jha, V.; Lameire, N.H.; Levin, N.W.; et al. International Society of Nephrology's 0by25 initiative for acute kidney injury (zero preventable deaths by 2025): A human rights case for nephrology. *Lancet* **2015**, *385*, 2616–2643. [CrossRef]
5. Sawhney, S.; Marks, A.; Fluck, N.; Levin, A.; McLernon, D.; Prescott, G.; Black, C. Post-discharge kidney function is associated with subsequent ten-year renal progression risk among survivors of acute kidney injury. *Kidney Int.* **2017**, *92*, 440–452. [CrossRef]
6. Ponce, D.; Balbi, A. Acute kidney injury: Risk factors and management challenges in developing countries. *Int. J. Nephrol. Renov. Dis.* **2016**, *9*, 193–200. [CrossRef]
7. Pavkov, M.E.; Harding, J.L.; Burrows, N.R. Trends in Hospitalizations for Acute Kidney Injury—United States, 2000–2014. *Morb. Mortal. Wkly. Rep.* **2018**, *67*, 289. [CrossRef]

8. United States Renal Data System. 2017. Available online: https://www.usrds.org/2017/download/v1_c05_AKI_17.pdf (accessed on 15 February 2019).
9. Mokdad, A.A.; Lopez, A.D.; Shahraz, S.; Lozano, R.; Mokdad, A.H.; Stanaway, J.; Murray, C.J.; Naghavi, M. Liver cirrhosis mortality in 187 countries between 1980 and 2010: A systematic analysis. *BMC Med.* **2014**, *12*, 145. [CrossRef] [PubMed]
10. McCauley, J.; Van Thiel, D.H.; Starzl, T.E.; Puschett, J.B. Acute and chronic renal failure in liver transplantation. *Nephron* **1990**, *55*, 121–128. [CrossRef] [PubMed]
11. Bilbao, I.; Charco, R.; Balsells, J.; Lazaro, J.L.; Hidalgo, E.; Llopart, L.; Murio, E.; Margarit, C. Risk factors for acute renal failure requiring dialysis after liver transplantation. *Clin. Transplant.* **1998**, *12*, 123–129.
12. Carmona, M.; Álvarez, M.; Marco, J.; Mahíllo, B.; Domínguez-Gil, B.; Núñez, J.R.; Matesanz, R. Global Organ Transplant Activities in 2015. Data from the Global Observatory on Donation and Transplantation (GODT). *Transplantation* **2017**, *101*, S29. [CrossRef]
13. White, S.L.; Hirth, R.; Mahillo, B.; Dominguez-Gil, B.; Delmonico, F.L.; Noel, L.; Chapman, J.; Matesanz, R.; Carmona, M.; Alvarez, M.; et al. The global diffusion of organ transplantation: Trends, drivers and policy implications. *Bull. World Health Organ.* **2014**, *92*, 826–835. [CrossRef]
14. Kim, W.H.; Lee, H.C.; Lim, L.; Ryu, H.G.; Jung, C.W. Intraoperative Oliguria with Decreased SvO Predicts Acute Kidney Injury after Living Donor Liver Transplantation. *J. Clin. Med.* **2018**, *8*, 29. [CrossRef] [PubMed]
15. Hamada, M.; Matsukawa, S.; Shimizu, S.; Kai, S.; Mizota, T. Acute kidney injury after pediatric liver transplantation: Incidence, risk factors, and association with outcome. *J. Anesth.* **2017**, *31*, 758–763. [CrossRef] [PubMed]
16. Nadkarni, G.N.; Chauhan, K.; Patel, A.; Saha, A.; Poojary, P.; Kamat, S.; Patel, S.; Ferrandino, R.; Konstantinidis, I.; Garimella, P.S.; et al. Temporal trends of dialysis requiring acute kidney injury after orthotopic cardiac and liver transplant hospitalizations. *BMC Nephrol.* **2017**, *18*, 244. [CrossRef] [PubMed]
17. Barri, Y.M.; Sanchez, E.Q.; Jennings, L.W.; Melton, L.B.; Hays, S.; Levy, M.F.; Klintmalm, G.B. Acute kidney injury following liver transplantation: Definition and outcome. *Liver Transplant.* **2009**, *15*, 475–483. [CrossRef] [PubMed]
18. Chen, J.; Singhapricha, T.; Hu, K.Q.; Hong, J.C.; Steadman, R.H.; Busuttil, R.W.; Xia, V.W. Postliver transplant acute renal injury and failure by the RIFLE criteria in patients with normal pretransplant serum creatinine concentrations: A matched study. *Transplantation* **2011**, *91*, 348–353. [CrossRef] [PubMed]
19. Hilmi, I.A.; Damian, D.; Al-Khafaji, A.; Planinsic, R.; Boucek, C.; Sakai, T.; Chang, C.C.; Kellum, J.A. Acute kidney injury following orthotopic liver transplantation: Incidence, risk factors, and effects on patient and graft outcomes. *Br. J. Anaesth.* **2015**, *114*, 919–926. [CrossRef]
20. Hilmi, I.A.; Damian, D.; Al-Khafaji, A.; Sakai, T.; Donaldson, J.; Winger, D.G.; Kellum, J.A. Acute kidney injury after orthotopic liver transplantation using living donor versus deceased donor grafts: A propensity score-matched analysis. *Liver Transplant.* **2015**, *21*, 1179–1185. [CrossRef]
21. Sun, K.; Hong, F.; Wang, Y.; Agopian, V.G.; Yan, M.; Busuttil, R.W.; Steadman, R.H.; Xia, V.W. Venovenous Bypass Is Associated With a Lower Incidence of Acute Kidney Injury After Liver Transplantation in Patients with Compromised Pretransplant Renal Function. *Anesth. Analg.* **2017**, *125*, 1463–1470. [CrossRef]
22. Wyatt, C.M.; Arons, R.R. The burden of acute renal failure in nonrenal solid organ transplantation. *Transplantation* **2004**, *78*, 1351–1355. [CrossRef] [PubMed]
23. Sanchez, E.Q.; Gonwa, T.A.; Levy, M.F.; Goldstein, R.M.; Mai, M.L.; Hays, S.R.; Melton, L.B.; Saracino, G.; Klintmalm, G.B. Preoperative and perioperative predictors of the need for renal replacement therapy after orthotopic liver transplantation. *Transplantation* **2004**, *78*, 1048–1054. [CrossRef] [PubMed]
24. Contreras, G.; Garces, G.; Quartin, A.A.; Cely, C.; LaGatta, M.A.; Barreto, G.A.; Roth, D.; Gomez, E. An epidemiologic study of early renal replacement therapy after orthotopic liver transplantation. *J. Am. Soc. Nephrol.* **2002**, *13*, 228–233.
25. Lebron Gallardo, M.; Herrera Gutierrez, M.E.; Seller Perez, G.; Curiel Balsera, E.; Fernandez Ortega, J.F.; Quesada Garcia, G. Risk factors for renal dysfunction in the postoperative course of liver transplant. *Liver Transplant.* **2004**, *10*, 1379–1385. [CrossRef]
26. Alvares-da-Silva, M.R.; Waechter, F.L.; Francisconi, C.F.; Barros, E.; Thome, F.; Traiber, C.; Fonseca, D.L.; Zingani, J.M.; Sampaio, J.A.; Pinto, R.D.; et al. Risk factors for postoperative acute renal failure at a new orthotopic liver transplantation program. *Transplant. Proc.* **1999**, *31*, 3050–3052. [CrossRef]

27.   Rossi, A.P.; Vella, J.P. Acute Kidney Disease After Liver and Heart Transplantation. *Transplantation* **2016**, *100*, 506–514. [CrossRef] [PubMed]

28.   Kandil, M.A.; Abouelenain, K.M.; Alsebaey, A.; Rashed, H.S.; Afifi, M.H.; Mahmoud, M.A.; Yassen, K.A. Impact of terlipressin infusion during and after live donor liver transplantation on incidence of acute kidney injury and neutrophil gelatinase-associated lipocalin serum levels: A randomized controlled trial. *Clin. Transplant.* **2017**, *31*, e13019. [CrossRef] [PubMed]

29.   Jochmans, I.; Meurisse, N.; Neyrinck, A.; Verhaegen, M.; Monbaliu, D.; Pirenne, J. Hepatic ischemia/reperfusion injury associates with acute kidney injury in liver transplantation: Prospective cohort study. *Liver Transplant.* **2017**, *23*, 634–644. [CrossRef]

30.   Zhou, Z.Q.; Fan, L.C.; Zhao, X.; Xia, W.; Luo, A.L.; Tian, Y.K.; Wang, X.R. Risk factors for acute kidney injury after orthotopic liver transplantation: A single-center data analysis. *J. Huazhong Univ. Sci. Technol. Med. Sci.* **2017**, *37*, 861–863. [CrossRef]

31.   Yoo, S.; Lee, H.J.; Lee, H.; Ryu, H.G. Association Between Perioperative Hyperglycemia or Glucose Variability and Postoperative Acute Kidney Injury After Liver Transplantation: A Retrospective Observational Study. *Anesth. Analg.* **2017**, *124*, 35–41. [CrossRef]

32.   O'Riordan, A.; Wong, V.; McQuillan, R.; McCormick, P.A.; Hegarty, J.E.; Watson, A.J. Acute renal disease, as defined by the RIFLE criteria, post-liver transplantation. *Am. J. Transplant.* **2007**, *7*, 168–176. [CrossRef]

33.   Xu, X.; Ling, Q.; Wei, Q.; Wu, J.; Gao, F.; He, Z.L.; Zhou, L.; Zheng, S.S. An effective model for predicting acute kidney injury after liver transplantation. *Hepatobiliary Pancreat. Dis. Int.* **2010**, *9*, 259–263.

34.   De Ataide, E.C.; Perales, S.R.; Bortoto, J.B.; Peres, M.A.O.; Filho, F.C.; Stucchi, R.S.B.; Udo, E.; Boin, I. Immunomodulation, Acute Renal Failure, and Complications of Basiliximab Use After Liver Transplantation: Analysis of 114 Patients and Literature Review. *Transplant. Proc.* **2017**, *49*, 852–857. [CrossRef] [PubMed]

35.   Zongyi, Y.; Baifeng, L.; Funian, Z.; Hao, L.; Xin, W. Risk factors of acute kidney injury after orthotopic liver transplantation in China. *Sci. Rep.* **2017**, *7*, 41555. [CrossRef]

36.   Croome, K.P.; Lee, D.D.; Croome, S.; Chadha, R.; Livingston, D.; Abader, P.; Keaveny, A.P.; Taner, C.B. The impact of post-reperfusion syndrome during liver transplantation using livers with significant macrosteatosis. *Am. J. Transplant.* **2019**. [CrossRef] [PubMed]

37.   De Haan, J.E.; Hoorn, E.J.; de Geus, H.R.H. Acute kidney injury after liver transplantation: Recent insights and future perspectives. *Best Pract. Res. Clin. Gastroenterol.* **2017**, *31*, 161–169. [CrossRef] [PubMed]

38.   Leithead, J.A.; Armstrong, M.J.; Corbett, C.; Andrew, M.; Kothari, C.; Gunson, B.K.; Muiesan, P.; Ferguson, J.W. Hepatic ischemia reperfusion injury is associated with acute kidney injury following donation after brain death liver transplantation. *Transpl. Int.* **2013**, *26*, 1116–1125. [CrossRef] [PubMed]

39.   Leithead, J.A.; Rajoriya, N.; Gunson, B.K.; Muiesan, P.; Ferguson, J.W. The evolving use of higher risk grafts is associated with an increased incidence of acute kidney injury after liver transplantation. *J. Hepatol.* **2014**, *60*, 1180–1186. [CrossRef] [PubMed]

40.   Lee, S.K.; Park, J.B.; Kim, S.J.; Choi, G.S.; Kim, D.J.; Kwon, C.H.; Joh, J.W. Early postoperative renal dysfunction in the adult living donor liver transplantation. *Transplant. Proc.* **2007**, *39*, 1517–1519. [CrossRef]

41.   Kundakci, A.; Pirat, A.; Komurcu, O.; Torgay, A.; Karakayali, H.; Arslan, G.; Haberal, M. Rifle criteria for acute kidney dysfunction following liver transplantation: Incidence and risk factors. *Transplant. Proc.* **2010**, *42*, 4171–4174. [CrossRef]

42.   Zhu, M.; Li, Y.; Xia, Q.; Wang, S.; Qiu, Y.; Che, M.; Dai, H.; Qian, J.; Ni, Z.; Axelsson, J.; et al. Strong impact of acute kidney injury on survival after liver transplantation. *Transplant. Proc.* **2010**, *42*, 3634–3638. [CrossRef] [PubMed]

43.   Karapanagiotou, A.; Kydona, C.; Dimitriadis, C.; Sgourou, K.; Giasnetsova, T.; Fouzas, I.; Imvrios, G.; Gritsi-Gerogianni, N. Acute kidney injury after orthotopic liver transplantation. *Transplant. Proc.* **2012**, *44*, 2727–2729. [CrossRef]

44.   Utsumi, M.; Umeda, Y.; Sadamori, H.; Nagasaka, T.; Takaki, A.; Matsuda, H.; Shinoura, S.; Yoshida, R.; Nobuoka, D.; Satoh, D.; et al. Risk factors for acute renal injury in living donor liver transplantation: Evaluation of the RIFLE criteria. *Transpl. Int.* **2013**, *26*, 842–852. [CrossRef] [PubMed]

45.   Romano, T.G.; Schmidtbauer, I.; Silva, F.M.; Pompilio, C.E.; D'Albuquerque, L.A.; Macedo, E. Role of MELD score and serum creatinine as prognostic tools for the development of acute kidney injury after liver transplantation. *PLoS ONE* **2013**, *8*, e64089. [CrossRef]

46. Klaus, F.; Keitel da Silva, C.; Meinerz, G.; Carvalho, L.M.; Goldani, J.C.; Cantisani, G.; Zanotelli, M.L.; Duro Garcia, V.; Keitel, E. Acute kidney injury after liver transplantation: Incidence and mortality. *Transplant. Proc.* **2014**, *46*, 1819–1821. [CrossRef] [PubMed]

47. Kim, J.M.; Jo, Y.Y.; Na, S.W.; Kim, S.I.; Choi, Y.S.; Kim, N.O.; Park, J.E.; Koh, S.O. The predictors for continuous renal replacement therapy in liver transplant recipients. *Transplant. Proc.* **2014**, *46*, 184–191. [CrossRef]

48. Karapanagiotou, A.; Dimitriadis, C.; Papadopoulos, S.; Kydona, C.; Kefsenidis, S.; Papanikolaou, V.; Gritsi-Gerogianni, N. Comparison of RIFLE and AKIN criteria in the evaluation of the frequency of acute kidney injury in post-liver transplantation patients. *Transplant. Proc.* **2014**, *46*, 3222–3227. [CrossRef] [PubMed]

49. Nadeem, A.; Salahuddin, N.; El Hazmi, A.; Joseph, M.; Bohlega, B.; Sallam, H.; Sheikh, Y.; Broering, D. Chloride-liberal fluids are associated with acute kidney injury after liver transplantation. *Crit. Care.* **2014**, *18*, 625. [CrossRef]

50. Yi, Z.; Mayorga, M.E.; Orman, E.S.; Wheeler, S.B.; Hayashi, P.H.; Barritt, A.S.T. Trends in Characteristics of Patients Listed for Liver Transplantation Will Lead to Higher Rates of Waitlist Removal Due to Clinical Deterioration. *Transplantation* **2017**, *101*, 2368–2374. [CrossRef]

51. Orman, E.S.; Barritt, A.S.T.; Wheeler, S.B.; Hayashi, P.H. Declining liver utilization for transplantation in the United States and the impact of donation after cardiac death. *Liver Transplant.* **2013**, *19*, 59–68. [CrossRef]

52. Chuang, F.R.; Lin, C.C.; Wang, P.H.; Cheng, Y.F.; Hsu, K.T.; Chen, Y.S.; Lee, C.H.; Chen, C.L. Acute renal failure after cadaveric related liver transplantation. *Transplant. Proc.* **2004**, *36*, 2328–2330. [CrossRef]

53. Cabezuelo, J.B.; Ramirez, P.; Rios, A.; Acosta, F.; Torres, D.; Sansano, T.; Pons, J.A.; Bru, M.; Montoya, M.; Bueno, F.S.; et al. Risk factors of acute renal failure after liver transplantation. *Kidney Int.* **2006**, *69*, 1073–1080. [CrossRef]

54. Rueggeberg, A.; Boehm, S.; Napieralski, F.; Mueller, A.R.; Neuhaus, P.; Falke, K.J.; Gerlach, H. Development of a risk stratification model for predicting acute renal failure in orthotopic liver transplantation recipients. *Anaesthesia* **2008**, *63*, 1174–1180. [CrossRef]

55. Portal, A.J.; McPhail, M.J.; Bruce, M.; Coltart, I.; Slack, A.; Sherwood, R.; Heaton, N.D.; Shawcross, D.; Wendon, J.A.; Heneghan, M.A. Neutrophil gelatinase–associated lipocalin predicts acute kidney injury in patients undergoing liver transplantation. *Liver Transplant.* **2010**, *16*, 1257–1266. [CrossRef]

56. Lee, J.P.; Heo, N.J.; Joo, K.W.; Yi, N.J.; Suh, K.S.; Moon, K.C.; Kim, S.G.; Kim, Y.S. Risk factors for consequent kidney impairment and differential impact of liver transplantation on renal function. *Nephrol. Dial. Transplant.* **2010**, *25*, 2772–2785. [CrossRef] [PubMed]

57. Ferreira, A.C.; Nolasco, F.; Carvalho, D.; Sampaio, S.; Baptista, A.; Pessegueiro, P.; Monteiro, E.; Mourao, L.; Barroso, E. Impact of RIFLE classification in liver transplantation. *Clin. Transplant.* **2010**, *24*, 394–400. [CrossRef] [PubMed]

58. Tinti, F.; Umbro, I.; Mecule, A.; Rossi, M.; Merli, M.; Nofroni, I.; Corradini, S.G.; Poli, L.; Pugliese, F.; Ruberto, F.; et al. RIFLE criteria and hepatic function in the assessment of acute renal failure in liver transplantation. *Transplant. Proc.* **2010**, *42*, 1233–1236. [CrossRef] [PubMed]

59. Umbro, I.; Tinti, F.; Mordenti, M.; Rossi, M.; Ianni, S.; Pugliese, F.; Ruberto, F.; Ginanni Corradini, S.; Nofroni, I.; Poli, L.; et al. Model for end-stage liver disease score versus simplified acute physiology score criteria in acute renal failure after liver transplantation. *Transplant. Proc.* **2011**, *43*, 1139–1141. [CrossRef] [PubMed]

60. Narciso, R.C.; Ferraz, L.R.; Mies, S.; Monte, J.C.; dos Santos, O.F.; Neto, M.C.; Rodrigues, C.J.; Batista, M.C.; Durao, M.S., Jr. Impact of acute kidney injury exposure period among liver transplantation patients. *BMC Nephrol.* **2013**, *14*, 43. [CrossRef]

61. Kirnap, M.; Colak, T.; Baskin, E.; Akdur, A.; Moray, G.; Arslan, G.; Haberal, M. Acute renal injury in liver transplant patients and its effect on patient survival. *Exp. Clin. Transplant.* **2014**, *12* (Suppl. 1), 156–158.

62. Lewandowska, L.; Matuszkiewicz-Rowinska, J.; Jayakumar, C.; Oldakowska-Jedynak, U.; Looney, S.; Galas, M.; Dutkiewicz, M.; Krawczyk, M.; Ramesh, G. Netrin-1 and semaphorin 3A predict the development of acute kidney injury in liver transplant patients. *PLoS ONE* **2014**, *9*, e107898. [CrossRef]

63. Barreto, A.G.; Daher, E.F.; Silva Junior, G.B.; Garcia, J.H.; Magalhaes, C.B.; Lima, J.M.; Viana, C.F.; Pereira, E.D. Risk factors for acute kidney injury and 30-day mortality after liver transplantation. *Ann. Hepatol.* **2015**, *14*, 688–694. [PubMed]

64. Park, M.H.; Shim, H.S.; Kim, W.H.; Kim, H.J.; Kim, D.J.; Lee, S.H.; Kim, C.S.; Gwak, M.S.; Kim, G.S. Clinical Risk Scoring Models for Prediction of Acute Kidney Injury after Living Donor Liver Transplantation: A Retrospective Observational Study. *PLoS ONE* **2015**, *10*, e0136230. [CrossRef] [PubMed]

65. Mukhtar, A.; Mahmoud, I.; Obayah, G.; Hasanin, A.; Aboul-Fetouh, F.; Dabous, H.; Bahaa, M.; Abdelaal, A.; Fathy, M.; El Meteini, M. Intraoperative terlipressin therapy reduces the incidence of postoperative acute kidney injury after living donor liver transplantation. *J. Cardiothorac. Vasc. Anesth.* **2015**, *29*, 678–683. [CrossRef] [PubMed]

66. Sang, B.H.; Bang, J.Y.; Song, J.G.; Hwang, G.S. Hypoalbuminemia within Two Postoperative Days Is an Independent Risk Factor for Acute Kidney Injury Following Living Donor Liver Transplantation: A Propensity Score Analysis of 998 Consecutive Patients. *Crit. Care Med.* **2015**, *43*, 2552–2561. [CrossRef] [PubMed]

67. Wyssusek, K.H.; Keys, A.L.; Yung, J.; Moloney, E.T.; Sivalingam, P.; Paul, S.K. Evaluation of perioperative predictors of acute kidney injury post orthotopic liver transplantation. *Anaesth. Intensive Care* **2015**, *43*, 757–763. [CrossRef] [PubMed]

68. Aksu Erdost, H.; Ozkardesler, S.; Ocmen, E.; Avkan-Oguz, V.; Akan, M.; Iyilikci, L.; Unek, T.; Ozbilgin, M.; Meseri Dalak, R.; Astarcioglu, I. Acute Renal Injury Evaluation After Liver Transplantation: With RIFLE Criteria. *Transplant. Proc.* **2015**, *47*, 1482–1487. [CrossRef]

69. Biancofiore, G.; Bindi, M.L.; Miccoli, M.; Cerutti, E.; Lavezzo, B.; Pucci, L.; Bisa, M.; Esposito, M.; Meacci, L.; Mozzo, R.; et al. Intravenous fenoldopam for early acute kidney injury after liver transplantation. *J. Anesth.* **2015**, *29*, 426–432. [CrossRef]

70. Jun, I.G.; Lee, B.; Kim, S.O.; Shin, W.J.; Bang, J.Y.; Song, J.G.; Song, G.W.; Lee, S.G.; Hwang, G.S. Comparison of acute kidney injury between ABO-compatible and ABO-incompatible living donor liver transplantation: A propensity matching analysis. *Liver Transplant.* **2016**, *22*, 1656–1665. [CrossRef]

71. Inoue, Y.; Soyama, A.; Takatsuki, M.; Hidaka, M.; Kinoshita, A.; Natsuda, K.; Baimakhanov, Z.; Kugiyama, T.; Adachi, T.; Kitasato, A.; et al. Does the development of chronic kidney disease and acute kidney injury affect the prognosis after living donor liver transplantation? *Clin. Transplant.* **2016**, *30*, 518–527. [CrossRef]

72. Erdost, H.A.; Ozkardesler, S.; Akan, M.; Iyilikci, L.; Unek, T.; Ocmen, E.; Dalak, R.M.; Astarcioglu, I. Comparison of the RIFLE, AKIN, and KDIGO Diagnostic Classifications for Acute Renal Injury in Patients Undergoing Liver Transplantation. *Transplant. Proc.* **2016**, *48*, 2112–2118. [CrossRef] [PubMed]

73. Kamei, H.; Onishi, Y.; Nakamura, T.; Ishigami, M.; Hamajima, N. Role of cytokine gene polymorphisms in acute and chronic kidney disease following liver transplantation. *Hepatol. Int.* **2016**, *10*, 665–672. [CrossRef] [PubMed]

74. Mizota, T.; Minamisawa, S.; Imanaka, Y.; Fukuda, K. Oliguria without serum creatinine increase after living donor liver transplantation is associated with adverse post-operative outcomes. *Acta Anaesthesiol. Scand.* **2016**, *60*, 874–881. [CrossRef] [PubMed]

75. Chae, M.S.; Lee, N.; Park, D.H.; Lee, J.; Jung, H.S.; Park, C.S.; Choi, J.H.; Hong, S.H. Influence of oxygen content immediately after graft reperfusion on occurrence of postoperative acute kidney injury in living donor liver transplantation. *Medicine* **2017**, *96*, e7626. [CrossRef] [PubMed]

76. Mizota, T.; Hamada, M.; Matsukawa, S.; Seo, H.; Tanaka, T.; Segawa, H. Relationship Between Intraoperative Hypotension and Acute Kidney Injury After Living Donor Liver Transplantation: A Retrospective Analysis. *J. Cardiothorac. Vasc. Anesth.* **2017**, *31*, 582–589. [CrossRef]

77. Trinh, E.; Alam, A.; Tchervenkov, J.; Cantarovich, M. Impact of acute kidney injury following liver transplantation on long-term outcomes. *Clin. Transplant.* **2017**, *31*, e12863. [CrossRef] [PubMed]

78. Kalisvaart, M.; de Haan, J.E.; Hesselink, D.A.; Polak, W.G.; Hansen, B.E.; JNM, I.J.; Gommers, D.; Metselaar, H.J.; de Jonge, J. The postreperfusion syndrome is associated with acute kidney injury following donation after brain death liver transplantation. *Transpl. Int.* **2017**, *30*, 660–669. [CrossRef] [PubMed]

79. Chen, X.; Ding, X.; Shen, B.; Teng, J.; Zou, J.; Wang, T.; Zhou, J.; Chen, N.; Zhang, B. Incidence and outcomes of acute kidney injury in patients with hepatocellular carcinoma after liver transplantation. *J. Cancer Res. Clin. Oncol.* **2017**, *143*, 1337–1346. [CrossRef]

80. Baron-Stefaniak, J.; Schiefer, J.; Miller, E.J.; Berlakovich, G.A.; Baron, D.M.; Faybik, P. Comparison of macrophage migration inhibitory factor and neutrophil gelatinase-associated lipocalin-2 to predict acute kidney injury after liver transplantation: An observational pilot study. *PLoS ONE* **2017**, *12*, e0183162. [CrossRef]

81. Paramesh, A.S.; Roayaie, S.; Doan, Y.; Schwartz, M.E.; Emre, S.; Fishbein, T.; Florman, S.; Gondolesi, G.E.; Krieger, N.; Ames, S.; et al. Post-liver transplant acute renal failure: Factors predicting development of end-stage renal disease. *Clin. Transplant.* **2004**, *18*, 94–99. [CrossRef]

82. Lima, E.Q.; Zanetta, D.M.; Castro, I.; Massarollo, P.C.; Mies, S.; Machado, M.M.; Yu, L. Risk factors for development of acute renal failure after liver transplantation. *Ren. Fail.* **2003**, *25*, 553–560. [CrossRef]

83. Leithead, J.A.; Armstrong, M.J.; Corbett, C.; Andrew, M.; Kothari, C.; Gunson, B.K.; Mirza, D.; Muiesan, P.; Ferguson, J.W. Split liver transplant recipients do not have an increased frequency of acute kidney injury. *Transpl. Int.* **2014**, *27*, 1125–1134. [CrossRef]

84. Moher, D.; Liberati, A.; Tetzlaff, J.; Altman, D.G. Preferred reporting items for systematic reviews and meta-analyses: The PRISMA statement. *PLoS Med.* **2009**, *6*, e1000097. [CrossRef] [PubMed]

85. Von Elm, E.; Altman, D.G.; Egger, M.; Pocock, S.J.; Gotzsche, P.C.; Vandenbroucke, J.P. The Strengthening the Reporting of Observational Studies in Epidemiology (STROBE) statement: Guidelines for reporting observational studies. *PLoS Med.* **2007**, *4*, e296. [CrossRef] [PubMed]

86. DerSimonian, R.; Laird, N. Meta-analysis in clinical trials. *Control. Clin. Trials* **1986**, *7*, 177–188. [CrossRef]

87. Higgins, J.P.; Thompson, S.G.; Deeks, J.J.; Altman, D.G. Measuring inconsistency in meta-analyses. *BMJ* **2003**, *327*, 557–560. [CrossRef] [PubMed]

88. Easterbrook, P.J.; Berlin, J.A.; Gopalan, R.; Matthews, D.R. Publication bias in clinical research. *Lancet* **1991**, *337*, 867–872. [CrossRef]

89. Hand, W.R.; Whiteley, J.R.; Epperson, T.I.; Tam, L.; Crego, H.; Wolf, B.; Chavin, K.D.; Taber, D.J. Hydroxyethyl starch and acute kidney injury in orthotopic liver transplantation: A single-center retrospective review. *Anesth. Analg.* **2015**, *120*, 619–626. [CrossRef]

90. Caragata, R.; Wyssusek, K.H.; Kruger, P. Acute kidney injury following liver transplantation: A systematic review of published predictive models. *Anaesth. Intensive Care* **2016**, *44*, 251–261. [CrossRef] [PubMed]

91. Agarwal, B.; Shaw, S.; Shankar Hari, M.; Burroughs, A.K.; Davenport, A. Continuous renal replacement therapy (CRRT) in patients with liver disease: Is circuit life different? *J. Hepatol.* **2009**, *51*, 504–509. [CrossRef]

92. Asch, W.S.; Bia, M.J. New Organ Allocation System for Combined Liver-Kidney Transplants and the Availability of Kidneys for Transplant to Patients with Stage 4-5 CKD. *Clin. J. Am. Soc. Nephrol.* **2017**, *12*, 848–852. [CrossRef]

93. Ojo, A.O. Renal disease in recipients of nonrenal solid organ transplantation. *Semin. Nephrol.* **2007**, *27*, 498–507. [CrossRef] [PubMed]

94. Biancofiore, G.; Pucci, L.; Cerutti, E.; Penno, G.; Pardini, E.; Esposito, M.; Bindi, L.; Pelati, E.; Romanelli, A.; Triscornia, S.; et al. Cystatin C as a marker of renal function immediately after liver transplantation. *Liver Transplant.* **2006**, *12*, 285–291. [CrossRef]

95. Huen, S.C.; Parikh, C.R. Predicting acute kidney injury after cardiac surgery: A systematic review. *Ann. Thorac. Surg.* **2012**, *93*, 337–347. [CrossRef] [PubMed]

96. Clajus, C.; Hanke, N.; Gottlieb, J.; Stadler, M.; Weismuller, T.J.; Strassburg, C.P.; Brocker, V.; Bara, C.; Lehner, F.; Drube, J.; et al. Renal comorbidity after solid organ and stem cell transplantation. *Am. J. Transplant.* **2012**, *12*, 1691–1699. [CrossRef]

97. Schlegel, A.; Linecker, M.; Kron, P.; Gyori, G.; De Oliveira, M.L.; Mullhaupt, B.; Clavien, P.A.; Dutkowski, P. Risk Assessment in High- and Low-MELD Liver Transplantation. *Am. J. Transplant.* **2017**, *17*, 1050–1063. [CrossRef] [PubMed]

98. Wadei, H.M.; Lee, D.D.; Croome, K.P.; Mai, M.L.; Golan, E.; Brotman, R.; Keaveny, A.P.; Taner, C.B. Early Allograft Dysfunction After Liver Transplantation Is Associated With Short- and Long-Term Kidney Function Impairment. *Am. J. Transplant.* **2016**, *16*, 850–859. [CrossRef]

99. Leithead, J.A.; Tariciotti, L.; Gunson, B.; Holt, A.; Isaac, J.; Mirza, D.F.; Bramhall, S.; Ferguson, J.W.; Muiesan, P. Donation after cardiac death liver transplant recipients have an increased frequency of acute kidney injury. *Am. J. Transplant.* **2012**, *12*, 965–975. [CrossRef] [PubMed]

100. Jo, S.K.; Rosner, M.H.; Okusa, M.D. Pharmacologic treatment of acute kidney injury: Why drugs haven't worked and what is on the horizon. *Clin. J. Am. Soc. Nephrol.* **2007**, *2*, 356–365. [CrossRef]

101. Valentino, K.L.; Gutierrez, M.; Sanchez, R.; Winship, M.J.; Shapiro, D.A. First clinical trial of a novel caspase inhibitor: Anti-apoptotic caspase inhibitor, IDN-6556, improves liver enzymes. *Int. J. Clin. Pharmacol. Ther.* **2003**, *41*, 441–449. [CrossRef]

Effect of Diabetes Mellitus on Acute Kidney Injury after Minimally Invasive Partial Nephrectomy: A Case-Matched Retrospective Analysis

Na Young Kim [1,†], Jung Hwa Hong [2,†], Dong Hoon Koh [3], Jongsoo Lee [4], Hoon Jae Nam [1] and So Yeon Kim [1,*]

[1] Department of Anesthesiology and Pain Medicine, Anesthesia and Pain Research Institute, Yonsei University College of Medicine, 50-1 Yonsei-ro, Seodaemun-gu, Seoul 03722, Korea; knnyyy@yuhs.ac (N.Y.K.); HJNAM90@yuhs.ac (H.J.N.)

[2] Department of Policy Research Affairs National Health Insurance Service Ilsan Hospital, 100 Ilsan-ro, Ilsandong-gu, Goyang, Gyeonggi-do 10444, Korea; jh_hong@nhimc.co.kr

[3] Department of Urology, Konyang University College of Medicine, 158 Gwanjeodong-ro, Daejeon 35365, Korea; urodhkoh@kyuh.ac.kr

[4] Department of Urology and Urological Science Institute, Yonsei University College of Medicine, 50-1 Yonsei-ro, Seodaemun-gu, Seoul 03722, Korea; JS1129@yuhs.ac

*   Correspondence: KIMSY326@yuhs.ac

† These authors contributed equally to this work.

Abstract: Postoperative acute kidney injury (AKI) is still a concern in partial nephrectomy (PN), even with the development of minimally invasive technique. We aimed to compare AKI incidence between patients with and without diabetes mellitus (DM) and to determine the predictive factors for postoperative AKI. This case-matched retrospective study included 884 patients with preoperative creatinine levels ≤1.4 mg/dL who underwent laparoscopic or robot-assisted laparoscopic PN between December 2005 and May 2018. Propensity score matching was employed to match patients with and without DM in a 1:3 ratio (101 and 303 patients, respectively). Of 884 patients, 20.4% had postoperative AKI. After propensity score matching, the incidence of postoperative AKI in DM and non-DM patients was 30.7% and 14.9%, respectively ($P < 0.001$). In multivariate analysis, male sex and warm ischemia time (WIT) >25 min were significantly associated with postoperative AKI in patients with and without DM. In patients with DM, hemoglobin A1c (HbA1c) >7% was a predictive factor for AKI, odds ratio (OR) = 4.59 (95% CI, 1.47–14.36). In conclusion, DM increased the risk of AKI after minimally invasive PN; male sex, longer WIT, and elevated HbA1c were independent risk factors for AKI in patients with DM.

Keywords: diabetes mellitus; acute kidney injury; nephrectomy; minimally invasive surgical procedures; risk factors

---

1. Introduction

Partial nephrectomy (PN) is the current gold standard treatment for small, localized renal tumors owing to reduced risk of acute and chronic kidney dysfunction compared with radical nephrectomy [1,2]. Nevertheless, the incidence rate of acute kidney injury (AKI) after PN is 12%–54% depending on the definition of AKI [2–4]. In case of robot assisted PN, the incidence of postoperative AKI was reported as 24%–27% [5,6]. Therefore, postoperative AKI remains a concern in minimally invasive PN, as parenchymal mass reduction and/or ischemic injury due to vascular clamping cannot be avoided [4].

Diabetes mellitus (DM) has an increasing global prevalence and is the leading cause of chronic kidney disease [7]. Moreover, patients with DM are at an increased risk of acute kidney dysfunction throughout their lifetime [8]. Furthermore, DM is a recognized risk factor for AKI in the postoperative setting, such as in cardiac [9] and non-cardiac surgeries [10,11]. Previous studies investigating risk factors for AKI in all patients who underwent PN did not distinguish the open technique from the minimally invasive approach [3,4,12–15]. Only one study evaluated the effect of warm ischemia time (WIT) on AKI in robot-assisted laparoscopic PN [5]. Therefore, data on risk factors for AKI after minimally invasive PN are limited. Furthermore, no study has determined whether patients with DM have an increased risk of AKI after minimally invasive PN. The present study aimed to compare the AKI incidence between patients with and without DM and to investigate the predictive factors for AKI in these patients after laparoscopic and robot-assisted laparoscopic PN.

2. Material and Methods

2.1. Patients

This case-matched retrospective analysis was performed after obtaining approval from the institutional review board and hospital research ethics committee (Yonsei University Health System, Seoul, Korea; IRB protocol No. 4-2018-0678, approved at August 29, 2018) with informed consent form from the patients being waived off. A total of 991 patients who underwent laparoscopic or robot-assisted laparoscopic PN between December 2005 and May 2018 were identified from the electronic medical records of a single institution, of which 58 were excluded owing to the type of operation; specifically, 18 patients underwent other combined procedures, whereas 5 and 35 patients were converted to open and radical nephrectomy, respectively. Furthermore, 20 patients with an American Society of Anesthesiologists (ASA) physical status ≥IV, 24 patients with an underlying chronic kidney disease or preoperative creatinine level >1.4 mg/dL, and 5 patients who underwent reoperation because of bleeding within 24 hours postoperatively were excluded from the analysis. Finally, 884 patients were identified, and propensity score matching was performed to match patients with and without DM in a 1:3 ratio (101 and 303 patients, respectively). In propensity score matching, hypertension, cerebrovascular disease, and coronary artery disease were used as covariates (Figure 1).

Standard general anesthesia was provided to all patients. Propofol, remifentanil, and rocuronium were used for anesthesia induction, whereas sevoflurane or desflurane and remifentanil were used for anesthesia maintenance. Administered colloid solution was 6% hydroxyethyl starch 130/0.4 (Volulyte® or Voluven®, Fresenius-Kabi, Seoul, Korea). Laparoscopic or robot-assisted laparoscopic PN was performed in accordance with our institution's protocol [16]. Tumor bed closure was performed using renorrhaphy with absorbable synthetic braided sutures or absorbable barbed sutures according to the surgeon's preference. In cases with calyceal opening, additional suturing was also performed to maintain watertightness.

2.2. Data Collection

All data were collected from electronic medical records. Demographic data included age, sex, body mass index, ASA physical status, and underlying diseases, such as diabetes controlled with oral medication or insulin, hypertension, cerebrovascular disease, and coronary artery disease. Cerebrovascular disease was defined as transient ischemic attack, stroke, history of carotid artery stent, and cerebral hemorrhage. Preoperative laboratory data included creatinine, hematocrit, and hemoglobin (Hb) A1c levels. Operative data included the type of operation, operative time, WIT, volume of intraoperatively administered fluid, intraoperative use of a colloid solution or packed red blood cells, and intraoperative urine output. Data on serum creatinine level and estimated glomerular filtration rate (eGFR) were collected before surgery, immediately after surgery, and at 1 day, 2 days, 1 month, and 3 months after surgery. The eGFR value was calculated using the Chronic Kidney Disease Epidemiology Collaboration equation.

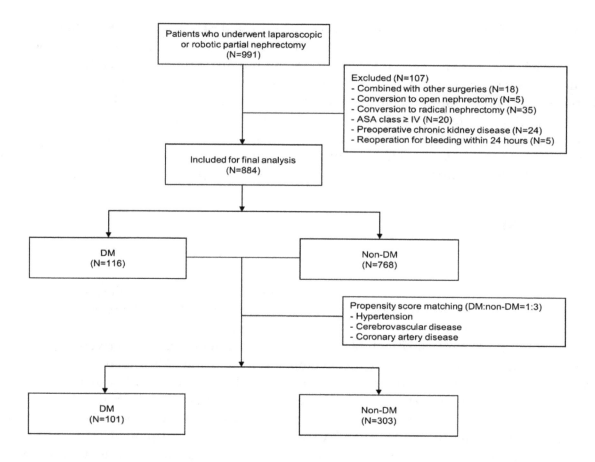

Figure 1. Flow diagram of patient selection. ASA—American Society of Anesthesiologists; DM—diabetes mellitus.

2.3. Primary and Secondary Outcomes

The primary outcome was comparison of AKI incidence between patients with and without DM after laparoscopic and robot-assisted laparoscopic PN. AKI was defined as an absolute increase in serum creatinine level by ≥0.3 mg/dL or ≥50% increase from the preoperative value within the first 48 h after surgery [17]. AKI was further categorized into three stages according to the acute kidney injury network classification: Stage 1, an increase in serum creatinine level ≥0.3 mg/dL or ≥150%–200% (1.5–2-fold) from the baseline value; stage 2, an increase in serum creatinine level >200%–300% (2–3-fold) from the baseline value; and stage 3, an increase in serum creatinine level >300% (3-fold) from the baseline value [17]. Additionally, we investigated predictive factors for AKI in patients with and without DM after laparoscopic and robot-assisted laparoscopic PN as the secondary outcome.

2.4. Statistical Analysis

Continuous variables are presented as mean (SD), whereas categorical variables are expressed as the number of patients in percentage. Continuous and categorical variables were evaluated using independent t-test and chi-squared test, respectively. Propensity score matching using a 1:3 ratio was performed to adjust the baseline characteristics of patients with and without DM. Multivariate logistic regression was employed to identify risk factors for AKI in patients with and without DM. A P value <0.05 was considered statistically significant. All statistical analyses were performed using SAS software version 9.4 (SAS Institute, Cary, NC, USA).

3. Results

In the analysis of all patients ($N = 884$) prior to matching, the incidence rate of AKI after minimally invasive PN was 20.4%, and the following variables were identified as independent risk factors for AKI (Table 1): Male sex, DM, longer operative duration, WIT >25 min, and higher intraoperative urine output.

Table 1. Univariate and multivariate analyses of risk factors for acute kidney injury after minimally invasive partial nephrectomy ($N = 884$).

Variables	Univariate		Multivariate	
	OR (95% CI)	P value	OR (95% CI)	P value
Age, year	0.99 (0.98–1.01)	0.292		
Male sex	3.84 (2.51–5.87)	<0.001	4.57 (2.40–8.72)	<0.001
Body mass index, kg/m²	1.02 (0.99–1.05)	0.151		
ASA physical status				
I	1			
II	0.95 (0.66–1.36)	0.772		
III	1.39 (0.74–2.63)	0.309		
Co-morbidities				
Diabetes mellitus	2.56 (1.68–3.92)	<0.001	2.85 (1.71–4.74)	<0.001
Hypertension	1.39 (0.99–1.95)	0.056	1.10 (0.73–1.65)	0.654
Cerebrovascular disease	1.19 (0.43–3.27)	0.738		
Coronary artery disease	2.20 (0.92–5.28)	0.077	1.39 (0.52–3.69)	0.507
Preoperative lab value				
Creatinine, mg/dL	7.07 (2.78–18.03)	<0.001	0.79 (0.20–3.09)	0.734
Hematocrit, %	1.06 (1.02–1.10)	0.002	1.00 (0.95–1.05)	0.912
Hemoglobin A1c				
≤7%	1			
>7%	1.63 (0.76–3.50)	0.214		
Type of operation				
Laparoscopic	1			
Robotic	0.98 (0.67–1.44)	0.907		
Operation time, 60 min increase	1.44 (1.30–1.61)	<0.001	1.26 (1.08–1.47)	0.003
Warm ischemia time				
≤25 min	1		1	
>25 min	3.25 (2.30–4.58)	<0.001	2.81 (1.92–4.10)	<0.001
Intraoperative I & O				
Fluid input, 500 mL increase	1.46 (1.30–1.65)	<0.001	1.09 (0.91–1.31)	0.349
Colloid administration	1.22 (0.88–1.70)	0.238		
RBC transfusion	2.61 (1.28–5.32)	0.008	1.72 (0.71–4.19)	0.230
Urine output, 100 mL increase	1.06 (1.02–1.10)	0.002	1.06 (1.02–1.11)	0.008
Blood loss, 300 mL increase	1.55 (1.33–1.80)	<0.001		

OR—odds ratio; CI—confidence interval; ASA—American Society of Anesthesiologists; RBC—red blood cells; I & O—input and output.

Among patients with a concomitant disease, only DM was shown to be a risk factor for AKI. Hence, we decided to investigate the effect of DM on AKI using propensity score matching. Prior to matching, the number of patients with DM who were older and had hypertension, cerebrovascular disease, and coronary artery disease was higher than that of patients without DM (Table 2). However, after matching, the demographic characteristics of patients with and without DM were similar except for the ASA physical status (Table 2) and the distribution of patients with and without DM was fairly uniform (Figure 2).

Table 2. Demographic characteristics after propensity score matching.

Variables	After Case Matching (N = 404)			Before Case Matching (N = 884)		
	DM (N = 101)	Non–DM (N = 303)	P value	DM (N = 116)	Non–DM (N = 768)	P value
Age, year	58.7 (9.2)	58.8 (9.6)	0.887	60.0 (9.8)	51.5 (12.5)	<0.001
Male sex	69 (68%)	182 (60%)	0.139	78 (67%)	472 (61%)	0.231
Body mass index, kg/m^2	26.8 (11.7)	25.0 (3.2)	0.131	26.6 (11.0)	24.6 (3.6)	0.065
ASA physical status			<0.001			<0.001
I	0	49 (16%)		0	295 (38%)	
II	91 (90%)	223 (74%)		100 (86%)	427 (56%)	
III	10 (10%)	31 (10%)		16 (14%)	46 (6%)	
Co-morbidities						
DM with oral medication	98 (97%)			113 (97%)		
DM with insulin	3 (3%)			3 (3%)		
Hypertension	68 (67%)	206 (68%)	0.902	83 (72%)	234 (30%)	<0.001
Cerebrovascular disease	4 (4%)	13 (4%)	>0.999	7 (6%)	15 (2%)	0.018
Coronary artery disease	4 (4%)	6 (2%)	0.276	8 (7%)	15 (2%)	0.006
Preoperative lab value						
Creatinine, mg/dL	0.8 (0.2)	0.8 (0.2)	0.821	0.8 (0.2)	0.8 (0.2)	0.530
Hematocrit, %	42.2 (5.1)	42.2 (4.5)	0.988	41.9 (5.1)	42.4 (4.4)	0.262
Hemoglobin A1c, %	7.3 (1.3)			7.3 (1.4)		
Type of operation			0.604			0.478
Laparoscopic	29 (29%)	79 (26%)		31 (27%)	182 (24%)	
Robotic	72 (71%)	224 (74%)		85 (73%)	586 (76%)	
Operation time, min	289.5 (78.3)	287.5 (98.0)	0.838	288.2 (78.2)	284.9 (91.2)	0.676
Warm ischemia time			0.952			0.511
≤25 min	64 (63%)	191 (63%)		72 (62%)	452 (59%)	
>25 min	37 (37%)	112 (37%)		44 (38%)	316 (41%)	
Intraoperative I & O						
Fluid input, mL	1793.5 (652.6)	1845.2 (658.8)	0.494	1812.9 (640.1)	1853.6 (652.8)	0.531
Patients administered with colloid, n	44 (44%)	125 (41%)	0.684	51 (44%)	326 (42%)	0.758
Patients transfused with RBC, n	7 (7%)	9 (3%)	0.135	10 (9%)	24 (3%)	0.009
Urine output, mL	583.7 (361.4)	563.7 (393.7)	0.652	609.6 (442.3)	593.9 (422.1)	0.710
Blood loss, mL	286.4 (337.7)	254.9 (303.4)	0.380	294.3 (336.8)	245.0 (288.6)	0.137

Values are presented as mean (SD) or number of patients (%). DM—diabetes mellitus; ASA—American Society of Anesthesiologists; RBC—red blood cells; I & O—input and output.

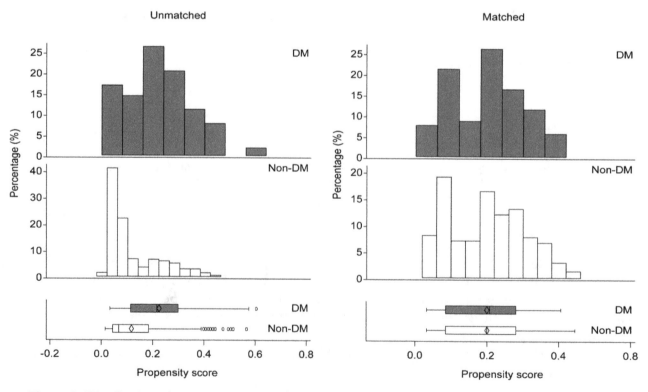

Figure 2. Distribution of propensity scores of patients with and without diabetes mellitus (DM) before and after matching. DM, Diabetes mellitus.

After matching, the incidence rate of postoperative AKI was significantly higher in patients with DM than in those without DM (total: 30.7% vs. 14.9%, $P < 0.001$; stage 1: 29.7% vs. 14.2%, $P < 0.001$; stage 2: 1.0% vs. 0.7%, $P > 0.999$) (Figure 3). No patient developed stage 3 of AKI.

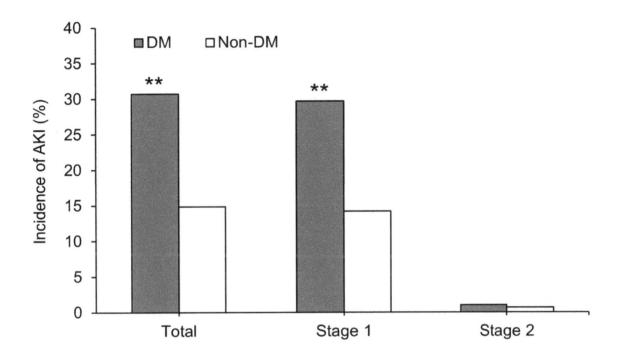

Figure 3. Incidence of acute kidney injury after minimally invasive partial nephrectomy according to the acute kidney injury network criteria. **$P < 0.001$ versus non-DM patients. DM, Diabetes mellitus; AKI, acute kidney injury; stage 1, increase in the serum creatinine level ≥0.3 mg/dL or ≥150%–200% (1.5–2-fold) from baseline; stage 2, increase in the serum creatinine level >200%–300% (2–3-fold) from baseline.

Results of the univariate and multivariate analyses of risk factors for AKI in patients with and without DM are summarized in Table 3. Male sex and WIT >25 min were determined to pose a significantly higher risk of postoperative AKI in patients with and without DM. In patients with DM, preoperative HbA1c >7% was a predictive factor for AKI: Odds ratio (OR) = 4.59 (95% confidence interval (CI), 1.47–14.36). When patients were classified according to DM and sex, the probabilities of AKI were as follows: Females without DM, OR = 1; females with DM, OR = 0.95 (95% CI: 0.16–5.59); males without DM, OR = 4.12 (95% CI: 1.32–12.86); and males with DM, OR = 14.46 (95% CI: 4.62–45.25) (Table 4).

The perioperative serum creatinine level and eGFR until three months after surgery are shown in Figure 4. Although no significant difference in serum creatinine level and eGFR was observed between patients with and without DM at each time point, there were significant intergroup differences over time ($P_{Group \times Time} = 0.016$ and 0.026, respectively).

Table 3. Univariate and multivariate analyses of risk factors for acute kidney injury after minimally invasive partial nephrectomy in patients with and without DM.

Variables	DM (N = 101) Univariate OR (95% CI)	P-value	Multivariate OR (95% CI)	P-value	Non-DM (N = 303) Univariate OR (95% CI)	P-value	Multivariate OR (95% CI)	P-value
Age, year	1.00 (0.96–1.05)	0.947			0.99 (0.96–1.03)	0.581		
Male sex	10.87 (2.41–49.18)	0.002	19.58 (2.47–155.35)	0.005	4.89 (2.00–11.99)	0.001	4.52 (1.32–15.48)	0.016
Body mass index, kg/m²	0.99 (0.96–1.04)	0.973			1.06 (0.96–1.17)	0.236		
ASA physical status								
I	1				1			
II	2.50 (0.67–9.36)				0.51 (0.24–1.12)	0.093		
III		0.174			0.38 (0.10–1.51)	0.170		
Co-morbidities								
Hypertension	2.03 (0.77–5.35)	0.154			1.10 (0.55–2.22)	0.787		
Cerebrovascular disease	0.74 (0.07–7.45)	0.802			1.10 (0.24–5.16)	0.900		
Coronary artery disease	7.39 (0.74–74.13)	0.089	10.41 (0.79–136.42)	0.074	0.45 (0.02–10.23)	0.616	0.39 (0.02–9.25)	0.557
Preoperative lab value								
Creatinine, mg/dL	21.28 (1.36–332.47)	0.029	5.46 (0.14–219.15)	0.367	7.37 (1.26–43.09)	0.027	0.25 (0.02–3.50)	0.301
Hematocrit, %	1.08 (0.99–1.18)	0.090	0.94 (0.83–1.08)	0.391	1.09 (1.02–1.18)	0.017	1.04 (0.95–1.13)	0.418
Hemoglobin A1c								
≤7%	1		1					
>7%	2.11 (0.89–5.01)	0.090	4.59 (1.47–14.36)	0.009				
Type of operation								
Laparoscopic	1				1			
Robotic	1.57 (0.59–4.19)	0.367			1.03 (0.49–2.16)	0.937		
Operation time, 60 min increase	1.35 (0.97–1.88)	0.077	1.24 (0.75–2.05)	0.408	1.45 (1.21–1.74)	<0.001	1.18 (0.90–1.56)	0.235
Warm ischemia time								
≤25 min	1		1				1	
>25 min	2.49 (1.04–5.94)	0.040	3.57 (1.17–10.94)	0.026	3.09 (1.59–6.01)	0.001	2.56 (1.24–5.26)	0.011
Intraoperative I & O								
Fluid input, 500 mL increase	1.31 (0.95–1.81)	0.101	0.93 (0.60–1.44)	0.752	1.63 (1.29–2.05)	<0.001	1.21 (0.87–1.68)	0.251
Colloid administration	1.33 (0.57–3.10)	0.516			0.92 (0.48–1.78)	0.805		
RBC transfusion	1.77 (0.37–8.42)	0.474	4.28 (0.40–46.09)	0.230	5.23 (1.35–20.33)	0.017	5.13 (0.96–27.42)	0.056
Urine output, 100 mL increase	0.91 (0.80–1.05)	0.185			1.07 (0.99–1.15)	0.097		
Blood loss, 300 mL increase	1.58 (1.07–2.33)	0.023			1.56 (1.20–2.04)	0.001		

OR, odds ratio; CI, confidence interval; ASA, American Society of Anesthesiologists; RBC, red blood cells; I & O, input and output.

Table 4. Incidence and odds ratio of acute kidney injury after minimally invasive partial nephrectomy based on the presence of DM and sex.

	Total patients, n	AKI incidence, n (%)	OR (95% CI)	*P* value
Non-DM female	121	8 (6.6%)	1	
DM female	32	2 (6.3%)	0.95 (0.16–5.59)	0.958
Non-DM male	182	37 (20.3%)	4.12 (1.32–12.86)	0.015
DM male	69	29 (42.0%)	14.46 (4.62–45.25)	<0.001

Values are presented as number of patients (%). AKI, acute kidney injury; OR, odds ratio; CI, confidence interval; DM, diabetes mellitus.

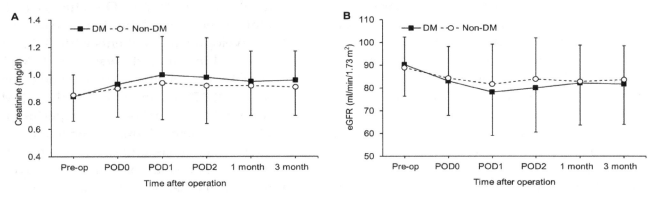

Figure 4. Changes in the serum creatinine level (**A**) and estimated glomerular filtration rate (**B**) until three months postoperatively. Values are presented as a mean (SD). No significant differences were observed between patients with and without DM at each time point. DM, Diabetes mellitus; eGFR, estimated glomerular filtration rate; Pre-op—preoperatively; POD0—postoperative day 0 (immediately after the operation); POD1—postoperative day 1—POD2, postoperative day 2.

4. Discussion

This is the first retrospective case-matched study to clarify whether patients with DM have an increased risk of AKI and evaluate risk factors for AKI in patients with and without DM after minimally invasive PN. The main findings were as follows: (1) DM was a strong predictive factor for AKI after minimally invasive PN. (2) The incidence rate of postoperative AKI was significantly higher in patients with DM than in those without DM, even after adjustment for other factors. (3) Male sex and WIT >25 min were predictive factors for AKI in both patients with and without DM. (4) Preoperative HbA1c >7% was a predictive factor for AKI in patients with DM

Although PN is associated with a reduced risk of postoperative AKI compared with radical nephrectomy owing to being a nephron-sparing surgery [15], the incidence rate of AKI after PN has been reported to be 12%–54% [2–4]. Although AKI incidence varies depending on the definition used, this incidence rate is definitely higher than that after non-cardiovascular surgery (1%–11%) [10,11]. In our study, the incidence rate of AKI in 884 patients who underwent laparoscopic or robot-assisted laparoscopic PN was 20.4%, which is comparable to the previously reported incidence rate of 24%–27% after robot-assisted laparoscopic PN [5,6]. Postoperative AKI is known as a high-risk factor for new-onset chronic kidney disease and is associated with increased morbidity and mortality after nephrectomy and non-cardiovascular surgery [10,11,18,19]. Therefore, attention should be paid to AKI after PN even with the development of the minimally invasive technique, and identification of patients at risk before surgery is important.

Several studies have investigated predictive factors for AKI after PN, which included open and minimally invasive techniques [3,4,12–15]. Longer WIT and operative duration as well as patient-related factors, such as old age, male sex, obesity, impaired preoperative kidney function, and history of hypertension were identified as risk factors for postoperative AKI [3,4,12–15,20,21]. In our study, which analyzed risk factors after minimally invasive PN only, WIT >25 min, longer operative duration, and patient-related factors, such as male sex, presence of DM, and high intraoperative urine output were revealed to be independent predictors of postoperative AKI. A previous study that included intraoperative urine output as one of the variables for analysis showed that a low urine output is a risk factor for AKI after PN [3]. The high urine output in the present study could be attributed to the use of diuretics typically prescribed by surgeons in difficult cases, which could be the reason for the different result in our study. As urine output in anesthetized patients has been proven to be a poor indicator of fluid balance and is not a predictive factor for AKI after general surgery [11], further studies on the relationship between intraoperative urine output and AKI after PN are required to establish a definite conclusion.

Although our study is the first to identify DM as a risk factor for AKI in PN, previous studies have already reported DM as a risk factor for AKI after general surgeries [10,11]. One study, which enrolled 7564 non-cardiovascular surgical patients and applied the same definition of AKI that we used, reported an OR of 1.51 (95% CI, 1.11–2.06) for AKI development in patients with DM [11]. In comparison, the OR for AKI development in patients with DM in our study was 2.85 (95% CI, 1.71–4.74). Moreover, even after adjustment for other factors by propensity score matching, the incidence rate of AKI was significantly higher in patients with DM (30.7%) than in those without DM (14.9%). Several experimental studies have indicated the susceptibility to renal ischemia/reperfusion (I/R) injury in DM [22–24]. Compared with the nondiabetic kidney, the diabetic kidney exhibited severe damage, including increased tubular cell apoptosis, tubulointerstitial fibrosis, and decreased tubular proliferation after renal I/R [22,23]. Moreover, reperfusion after renal ischemia was markedly delayed in diabetic mice than that in nondiabetic mice [24]. Therefore, the combination of these factors might have made patients with DM more susceptible to AKI in our study.

WIT is recognized as a strong contributing factor for AKI after PN [3–5,12,13,20,21]. WIT >25 min results in irreversible damage that is diffusely distributed throughout the operated kidney, even at six months after PN [25]. Porpiglia and colleagues [26] reported that every minute of warm ischemia could diminish the postoperative kidney function; moreover, they identified 25 min as a safe cut-off for WIT in laparoscopic PN. In line with previous results, WIT > 25 min was a predictive factor for AKI in patients with and without DM.

Previous studies showed that male sex is a risk factor for AKI after PN as well as general surgery [10,12,14,20,27]. Consistent with prior results, we observed a significantly higher risk of postoperative AKI among male patients with and without DM. Sexual dimorphism exists in renal I/R injury, and sex hormones (i.e., ratio of testosterone to estrogen) are considered as the primary factor. Park and colleagues [28] showed that the presence of testosterone rather than the absence of estrogen is crucial in sex difference with respect to susceptibility to renal I/R injury via an increase in inflammation and functional injury to the kidney. Moreover, estrogen displayed a protective effect against renal I/R injury via activation of nitric oxide synthases, inhibition of endothelin-1 production, and depression of the renal sympathetic nervous system [28–30]. Thus, the combination of male sex and DM might have resulted in synergistic effects, and this might have led to our result that male patients with DM had approximately 14 times higher risk of developing AKI than female patients without DM.

HbA1c measurement is a standard method for assessing blood glucose management in patients with DM and it reflects the average blood glucose level over the past 2–3 months. The patients with an HbA1c level of 7% or more had a significantly increased risk of renal failure as well as cerebrovascular accidents, wound infection, and hospital death after coronary artery bypass surgery [31]. However, no study has determined whether elevated preoperative HbA1c increases AKI after PN. Our study is the first to demonstrate that preoperative HbA1c >7% was associated with increased risk for AKI after minimally invasive PN in patients with DM.

The present study has limitations, its main drawback being its retrospective observational nature; thus, it is susceptible to bias and other confounding factors. The baseline difference between patients with and without DM can confound analyses of AKI incidence and risk factors for AKI. In fact, prior to matching, the number of patients with DM who were older and had hypertension, cerebrovascular disease, and coronary artery disease was higher than that of patients without DM; however, these data were adjusted after propensity score matching. Although this study cannot replace a randomized trial, propensity score matching is a powerful tool for adjusting for confounding variables and reducing selection bias [32]. Therefore, this study is valuable in that it is the first study to compare patients with and without DM with respect to postoperative AKI using propensity score matching. Second, long-term functional outcomes of patients with AKI were not evaluated in the current study. Since postoperative AKI is known as a high-risk factor for new-onset chronic kidney disease [19], long-term follow-up studies are required.

In conclusion, patients with DM had an increased risk of developing AKI after minimally invasive PN, even after adjustment for other factors. Male patients with DM were most susceptible to AKI. WIT >25 min and preoperative HbA1c >7% were associated with AKI in patients with DM. Therefore, caution should be taken to reduce WIT during minimally invasive PN, especially in male patients with DM combined with elevated preoperative HbA1c.

Author Contributions: N.Y.K and J.H.H. contributed equally to this work. N.Y.K. and J.H.H. contributed to study design and conduct, data analysis, and manuscript writing. D.H.K, contributed to methodology and project administration. J.L. contributed to investigation. H.J.N. participated in data curation. S.Y.K. participated as the corresponding author and supervised the overall study and drafting of the manuscript.

References

1. Lau, W.K.; Blute, M.L.; Weaver, A.L.; Torres, V.E.; Zincke, H. Matched comparison of radical nephrectomy vs nephron-sparing surgery in patients with unilateral renal cell carcinoma and a normal contralateral kidney. *Mayo Clin. Proc.* **2000**, *75*, 1236–1242. [CrossRef] [PubMed]

2. Suer, E.; Burgu, B.; Gokce, M.I.; Turkolmez, K.; Beduk, Y.; Baltaci, S. Comparison of radical and partial nephrectomy in terms of renal function: A retrospective cohort study. *Scand. J. Urol. Nephrol.* **2011**, *45*, 24–29. [CrossRef]

3. Rajan, S.; Babazade, R.; Govindarajan, S.R.; Pal, R.; You, J.; Mascha, E.J.; Khanna, A.; Yang, M.; Marcano, F.D.; Singh, A.K.; et al. Perioperative factors associated with acute kidney injury after partial nephrectomy. *Br. J. Anaesth.* **2016**, *116*, 70–76. [CrossRef]

4. Zhang, Z.; Zhao, J.; Dong, W.; Remer, E.; Li, J.; Demirjian, S.; Zabell, J.; Campbell, S.C. Acute kidney injury after partial nephrectomy: Role of parenchymal mass reduction and ischemia and impact on subsequent functional recovery. *Eur. Urol.* **2016**, *69*, 745–752. [CrossRef] [PubMed]

5. Rosen, D.C.; Kannappan, M.; Paulucci, D.J.; Beksac, A.T.; Attallah, K.; Abaza, R.; Eun, D.D.; Bhandari, A.; Hemal, A.K.; Porter, J.; et al. Reevaluating warm ischemia time as a predictor of renal function outcomes after robotic partial nephrectomy. *Urology* **2018**, *120*, 156–161. [CrossRef]

6. Lee, B.; Lee, S.Y.; Kim, N.Y.; Rha, K.H.; Choi, Y.D.; Park, S.; Kim, S.Y. Effect of ulinastatin on postoperative renal function in patients undergoing robot-assisted laparoscopic partial nephrectomy: A randomized trial. *Surg. Endosc.* **2017**, *31*, 3728–3736. [CrossRef]

7. National Kidney, F. Kdoqi clinical practice guideline for diabetes and ckd: 2012 update. *Am. J. Kidney Dis.* **2012**, *60*, 850–886.

8. Girman, C.J.; Kou, T.D.; Brodovicz, K.; Alexander, C.M.; O'Neill, E.A.; Engel, S.; Williams-Herman, D.E.; Katz, L. Risk of acute renal failure in patients with type 2 diabetes mellitus. *Diabet. Med.* **2012**, *29*, 614–621. [CrossRef] [PubMed]

9. Wang, Y.; Bellomo, R. Cardiac surgery-associated acute kidney injury: Risk factors, pathophysiology and treatment. *Nat. Rev. Nephrol.* **2017**, *13*, 697–711. [CrossRef]

10. Kheterpal, S.; Tremper, K.K.; Heung, M.; Rosenberg, A.L.; Englesbe, M.; Shanks, A.M.; Campbell, D.A., Jr. Development and validation of an acute kidney injury risk index for patients undergoing general surgery: Results from a national data set. *Anesthesiology* **2009**, *110*, 505–515. [CrossRef] [PubMed]

11. Pourafkari, L.; Arora, P.; Porhomayon, J.; Dosluoglu, H.H.; Arora, P.; Nader, N.D. Acute kidney injury after non-cardiovascular surgery: Risk factors and impact on development of chronic kidney disease and long-term mortality. *Curr. Med. Res. Opin.* **2018**, *34*, 1829–1837. [CrossRef] [PubMed]

12. Lane, B.R.; Babineau, D.C.; Poggio, E.D.; Weight, C.J.; Larson, B.T.; Gill, I.S.; Novick, A.C. Factors predicting renal functional outcome after partial nephrectomy. *J. Urol.* **2008**, *180*, 2363–2368. [CrossRef] [PubMed]

13. Volpe, A.; Blute, M.L.; Ficarra, V.; Gill, I.S.; Kutikov, A.; Porpiglia, F.; Rogers, C.; Touijer, K.A.; Van Poppel, H.; Thompson, R.H. Renal ischemia and function after partial nephrectomy: A collaborative review of the literature. *Eur. Urol.* **2015**, *68*, 61–74. [CrossRef]

14. Schmid, M.; Krishna, N.; Ravi, P.; Meyer, C.P.; Becker, A.; Dalela, D.; Sood, A.; Chun, F.K.; Kibel, A.S.; Menon, M.; et al. Trends of acute kidney injury after radical or partial nephrectomy for renal cell carcinoma. *Urol. Oncol.* **2016**, *34*, 293.e1–293.e10. [CrossRef] [PubMed]

15. Schmid, M.; Abd-El-Barr, A.E.; Gandaglia, G.; Sood, A.; Olugbade, K., Jr.; Ruhotina, N.; Sammon, J.D.; Varda, B.; Chang, S.L.; Kibel, A.S.; et al. Predictors of 30-day acute kidney injury following radical and partial nephrectomy for renal cell carcinoma. *Urol. Oncol.* **2014**, *32*, 1259–1266. [CrossRef]

16. Jeong, W.; Park, S.Y.; Lorenzo, E.I.; Oh, C.K.; Han, W.K.; Rha, K.H. Laparoscopic partial nephrectomy versus robot-assisted laparoscopic partial nephrectomy. *J Endourol.* **2009**, *23*, 1457–1460. [CrossRef] [PubMed]

17. Mehta, R.L.; Kellum, J.A.; Shah, S.V.; Molitoris, B.A.; Ronco, C.; Warnock, D.G.; Levin, A. Acute kidney injury network: Report of an initiative to improve outcomes in acute kidney injury. *Crit Care.* **2007**, *11*, R31. [CrossRef] [PubMed]

18. Weight, C.J.; Larson, B.T.; Fergany, A.F.; Gao, T.; Lane, B.R.; Campbell, S.C.; Kaouk, J.H.; Klein, E.A.; Novick, A.C. Nephrectomy induced chronic renal insufficiency is associated with increased risk of cardiovascular death and death from any cause in patients with localized ct1b renal masses. *J. Urol.* **2010**, *183*, 1317–1323. [CrossRef]

19. Cho, A.; Lee, J.E.; Kwon, G.Y.; Huh, W.; Lee, H.M.; Kim, Y.G.; Kim, D.J.; Oh, H.Y.; Choi, H.Y. Post-operative acute kidney injury in patients with renal cell carcinoma is a potent risk factor for new-onset chronic kidney disease after radical nephrectomy. *Nephrol. Dial. Transplant.* **2011**, *26*, 3496–3501. [CrossRef] [PubMed]

20. Zaher Bahouth, E.S.; Nativ, O.; Halachmi, S.; Moskovitz, B.; Abassi, Z.; Nativ, O. Relationship between clinical factors and the occurrence of post-operative acute kidney injury in patients undergoing nephron-sparing surgery. *JMCM* **2018**, *1*, 47–50.

21. Nativ, O.; Bahouth, Z.; Sabo, E.; Halachmi, S.; Moskovitz, B.; Hellou, E.G.; Abassi, Z.; Nativ, O. Method used for tumor bed closure (suture vs. Sealant), ischemia time and duration of surgery are independent predictors of post-nephron sparing surgery acute kidney injury. *Urol. Int.* **2018**, *101*, 184–189. [CrossRef] [PubMed]

22. Nakazawa, J.; Isshiki, K.; Sugimoto, T.; Araki, S.; Kume, S.; Yokomaku, Y.; Chin-Kanasaki, M.; Sakaguchi, M.; Koya, D.; Haneda, M.; et al. Renoprotective effects of asialoerythropoietin in diabetic mice against ischaemia-reperfusion-induced acute kidney injury. *Nephrology* **2010**, *15*, 93–101. [CrossRef] [PubMed]

23. Peng, J.; Li, X.; Zhang, D.; Chen, J.K.; Su, Y.; Smith, S.B.; Dong, Z. Hyperglycemia, p53, and mitochondrial pathway of apoptosis are involved in the susceptibility of diabetic models to ischemic acute kidney injury. *Kidney Int.* **2015**, *87*, 137–150. [CrossRef] [PubMed]

24. Shi, H.; Patschan, D.; Epstein, T.; Goligorsky, M.S.; Winaver, J. Delayed recovery of renal regional blood flow in diabetic mice subjected to acute ischemic kidney injury. *Am. J. Physiol. Renal Physiol.* **2007**, *293*, F1512–F1517. [CrossRef] [PubMed]

25. Funahashi, Y.; Hattori, R.; Yamamoto, T.; Kamihira, O.; Kato, K.; Gotoh, M. Ischemic renal damage after nephron-sparing surgery in patients with normal contralateral kidney. *Eur. Urol.* **2009**, *55*, 209–215. [CrossRef] [PubMed]

26. Porpiglia, F.; Fiori, C.; Bertolo, R.; Angusti, T.; Piccoli, G.B.; Podio, V.; Russo, R. The effects of warm ischaemia time on renal function after laparoscopic partial nephrectomy in patients with normal contralateral kidney. *World J. Urol.* **2012**, *30*, 257–263. [CrossRef] [PubMed]

27. Bell, S.; Dekker, F.W.; Vadiveloo, T.; Marwick, C.; Deshmukh, H.; Donnan, P.T.; Van Diepen, M. Risk of postoperative acute kidney injury in patients undergoing orthopaedic surgery—development and validation of a risk score and effect of acute kidney injury on survival: Observational cohort study. *BMJ* **2015**, *351*, h5639. [CrossRef]

28. Park, K.M.; Kim, J.I.; Ahn, Y.; Bonventre, A.J.; Bonventre, J.V. Testosterone is responsible for enhanced susceptibility of males to ischemic renal injury. *J. Biol. Chem.* **2004**, *279*, 52282–52292. [CrossRef]

29. Muller, V.; Losonczy, G.; Heemann, U.; Vannay, A.; Fekete, A.; Reusz, G.; Tulassay, T.; Szabo, A.J. Sexual dimorphism in renal ischemia-reperfusion injury in rats: Possible role of endothelin. *Kidney Int.* **2002**, *62*, 1364–1371. [CrossRef]

30. Tanaka, R.; Tsutsui, H.; Ohkita, M.; Takaoka, M.; Yukimura, T.; Matsumura, Y. Sex differences in ischemia/reperfusion-induced acute kidney injury are dependent on the renal sympathetic nervous system. *Eur. J. Pharmacol.* **2013**, *714*, 397–404. [CrossRef]

31. Halkos, M.E.; Puskas, J.D.; Lattouf, O.M.; Kilgo, P.; Kerendi, F.; Song, H.K.; Guyton, R.A.; Thourani, V.H. Elevated preoperative hemoglobin a1c level is predictive of adverse events after coronary artery bypass surgery. *J. Thorac. Cardiovasc. Surg.* **2008**, *136*, 631–640. [CrossRef]

32. Morgan, C.J. Reducing bias using propensity score matching. *J. Nucl. Cardiol.* **2018**, *25*, 404–406. [CrossRef]

15

Acute Kidney Injury Adjusted for Parenchymal Mass Reduction and Long-Term Renal Function after Partial Nephrectomy

Hyun-Kyu Yoon [1], Ho-Jin Lee [1], Seokha Yoo [1], Sun-Kyung Park [1], Yongsuk Kwon [1], Kwanghoon Jun [1], Chang Wook Jeong [2] and Won Ho Kim [1,*]

[1]   Department of Anesthesiology and Pain Medicine, Seoul National University Hospital, Seoul National University College of Medicine, Seoul 03080, Korea; hyunkyu18@gmail.com (H.-K.Y.); zenerdiode03@gmail.com (H.-J.L.); muroki22@gmail.com (S.Y.); mayskpark@gmail.com (S.-K.P.); ulsan-no8@hanmail.net (Y.K.); tonyjj88@gmail.com (K.J.)

[2]   Department of Urology, Seoul National University Hospital, Seoul National University College of Medicine, Seoul 03080, Korea; drboss@korea.com

*   Correspondence: wonhokim@snu.ac.kr

Abstract: We sought to evaluate the association of postoperative acute kidney injury (AKI) adjusted for parenchymal mass reduction with long-term renal function in patients undergoing partial nephrectomy. A total of 629 patients undergoing partial nephrectomy were reviewed. Postoperative AKI was defined by the Kidney Disease: Improving Global Outcomes (KDIGO) serum creatinine criteria, by using either the unadjusted or adjusted baseline serum creatinine level, accounting for renal parenchymal mass reduction. Estimated glomerular filtration rates (eGFRs) were followed up to 61 months (median 28 months) after surgery. The primary outcome was the functional change ratio (FCR) of eGFR calculated by the ratio of the most recent follow-up value, at least 24 months after surgery, to eGFR at 3–12 months after surgery. Multivariable linear regression analysis was performed to evaluate whether unadjusted or adjusted AKI was an independent predictor of FCR. As a sensitivity analysis, functional recovery at 3–12 months after surgery compared to the preoperative baseline was analyzed. Median parenchymal mass reduction was 11%. Unadjusted AKI occurred in 16.5% (104/625) and adjusted AKI occurred in 8.6% (54/629). AKI using adjusted baseline creatinine was significantly associated with a long-term FCR ($\beta = -0.129 \pm 0.026$, $p < 0.001$), while unadjusted AKI was not. Adjusted AKI was also a significant predictor of functional recovery ($\beta = -0.243 \pm 0.106$, $p = 0.023$), while unadjusted AKI was not. AKI adjusted for the parenchymal mass reduction was significantly associated with a long-term functional decline after partial nephrectomy. A creatinine increase due to remaining parenchymal ischemic injury may be important in order to predict long-term renal functional outcomes after partial nephrectomy.

Keywords: acute kidney injury; partial nephrectomy; parenchymal mass reduction; ischemia

1. Introduction

Acute kidney injury (AKI) frequently occurs after partial nephrectomy, with an incidence of up to 54% [1,2]. Furthermore, renal function gradually declines and chronic renal insufficiency may develop after partial nephrectomy [3]. A new baseline estimated glomerular filtration rate (eGFR) after early postoperative recovery following partial nephrectomy can impact survival after nephrectomy [4]. As a postoperative AKI is associated with the development of chronic kidney disease (CKD) [5], the AKI after a nephrectomy could also be associated with poor long-term renal function. However, the potential impact of an AKI after a partial nephrectomy on long-term renal function has been debated.

Several studies investigated the impact of AKI after radical or partial nephrectomies, with controversy resulting [2,6–8]. Studies of radical nephrectomy reported that AKIs are associated with new-onset CKD [7,8], while studies of partial nephrectomy reported inconsistent results [2,6].

Furthermore, there remains uncertainty regarding how to diagnose AKI after partial nephrectomy. An AKI is diagnosed by the degree of serum creatinine elevation according to clinical criteria, such as the Kidney Disease: Improving Global Outcomes (KDIGO) criteria [9]. However, an AKI after nephrectomy is different from other surgeries, because postoperative serum creatinine elevation could be due to the parenchymal mass reduction by surgical resection as well as ischemic injury of the remaining renal nephrons [2,4,10]. Therefore, conventional criteria which do not consider the parenchymal mass reduction by partial nephrectomy could overestimate the incidence and severity of AKIs. In light of that, a recent study proposed new criteria for AKI after partial nephrectomy, which use an adjusted creatinine measurement as a postoperative baseline to determine AKI. Adjusted baseline creatinine was determined as the projection of the creatinine value after correcting it for the creatinine elevation due to the effect of parenchymal mass reduction [2]. There was a significant association between the renal functional recovery after surgery and AKI, determined by their proposed criteria, using adjusted baseline creatinine, but not for the AKIs determined by conventional criteria. However, another study using similar methodology reported no association between AKIs adjusted for parenchymal mass reduction and long-term renal function after partial nephrectomy [6].

As such, the diagnosis of AKI and the influence of AKI on long-term renal function after partial nephrectomy, are still not clear. Therefore, we attempted to investigate the relationship between AKI after partial nephrectomy and long-term renal outcomes in our cohort. To evaluate AKI adjusted for the parenchymal mass reduction, we compared the association between AKI and postoperative long-term renal function by using both AKIs determined by unadjusted and adjusted baseline serum creatinine, accounting for parenchymal mass reduction. Previous studies investigated the long-term renal function after partial nephrectomy by measuring functional recovery and functional change ratio (FCR) (Figure 1) [2,6]. These outcomes measure the ratio of glomerular filtration rate (GFR) at different time points after surgery. We compared long-term renal function regarding two outcomes of functional recovery and FCR.

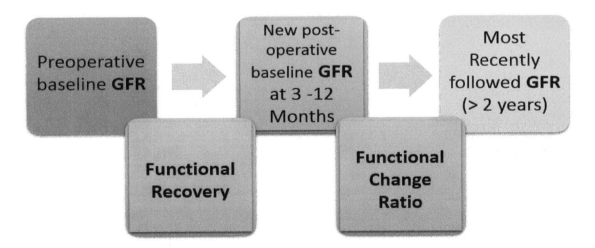

Figure 1. Study outcomes and time points of measurement. Functional recovery was measured as the ratio of glomerular filtration rate (GFR) at 3–12 months to preoperative baseline GFR. Functional change ratio was calculated as the ratio of most recent GFR to a new postoperative baseline GFR at 3–12 months. Preoperative baseline GFR was used as a baseline to calculate the outcome of functional recovery and a new post-operative baseline GFR at 3–12 months was used as a baseline to calculate the outcome of functional change ratio.

2. Materials and Methods

2.1. Study Population

This single-center retrospective observational study was approved by the institutional review board of Seoul National University Hospital (1904-060-1026). Written informed consent was waived due to the retrospective nature of the present study. We reviewed electronic medical records of the patients who were ≥18 years old; had a renal mass and underwent partial nephrectomy, regardless of surgical techniques; and had a contralateral kidney between 2010 and 2014. Among the 639 patients who underwent partial nephrectomy, 629 patients were included in the final analysis, after excluding the patients without a preoperative, computed tomography (CT), coronal reconstruction image ($n = 10$).

2.2. Surgical and Anesthesia Procedure

Partial nephrectomies by open, laparoscopic and robot-assisted techniques were included in our analysis. Decisions regarding the type of surgical approach and use of warm versus cold ischemia were made based on the tumor characteristics. Surgical resection was performed after clamping the main renal artery or arteries. The renal vein was clamped selectively. Saline ice slush was used for cold ischemia. Anesthesia was induced and maintained by sevoflurane, desflurane or total intravenous anesthesia with propofol and remifentanil. All patients received an intraoperative 20 g mannitol infusion within 30 min before vascular clamping. For significant surgical bleeding, hydroxyethyl starch was administered to expand the intravascular volume and red blood cells were transfused to maintain the intraoperative hematocrit >24%.

2.3. Patient Data and Outcome Measurements

Demographic, baseline characteristics and surgery-related parameters that were known to be associated with renal function after nephrectomy were extracted from our electronic medical records (Table 1) [1,2,6,11–13]. Serum creatinine values measured 3 to 60 months after surgery were collected. GFR estimates were based on the equation in [14].

Table 1. Patient characteristics and perioperative parameters according to acute kidney injury adjusted for parenchymal mass reduction.

Characteristic	Adjusted AKI	No AKI	p-Value
Patient population, n	54 (8.6)	575 (91.4)	
Demographic data			
Age, yr	61 (51–67)	54 (46–65)	0.020
Female, n	3 (5.6)	176 (30.6)	<0.001
Body-mass index, kg/m^2	24.2 (22.5–26.7)	24.6 (22.6–26.7)	0.599
Background medical status			
Hypertension, n	27 (50.0)	202 (35.1)	0.030
Diabetes mellitus, n	9 (16.7)	75 (13.0)	0.409
Cerebrovascular accident, n	1 (1.9)	14 (2.4)	0.781
Angina pectoris, n	2 (3.7)	4 (0.7)	0.087
Preoperative hemoglobin, g/dL	14.0 (11.1–15.2)	14.1 (12.9–15.0)	0.147
Preoperative serum albumin level, g/dL	4.3 (3.9–4.5)	4.5 (4.2–4.6)	0.001
Preoperative proteinuria, n	8 (14.8)	27 (4.7)	0.007
Unilateral kidney, n	8 (14.8)	51 (8.9)	0.147
Operation and anesthesia details			
Surgery type, n			0.965
Laparoscopic	1 (1.9)	31 (5.4)	
Robot-assisted	6 (11.1)	122 (21.2)	
Open	47 (87.0)	422 (73.4)	
Clinical stage, n			<0.001

Table 1. *Cont.*

Characteristic	Adjusted AKI	No AKI	*p*-Value
T1a/T1b	35 (64.8)/12 (22.2)	496 (86.3)/62 (10.8)	
T2a/T2b	3 (5.6)/2 (3.7)	14 (2.4)/2 (0.3)	
T3a/T3b/T3c	1 (1.9)/1 (1.9)/0	1 (0.2)/0/0	
N 0/1	51 (94.4)/3 (5.6)	571 (99.3)/4 (0.7)	0.016
M 0/1	51 (94.4)/3 (5.6)	567 (98.6)/8 (1.4)	0.060
R.E.N.A.L. score	7 (7–8)	6 (5–7)	<0.001
Low (4–6)	9 (16.7)	390 (67.8)	
Intermediate (7–9)	42 (77.8)	179 (31.1)	
High (10–12)	3 (5.6)	6 (1.0)	
Tumor maximal diameter, cm	2.5 (2.0–4.0)	2.3 (1.5–3.5)	0.038
Operation time, min	150 (120–206)	140 (107–180)	0.113
Warm ischemia, *n*	51 (94.4)	548 (95.3)	0.736
Cold ischemia, *n*	3 (5.6)	27 (4.7)	0.736
Renal ischemic time, min	30 (24–42)	24 (17–30)	<0.001
Warm ischemic time, min	28 (24–42)	24 (18–30)	<0.001
Cold ischemic time, min	38 (30–38)	31 (17–39)	0.387
Estimated parenchymal volume preservation, %	89 (85–90)	89 (88–90)	0.623
Anesthesia technique			0.113
Total intravenous agent, *n*	50 (92.6)	483 (84.0)	
Inhalational agent, *n*	4 (7.4)	92 (16.0)	
Intraoperative vasopressor use, *n*	7 (16.3)	66 (12.0)	0.467
Bleeding and transfusion amount			
pRBC transfusion, *n*	10 (18.5)	20 (3.5)	<0.001
Estimated blood loss, mL	300 (200–600)	200 (100–350)	<0.001
Input and output during surgery			
Crystalloid administration, mL	1150 (800–1700)	1200 (800–1700)	0.653
Colloid administration, mL	0 (0–500)	0 (0–400)	0.486

Data are presented as median (interquartile range) or number (%). AKI = acute kidney injury; R.E.N.A.L. = radius, exophytic/endophytic properties, nearness of tumor to collecting system or sinus, anterior/posterior, hilar, location relative to polar lines; pRBC = packed red blood cell.

The primary outcome was a long-term FCR of GFR, which was defined as the most recent GFR/new baseline GFR after surgery [7]. New baseline GFR was defined as the latest value available during 3–12 months. Renal function is expected to recover a little after the sudden drop following partial nephrectomy, and the recovering GFR was defined as the new baseline GFR. This period of 3–12 months was chosen because individual follow-up duration varied and according to a previous study [6]. The most recent GFR collected was the GFR of at least 24 months after surgery. One secondary outcome was functional recovery from renal ischemia [2]. Functional recovery was calculated as the ratio of the percentage of function saved to the percent of parenchymal volume saved. The percentage of function saved was determined as the ratio of eGFR at 3–12 months after nephrectomy to the preoperative baseline eGFR. The summary and time points for these outcomes are shown in Figure 1. Outcome definitions and time points were selected to be the same as previous studies to compare results in the same time period [2,6].

Postoperative unadjusted AKI was defined by the creatinine criteria of KDIGO, which was determined according to the maximal change in serum creatinine level during the first seven postoperative days (stage 1, stage 2 and stage 3: 1.5–1.9, 2: 2–2.9 and a more than three-fold increase of preoperative baseline serum creatinine, respectively) [9,15]. The most recent serum creatinine level measured before surgery was used as the baseline. Adjusted AKI was defined by using the concept of previous studies [2,4], which set a new baseline adjusted creatinine after removing the contribution of parenchymal mass reduction and compared the postoperative peak serum creatinine level to the new baseline. We calculated the baseline adjusted creatinine by using the percentage of functional volume preservation (PFVP) based on the measurements on the preoperative CT image (Figure 2) [16,17]. The details of our calculation were described in Supplemental Text S1. By using the adjusted baseline, adjusted AKI was determined again using the same KDIGO criteria.

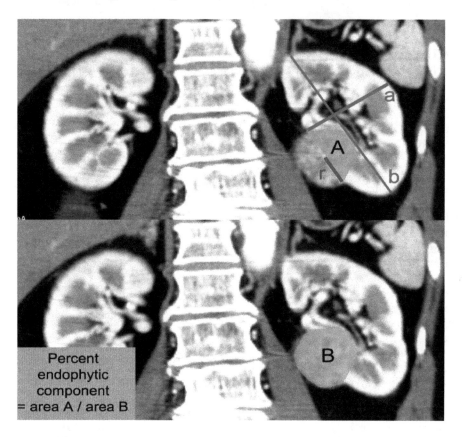

Figure 2. Measurements of the study. Kidney volume was estimated as cylindrical volume using the short (**a**) and long diameter (**b**) of the kidney on the three-dimensional computerized tomography (CT) image. The tumor volume was estimated as a ball with its radius of maximal tumor radius (r). Percent endophytic component was measured as a percentage ratio of endophytic tumor area (**A**) to whole tumor area (**B**) on the CT image where the maximal tumor area was observed.

2.4. Statistical Analysis

SPSS software version 25.0 (IBM Corp., Armonk, NY, USA) and STATA/MP version 15.1 (StataCorp, College Station, TX, USA) were used to analyze the data. For all analyses, $p < 0.05$ was considered statistically significant. The Kolmogorov-Smirnov test was used to determine the normality of the data. All following analyses were performed separately for adjusted and unadjusted AKIs.

Firstly, baseline patient and surgical characteristics were compared between patients with and without adjusted AKIs. Mann–Whitney tests were used for continuous variables, and the chi-square test or Fisher's exact test was used to compare incidence variables according to their expected counts.

Secondly, we performed a multivariable linear regression analysis to elucidate significant predictors of the long-term FCR from the new baseline GFR after surgery to the most recent follow-up. Unadjusted and adjusted AKI stages were entered alternatively as a covariate to evaluate the association between AKI and FCR. Neither stepwise variable selection nor univariable screening was performed.

Thirdly, multivariable linear regression was performed to identify independent risk factors of the functional recovery during 3–12 months after partial nephrectomy. Unadjusted and adjusted AKI stages were considered the potential predictor alternatively.

Fourthly, univariable Spearman correlation analyses were performed to assess the relationships between the stages of adjusted AKIs and the longitudinal FCR.

3. Results

Demographics and perioperative parameters are compared between adjusted AKI and no-AKI in Table 1 and between unadjusted AKI and no-AKI in supplemental Table S1. Baseline renal function is compared in supplemental Table S2. The incidence of unadjusted AKI was 16.5% ($n = 104/629$) (stage 1: $n = 88$ (14.0%); stage 2 or 3: $n = 16$ (2.5%)). The incidence of adjusted AKI was 8.6% ($n = 54/629$) (stage 1: $n = 40$ (6.4%); stage 2 or 3: $n = 14$ (2.2%)). Among all patients, only 19 patients (3.0%) required any renal replacement therapy during the postoperative hospital stay.

The median patient age was 54 years and the median parenchyma volume preservation was 89%. The median follow-up times for renal function were 27 and 28 months for patients with and without adjusted AKI (up to 61 months). The median FCR was 1.0 in patients without AKIs; and 0.92, 0.79 and 0.45 for patients with stage 1, 2 and 3 adjusted AKIs, respectively. The median functional recovery was 99% in patients without AKI; and 93%, 81% and 67% for patients with stage 1, 2 and 3 adjusted AKIs. There was no immediate postoperative mortality in our retrospective cohort. During the whole follow-up period, there were 17 (2.7%) cases of mortality from any cause and 13 (2.1%) cases of mortality from renal cell carcinoma.

Table 2 shows the results of multivariable linear regression analysis for FCR after partial nephrectomy. Postoperative adjusted AKI was identified as an independent risk factor for FCR of the most recent follow-up ($\beta = -0.129 \pm 0.026$, $p < 0.001$), while unadjusted AKI was not. Performance of our multivariable prediction in terms of R^2 was 0.10 and there was no significant multicollinearity between covariates. Figure 3 shows the distribution of FCR across the adjusted AKI stages. There was a significant correlation between FCR and adjusted AKI stages ($p < 0.001$, correlation coefficient -0.241).

Table 2. Multivariable linear regression analysis of functional change ratio after partial nephrectomy.

Variable	$\beta \pm$ Standard Error	p-Value	VIF
Age, per 10 yr	0.003 ± 0.009	0.741	1.48
Male	-0.014 ± 0.024	0.556	1.34
Body-mass index, kg/m^2	0.008 ± 0.003	0.107	1.16
Hypertension	-0.011 ± 0.022	0.622	1.28
Diabetes mellitus	0.016 ± 0.030	0.608	1.14
Preoperative hemoglobin concentration, g/dL	0.014 ± 0.007	0.051	1.56
Preoperative albumin level, g/dL	0.065 ± 0.026	0.011	1.41
Preoperative proteinuria	-0.147 ± 0.054	0.007	1.23
Preoperative estimated glomerular filtration rate, mL/min/1.73 m^2	0.001 ± 0.001	0.160	1.13
Surgery type, open versus minimal invasive surgery	-0.014 ± 0.023	0.555	1.20
Renal ischemia time, per 10 min	-0.026 ± 0.009	0.008	1.21
Ischemia type (cold)	0.036 ± 0.047	0.444	1.06
Maximal diameter of renal mass, cm	-0.005 ± 0.007	0.410	1.16
Adjusted acute kidney injury grade *	-0.129 ± 0.026	<0.001	1.10
OR unadjusted acute kidney injury grade	-0.011 ± 0.020	0.573	1.32

VIF = variance inflation factor. * Adjusted acute kidney injury was determined based on adjusted baseline creatinine value accounting for parenchymal mass reduction. Functional change ratio was determined as the ratio of most recent glomerular filtration rate (GFR) (at least 24 months after surgery) to GFR at 3 to 12 months.

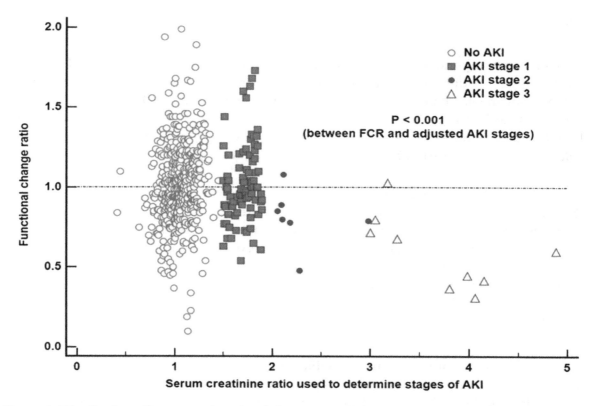

Figure 3. Distribution of long-term functional change ratio (FCR) across the different serum creatinine ratios used to determine acute kidney injury (AKI) stages. There was a significant correlation between FCR and adjusted AKI stages ($p < 0.001$).

As a sensitivity analysis, the association between functional recovery from ischemia at 3–12 months after partial nephrectomy was evaluated (Table 3). In the multivariable linear regression analysis, adjusted AKI stage was significantly associated with subsequent functional recovery ($\beta = -0.243 \pm 0.106$, $p = 0.023$), while unadjusted AKI stage classified by the standard criteria failed to associate.

Table 3. Multivariable linear regression analysis of functional recovery from ischemia at 3–12 months after partial nephrectomy.

Variable	$\beta \pm$ **Standard Error**	p-**Value**	**VIF**
Age, per 10 yr	-0.019 ± 0.049	0.706	1.48
Male	-0.186 ± 0.130	0.152	1.31
Body-mass index, kg/m^2	-0.024 ± 0.017	0.162	1.17
Hypertension	-0.027 ± 0.122	0.826	1.27
Diabetes mellitus	-0.073 ± 0.166	0.663	1.14
Preoperative hemoglobin concentration, g/dL	0.020 ± 0.041	0.631	1.55
Preoperative albumin level, g/dL	0.130 ± 0.136	0.338	1.29
Preoperative estimated glomerular filtration rate, mL/min/1.73 m^2	0.001 ± 0.003	0.726	1.25
Renal ischemia time, per 10 min	-0.057 ± 0.048	0.236	1.17
Ischemia type (cold)	0.774 ± 0.262	0.003	1.06
Maximal diameter of renal mass, cm	-0.230 ± 0.037	<0.001	1.23
Adjusted acute kidney injury stage *	-0.243 ± 0.106	0.023	1.28
OR unadjusted acute kidney injury stage	-0.177 ± 0.118	0.137	1.15

VIF = variance inflation factor. Functional recovery was calculated as the ratio of the percentage of function saved to the percentage of parenchymal volume saved. * Adjusted acute kidney injury was determined based on adjusted baseline creatinine value accounting for parenchymal mass reduction. Percent function saved was determined as the ratio of estimated glomerular filtration rate (eGFR) at 3–12 months after nephrectomy to preoperative baseline eGFR.

4. Discussion

We evaluated the association between AKI after partial nephrectomy, and long-term renal function. To account for the nephron mass reduction when diagnosing AKI, we determined AKI in two ways: using either unadjusted or adjusted baseline creatinine. Adjusted AKI after partial nephrectomy was a significant predictor of long-term FCR, but was not for unadjusted AKI. This significant association was consistent for both outcomes of FCR of at least two years after surgery and functional recovery of 3–12 months after partial nephrectomy.

AKI may be important for the long-term renal function only when it reflects true acute ischemic injury of the remaining renal nephrons. Efforts to reduce this ischemic injury may mitigate long-term renal dysfunction, thereby improving patient outcomes.

Partial nephrectomy has been regarded as standard therapy for patients with localized renal cancer [18]. Nevertheless, using the conventional diagnostic criteria of AKI, the incidence of AKI after partial nephrectomy was reported to be as high as 39%–54% [1,2]. Renal functional decline after partial nephrectomy is due to incomplete recovery of the remaining kidney from ischemic insult and parenchymal volume loss due to renal resection [4,19]. In surgeries other than nephrectomy, AKI is closely associated with the development of CKD and increased mortality [5,20,21]. However, for partial nephrectomy, this association has not been clearly ascertained. Previous studies reported varying results [2,6–8], possibly due to the difficulty there is to diagnose the pure renal parenchymal injury, and different study outcomes measuring long-term renal function at a varying intervals from nephrectomy.

Therefore, accurate diagnosis of AKI after partial nephrectomy is important, to evaluate the true impact of AKI on long-term renal function after nephrectomy. However, conventional AKI criteria simply compare the preoperative baseline creatinine level with postoperative values, not considering the aforementioned two components [2,9]. Although both of those two components could contribute to the long-term renal outcomes, our analysis indicated that the ischemic injury of the remaining kidney is more important for long-term renal prognosis.

We estimated PFVP according to a previous method which measures the renal volume on the CT images using a cylinder volume ratio method [16]. Although this is a simple and easy estimation of kidney volume, this could be inaccurate. We calculated adjusted baseline serum creatinine and eGFR by using this estimated PFVP under the assumption that endophytic components of the kidney lose functioning nephrons due to surgical resection. However, previous studies of partial nephrectomy used volumetric analysis using pre and postoperative CT images, which could be more accurate [2,6,22]. The spherical cap surface model used only the preoperative CT image to measure PFVP like our study [17]. However, they calculated the volume of normal parenchyma removed during surgery, which was not considered in our calculation. Although not available in our data, the surgeon's visual assessment of parenchymal preserved volume was reported to be strongly associated with measured values [23]. Preoperative assessment of PFVP based on preoperative imaging provided similar predictive capacity to the surgeon's assessment [24]. Our study results should be interpreted under these limitations.

There have been two studies investigating the association between AKI and long-term renal function after partial nephrectomy [2,6]. Both studies used a volumetric analysis of pre and postoperative CT images. Zhang et al. defined adjusted AKI according to projected serum creatinine as a new baseline and reported a significant association between AKI using a creatinine-adjusted baseline, and early renal functional recovery after partial nephrectomy [2]. This study used functional recovery at 3–12 months after partial nephrectomy and the preoperative baseline. The median parenchymal mass reduction was 11% and cold ischemia was used 53% of the time. However, in another study, which evaluated FCR at least after 12 months after partial nephrectomy compared to the postoperative, new baseline at 3–12 months after surgery, reported no significant association between adjusted AKI stages and FCR [6]. The median parenchymal mass reduction was 20% and cold ischemia was used 47% of the time. Although adjusted AKI was used in both studies, varying follow-up duration and different baseline of renal function could yield different results. Different sizes of the tumors, degrees of parenchymal resection, the incidence of cold ischemia, ischemic time and tumor complexity, could influence long-term renal function after partial nephrectomy. A patient cohort with shorter ischemic time and higher incidence of cold ischemia may lead to relatively good long-term renal function, and a population with a longer ischemic time and low incidence of cold ischemia may yield poor long-term renal function, which could discriminate the influence of AKI. We used the same outcomes as those two studies for a valid comparison.

For the patients undergoing unilateral radical nephrectomy, there have been only two studies, which reported a significant association between postoperative AKI and progressive CKD [7,8]. The incidence of AKI was rather high, up to 49.1%, and the association was strong, with a three to four-fold higher risk, although CKD was defined differently between the two studies. Further prospective studies are required to validate this association.

Although functional recovery after partial nephrectomy is mainly determined by parenchymal volume preservation [22], we demonstrated that ischemic insult of the remaining kidney could also affect the functional outcome substantially if ischemic time is prolonged. Efforts have been made to reduce renal injury after partial nephrectomy. The effects of pharmacological agents, such as mannitol and dopamine, have been questioned [25,26]. Cold ischemia is known to be effective in restoring renal function after partial nephrectomy [27]. However, cold ischemia was not significant in the present study, possibly due to its low incidence in our cohort. Recently, zero ischemia partial nephrectomy or selective arterial clamping has been suggested [28,29]. Remote ischemic conditioning using transient limb ischemia was suggested to reduce short-term renal functional impairment after a laparoscopic partial nephrectomy [30,31]. A previous pilot study reported combined treatment of ketorolac and remote ischemic conditioning in patients undergoing partial nephrectomy reduced the incidence of AKI [32]. Hydrogen sulfide was effective in attenuating prolonged warm renal ischemia-reperfusion injury in a previous animal study [33]. However, the incidence of AKI and CKD after partial nephrectomy was still high. Further studies for these interventions may consider the outcome of AKI based on adjusted creatinine.

Most of the significant predictors for new-onset CKD are consistent with previous studies. Although unmodifiable, preoperative proteinuria is a known predictor [1,11,34], which was consistent with our results. Renal ischemic time [1,34,35] should be reduced and cold ischemia can be applied during renal mass resection to reduce renal injury, despite existing controversy [4,36,37].

This study has several limitations. Firstly, our study was a retrospective study of a single tertiary care center. Unknown and unmeasured biases could have affected our results. Open and minimally invasive surgeries are mixed in our population. Missing values of long-term renal function jeopardize the validity of our results. Secondly, as mentioned earlier, our estimation of adjusted baseline creatinine or eGFR has limitations. Further studies are required to support our results with validated volumetric analysis. Thirdly, we included patients who have bilateral kidneys in our analysis. Although all patients underwent partial nephrectomy, the adjustment of baseline creatinine could be more inaccurate in a patient with bilateral kidneys compared to one with a single kidney.

5. Conclusions

By using baseline creatinine corrected for parenchymal mass reduction based on our simple measurements on preoperative CT, AKI adjusted for the renal parenchymal mass reduction was a significant predictor of long-term renal function for at least two years after surgery, while unadjusted AKI was not. We demonstrated this association by using two different outcomes that previous studies used. Our study suggests the prognostic implication of acute injury of remaining renal parenchyma during partial nephrectomy, in regard to long-term renal function. Efforts to reduce the remaining renal parenchymal injury may contribute to mitigate the risk of long-term deterioration in renal function after partial nephrectomy. However, prospective trials with validated renal volume measurements are required.

Supplementary Materials:
Supplemental Text S1. Calculation of adjusted preoperative estimated glomerular filtration rate and adjusted serum creatinine in partial nephrectomy. Supplemental Table S1. Patient characteristics and perioperative parameters according to acute kidney injury using unadjusted preoperative baseline creatinine. Supplemental Table S2. Comparison of baseline renal function and the rates of surgical complications between those with and without adjusted acute kidney injury.

Author Contributions: H.-K.Y.: data curation, formal analysis and writing—original draft preparation; H.-J.L.: data curation, and writing—review and editing; S.Y., S.-K.P., Y.K. and K.J.: writing review and editing; C.W.J.: data curation and writing—review and editing; W.H.K.: conceptualization, data curation, formal analysis, investigation, methodology, software, visualization and writing—original draft preparation.

Acknowledgments: The authors would like to thank our institutional statistical support team (Medical Research Collaborating Center, MRCC, mrss.snuh.org) for their assistance with statistical analysis.

References

1. Rajan, S.; Babazade, R.; Govindarajan, S.R.; Pal, R.; You, J.; Mascha, E.J.; Khanna, A.; Yang, M.; Marcano, F.D.; Singh, A.K.; et al. Perioperative factors associated with acute kidney injury after partial nephrectomy. *Br. J. Anaesth.* **2016**, *116*, 70–76. [CrossRef] [PubMed]

2. Zhang, Z.; Zhao, J.; Dong, W.; Remer, E.; Li, J.; Demirjian, S.; Zabell, J.; Campbell, S.C. Acute Kidney Injury after Partial Nephrectomy: Role of Parenchymal Mass Reduction and Ischemia and Impact on Subsequent Functional Recovery. *Eur. Urol.* **2016**, *69*, 745–752. [CrossRef] [PubMed]

3. Weight, C.J.; Larson, B.T.; Fergany, A.F.; Gao, T.; Lane, B.R.; Campbell, S.C.; Kaouk, J.H.; Klein, E.A.; Novick, A.C. Nephrectomy induced chronic renal insufficiency is associated with increased risk of cardiovascular death and death from any cause in patients with localized cT1b renal masses. *J. Urol.* **2010**, *183*, 1317–1323. [CrossRef] [PubMed]

4. Mir, M.C.; Ercole, C.; Takagi, T.; Zhang, Z.; Velet, L.; Remer, E.M.; Demirjian, S.; Campbell, S.C. Decline in renal function after partial nephrectomy: Etiology and prevention. *J. Urol.* **2015**, *193*, 1889–1898. [CrossRef] [PubMed]

5. Chawla, L.S.; Eggers, P.W.; Star, R.A.; Kimmel, P.L. Acute kidney injury and chronic kidney disease as interconnected syndromes. *N. Engl. J. Med.* **2014**, *371*, 58–66. [CrossRef] [PubMed]

6. Zabell, J.; Isharwal, S.; Dong, W.; Abraham, J.; Wu, J.; Suk-Ouichai, C.; Palacios, D.A.; Remer, E.; Li, J.; Campbell, S.C. Acute Kidney Injury after Partial Nephrectomy of Solitary Kidneys: Impact on Long-Term Stability of Renal Function. *J. Urol.* **2018**, *200*, 1295–1301. [CrossRef]

7. Cho, A.; Lee, J.E.; Kwon, G.Y.; Huh, W.; Lee, H.M.; Kim, Y.G.; Kim, D.J.; Oh, H.Y.; Choi, H.Y. Post-operative acute kidney injury in patients with renal cell carcinoma is a potent risk factor for new-onset chronic kidney disease after radical nephrectomy. *Nephrol. Dial. Transplant.* **2011**, *26*, 3496–3501. [CrossRef]

8. Garofalo, C.; Liberti, M.E.; Russo, D.; Russo, L.; Fuiano, G.; Cianfrone, P.; Conte, G.; De Nicola, L.; Minutolo, R.; Borrelli, S. Effect of post-nephrectomy acute kidney injury on renal outcome: A retrospective long-term study. *World J. Urol.* **2018**, *36*, 59–63. [CrossRef]

9. Thomas, M.E.; Blaine, C.; Dawnay, A.; Devonald, M.A.; Ftouh, S.; Laing, C.; Latchem, S.; Lewington, A.; Milford, D.V.; Ostermann, M. The definition of acute kidney injury and its use in practice. *Kidney Int.* **2015**, *87*, 62–73. [CrossRef]

10. Chapman, D.; Moore, R.; Klarenbach, S.; Braam, B. Residual renal function after partial or radical nephrectomy for renal cell carcinoma. *Can. Urol. Assoc. J.* **2010**, *4*, 337–343. [CrossRef]

11. Tachibana, H.; Kondo, T.; Takagi, T.; Okumi, M.; Tanabe, K. Impact of preoperative proteinuria on renal functional outcomes after open partial nephrectomy in patients with a solitary kidney. *Investig. Clin. Urol.* **2017**, *58*, 409–415. [CrossRef] [PubMed]

12. Martín, O.D.; Bravo, H.; Arias, M.; Dallos, D.; Quiroz, Y.; Medina, L.G.; Cacciamani, G.E.; Carlini, R.G. Determinant factors for chronic kidney disease after partial nephrectomy. *Oncoscience* **2018**, *5*, 13–20. [PubMed]

13. Kim, N.Y.; Hong, J.H.; Koh, D.H.; Lee, J.; Nam, H.J.; Kim, S.Y. Effect of Diabetes Mellitus on Acute Kidney Injury after Minimally Invasive Partial Nephrectomy: A Case-Matched Retrospective Analysis. *J. Clin. Med.* **2019**, *8*, 468. [CrossRef] [PubMed]

14. Levey, A.S.; Bosch, J.P.; Lewis, J.B.; Greene, T.; Rogers, N.; Roth, D. A more accurate method to estimate glomerular filtration rate from serum creatinine: A new prediction equation. Modification of Diet in Renal Disease Study Group. *Ann. Intern. Med.* **1999**, *130*, 461–470. [CrossRef] [PubMed]
15. Shin, S.R.; Kim, W.H.; Kim, D.J.; Shin, I.W.; Sohn, J.T. Prediction and Prevention of Acute Kidney Injury after Cardiac Surgery. *BioMed Res. Int.* **2016**, *2016*, 2985148. [CrossRef] [PubMed]
16. Simmons, M.N.; Fergany, A.F.; Campbell, S.C. Effect of parenchymal volume preservation on kidney function after partial nephrectomy. *J. Urol.* **2011**, *186*, 405–410. [CrossRef]
17. Ding, Y.; Kong, W.; Zhang, J.; Dong, B.; Chen, Y.; Xue, W.; Liu, D.; Huang, Y. Spherical cap surface model: A novel method for predicting renal function after partial nephrectomy. *Int. J. Urol.* **2016**, *23*, 667–672. [CrossRef] [PubMed]
18. Campbell, S.; Uzzo, R.G.; Allaf, M.E.; Bass, E.B.; Cadeddu, J.A.; Chang, A.; Clark, P.E.; Davis, B.J.; Derweesh, I.H.; Giambarresi, L.; et al. Renal Mass and Localized Renal Cancer: AUA Guideline. *J. Urol.* **2017**, *198*, 520–529. [CrossRef]
19. McIntosh, A.G.; Parker, D.C.; Egleston, B.L.; Uzzo, R.G.; Haseebuddin, M.; Joshi, S.S.; Viterbo, R.; Greenberg, R.E.; Chen, D.Y.T.; Smaldone, M.C.; et al. Prediction of significant estimated glomerular filtration rate decline after renal unit removal to aid in the clinical choice between radical and partial nephrectomy in patients with a renal mass and normal renal function. *BJU Int.* **2019**. [CrossRef]
20. Coca, S.G.; Singanamala, S.; Parikh, C.R. Chronic kidney disease after acute kidney injury: A systematic review and meta-analysis. *Kidney Int.* **2012**, *81*, 442–448. [CrossRef]
21. Chertow, G.M.; Burdick, E.; Honour, M.; Bonventre, J.V.; Bates, D.W. Acute kidney injury, mortality, length of stay, and costs in hospitalized patients. *J. Am. Soc. Nephrol.* **2005**, *16*, 3365–3370. [CrossRef] [PubMed]
22. Mir, M.C.; Campbell, R.A.; Sharma, N.; Remer, E.M.; Li, J.; Demirjian, S.; Kaouk, J.; Campbell, S.C. Parenchymal volume preservation and ischemia during partial nephrectomy: Functional and volumetric analysis. *Urology* **2013**, *82*, 263–268. [CrossRef] [PubMed]
23. Tobert, C.M.; Takagi, T.; Liss, M.A.; Lee, H.; Derweesh, I.H.; Campbell, S.C.; Lane, B.R. Multicenter Validation of Surgeon Assessment of Renal Preservation in Comparison to Measurement with 3D Image Analysis. *Urology* **2015**, *86*, 534–538. [CrossRef] [PubMed]
24. Klingler, M.J.; Babitz, S.K.; Kutikov, A.; Campi, R.; Hatzichristodoulou, G.; Sanguedolce, F.; Brookman-May, S.; Akdogan, B.; Capitanio, U.; Roscigno, M.; et al. Assessment of volume preservation performed before or after partial nephrectomy accurately predicts postoperative renal function: Results from a prospective multicenter study. *Urol. Oncol.* **2019**, *37*, 33–39. [CrossRef] [PubMed]
25. Cosentino, M.; Breda, A.; Sanguedolce, F.; Landman, J.; Stolzenburg, J.U.; Verze, P.; Rassweiler, J.; Van Poppel, H.; Klingler, H.C.; Janetschek, G.; et al. The use of mannitol in partial and live donor nephrectomy: An international survey. *World J. Urol.* **2013**, *31*, 977–982. [CrossRef] [PubMed]
26. O'Hara, J.F.; Hsu, T.H., Jr.; Sprung, J.; Cywinski, J.B.; Rolin, H.A.; Novick, A.C. The effect of dopamine on renal function in solitary partial nephrectomy surgery. *J. Urol.* **2002**, *167*, 24–28. [CrossRef]
27. Mir, M.C.; Takagi, T.; Campbell, R.A.; Sharma, N.; Remer, E.M.; Li, J.; Demirjian, S.; Stein, R.; Kaouk, J.; Campbell, S.C. Poorly functioning kidneys recover from ischemia after partial nephrectomy as well as strongly functioning kidneys. *J. Urol.* **2014**, *192*, 665–670. [CrossRef]
28. Hung, A.J.; Cai, J.; Simmons, M.N.; Gill, I.S. "Trifecta" in partial nephrectomy. *J. Urol.* **2013**, *189*, 36–42. [CrossRef]
29. Paulucci, D.J.; Rosen, D.C.; Sfakianos, J.P.; Whalen, M.J.; Abaza, R.; Eun, D.D.; Krane, L.S.; Hemal, A.K.; Badani, K.K. Selective arterial clamping does not improve outcomes in robot-assisted partial nephrectomy: A propensity-score analysis of patients without impaired renal function. *BJU Int.* **2017**, *119*, 430–435. [CrossRef]
30. Huang, J.; Chen, Y.; Dong, B.; Kong, W.; Zhang, J.; Xue, W.; Liu, D.; Huang, Y. Effect of remote ischaemic preconditioning on renal protection in patients undergoing laparoscopic partial nephrectomy: A 'blinded' randomised controlled trial. *BJU Int.* **2013**, *112*, 74–80. [CrossRef]
31. Hur, M.; Park, S.K.; Shin, J.; Choi, J.Y.; Yoo, S.; Kim, W.H.; Kim, J.T. The effect of remote ischemic preconditioning on serum creatinine in patients undergoing partial nephrectomy: A study protocol for a randomized controlled trial. *Trials* **2018**, *19*, 473. [CrossRef] [PubMed]
32. Kil, H.K.; Kim, J.Y.; Choi, Y.D.; Lee, H.S.; Kim, T.K.; Kim, J.E. Effect of Combined Treatment of Ketorolac and Remote Ischemic Preconditioning on Renal Ischemia-Reperfusion Injury in Patients Undergoing Partial

Nephrectomy: Pilot Study. *J. Clin. Med.* **2018**, *7*, 470. [CrossRef] [PubMed]

33. Zhu, J.X.; Kalbfleisch, M.; Yang, Y.X.; Bihari, R.; Lobb, I.; Davison, M.; Mok, A.; Cepinskas, G.; Lawendy, A.-R.; Sener, A. Detrimental effects of prolonged warm renal ischaemia-reperfusion injury are abrogated by supplemental hydrogen sulphide: An analysis using real-time intravital microscopy and polymerase chain reaction. *BJU Int.* **2012**, *110*, E1218–E1227. [CrossRef] [PubMed]

34. Porpiglia, F.; Renard, J.; Billia, M.; Musso, F.; Volpe, A.; Burruni, R.; Terrone, C.; Colla, L.; Piccoli, G.; Podio, V.; et al. Is renal warm ischemia over 30 min during laparoscopic partial nephrectomy possible? One-year results of a prospective study. *Eur. Urol.* **2007**, *52*, 1170–1178. [CrossRef] [PubMed]

35. Funahashi, Y.; Hattori, R.; Yamamoto, T.; Kamihira, O.; Kato, K.; Gotoh, M. Ischemic renal damage after nephron-sparing surgery in patients with normal contralateral kidney. *Eur. Urol.* **2009**, *55*, 209–215. [CrossRef] [PubMed]

36. Lane, B.R.; Russo, P.; Uzzo, R.G.; Hernandez, A.V.; Boorjian, S.A.; Thompson, R.H.; Fergany, A.F.; Love, T.E.; Campbell, S.C. Comparison of cold and warm ischemia during partial nephrectomy in 660 solitary kidneys reveals predominant role of nonmodifiable factors in determining ultimate renal function. *J. Urol.* **2011**, *185*, 421–427. [CrossRef] [PubMed]

37. Lee, H.; Song, B.D.; Byun, S.S.; Lee, S.E.; Hong, S.K. Impact of warm ischaemia time on postoperative renal function after partial nephrectomy for clinical T1 renal cell carcinoma: A propensity score-matched study. *BJU Int.* **2018**, *121*, 46–52. [CrossRef] [PubMed]

16

Utility of Novel Cardiorenal Biomarkers in the Prediction and Early Detection of Congestive Kidney Injury Following Cardiac Surgery

Jason G. E. Zelt [1], Lisa M. Mielniczuk [1,2], Peter P. Liu [2], Jean-Yves Dupuis [4], Sharon Chih [2], Ayub Akbari [3] and Louise Y. Sun [4,5,*]

[1] Department of Cellular and Molecular Medicine, Faculty of Medicine, University of Ottawa, Ottawa, ON K1H8M5, Canada; jzelt@ottawaheart.ca (J.G.E.Z.); LMielniczuk@ottawaheart.ca (L.M.M.)

[2] Division of Cardiology, Department of Medicine, University of Ottawa Heart Institute, 40 Ruskin Street Ottawa, ON K1Y 4W7, Canada; pliu@ottawaheart.ca (P.P.L.); schih@ottawaheart.ca (S.C.)

[3] Division of Nephrology, Department of Medicine, The Ottawa Hospital, 1967 Riverside Dr., Ottawa, ON K1H 7W9, Canada; aakbari@toh.ca

[4] Division of Cardiac Anesthesiology, Department of Anesthesiology and Pain Medicine, University of Ottawa Heart Institute, 40 Ruskin Street, Ottawa, ON K1Y 4W7, Canada; jydupuis@ottawaheart.ca

[5] School of Epidemiology and Public Health, University of Ottawa, 600 Peter Morand Crescent, Ottawa, ON K1G 5Z3, Canada

* Correspondence: lsun@ottawaheart.ca

Abstract: Acute Kidney Injury (AKI) in the context of right ventricular failure (RVF) is thought to be largely congestive in nature. This study assessed the utility of biomarkers high sensitivity cardiac troponin T (hs-cTnT), N-Terminal Pro-B-Type Natriuretic Peptide (NT-proBNP), and neutrophil gelatinase-associated lipocalin (NGAL) for prediction and early detection of congestive AKI (c-AKI) following cardiac surgery. This prospective nested case-control study recruited 350 consecutive patients undergoing elective cardiac surgery requiring cardiopulmonary bypass. Cases were patients who developed (1) AKI (2) new or worsening RVF, or (3) c-AKI. Controls were patients free of these complications. Biomarker levels were measured at baseline after anesthesia induction and immediately postoperatively. Patients with c-AKI had increased mean duration of mechanical ventilation and length of stay in hospital and in the intensive care unit ($p < 0.01$). For prediction of c-AKI, baseline NT-proBNP yielded an area under the curve (AUC) of 0.74 (95% CI, 0.60–0.89). For early detection of c-AKI, postoperative NT-proBNP yielded an AUC of 0.78 (0.66–0.91), postoperative hs-cTnT yielded an AUC of 0.75 (0.58–0.92), and Δhs-cTnT yielded an AUC of 0.80 (0.64–0.96). The addition of baseline creatinine to Δhs-cTnT improved the AUC to 0.87 (0.76–0.99), and addition of diabetes improved the AUC to 0.93 (0.88–0.99). Δhs-cTnT alone, or in combination with baseline creatinine or diabetes, detects c-AKI with high accuracy following cardiac surgery.

Keywords: cardiac surgery; biomarkers; right heart failure; congestive acute kidney injury; venous congestion

1. Introduction

Right ventricular failure (RVF) is associated with significant morbidity and mortality following cardiac surgery [1,2]. Acute RVF is present in up to 50% of patients with postoperative hemodynamic instability [3] and is associated with difficult separation from cardiopulmonary bypass (CPB) [4], up to 75% increase in operative mortality as well as poor late survival [5,6]. Acute kidney injury (AKI) is a common sequela of RVF, which further complicates the management of RVF and portends a worsening prognosis. AKI occurs in up to 30% of cardiac surgical patients, of whom 1–2% require renal replacement therapy [7,8]. Management of perioperative AKI is primarily focused on maintenance of renal perfusion pressure and treatment of hypovolemia [9,10]. However, in the presence of RVF, AKI worsens with fluid administration and improves only with fluid removal [2]. This congestive form of AKI (c-AKI) is both difficult to diagnose and treat, especially as the cause of c-AKI is often not readily apparent and it is difficult to diagnose using current clinical criteria. Current diagnosis of AKI relies on measures of glomerular filtration such as serum creatinine, which is insensitive and lags behind actual renal injury; leading to delayed diagnosis and unfavourable outcomes [11,12]. Hemodilution, especially during the immediate postoperative period, may further confound creatinine-based diagnosis of AKI [13]. The paucity of early predictive biomarkers is one purported reason for the failure of recent prevention and treatment clinical trials for cardiac surgery induced AKI [14].

The pathogenesis of cardiac surgery induced AKI is multifactorial including many interrelated, and largely non-modifiable, injury pathways. However, venous congestion-induced AKI may potentially be reversed through diuretic and vasodilator based preventative and early treatment strategies. Contrary to popular belief [15], central venous pressure (CVP) is a poor indicator of circulating blood volume and fluid responsiveness [16,17]. Hence, there remains a need for better identification of patients who are most likely to benefit from early decongestive therapy.

Cardiac and renal biomarkers such as high sensitivity cardiac troponin T (hs-cTnT), N-Terminal Pro-B-Type Natriuretic Peptide (NT-proBNP), and neutrophil gelatinase-associated lipocalin (NGAL) are excellent prognosticators in patients with RVF and/or AKI [18–25]. These biomarkers provide direct cellular insight into cardiorenal physiology and may enable early identification of patients who are already in a congestive state prior to development of clinical consequences of venous congestion. However, the timing and pattern of release of these biomarkers are unknown in the setting of c-AKI with an acutely failing right ventricle (RV). An in-depth understanding of these biomarker patterns may enable identification of high-risk patients for intensive monitoring and early treatment. The objective of this study was to evaluate the utility of NT-proBNP, hs-cTnT, and NGAL for prediction and early detection of c-AKI following cardiac surgery.

2. Methods

The research ethics board of the University of Ottawa Heart Institute (UOHI) approved this prospective nested case-control study (protocol #: 2015049401H). Written informed consent was obtained from all participants prior to enrolment.

2.1. Patients

We recruited 350 consecutive consenting patients aged 18 years or older, who underwent major elective cardiac surgery requiring CPB at UOHI between 29 September 2015 and 21 February 2017. Exclusion criteria included end stage renal disease (glomerular filtration rate [GFR] <15 mL/min or dialysis dependence), history of renal transplantation, solitary kidney, emergent operative status, off pump procedures, procedures involving circulatory arrest, heart transplantation, and left ventricular assist device implantation.

2.2. Outcomes

The primary outcome was c-AKI, defined by AKI in the presence of postoperative RVF (definition of c-AKI is detailed in Supplemental Table S1). The secondary outcomes were non-congestive AKI, RVF, duration of mechanical ventilation, intensive care unit (ICU) and hospital lengths of stay and in-hospital mortality. AKI was defined by the Acute Kidney Injury Network (AKIN) criteria [26] as >50% relative or >26 μmol/L absolute rise in serum creatinine above preoperative value within 48 h of surgery, or new onset dialysis. Postoperative RVF was defined as new or worsening RVF satisfying published criteria A and/or B [27,28] post separation from CPB and until postoperative day 2 (Supplemental Table S1). Pulmonary artery catheterization is practiced routinely for patients undergoing cardiac surgery at our institution.

A.   Combined Clinical and Echocardiographic: [28,29]

    i.   Difficult separation from CPB, characterized by

        1.   Concurrent use of $\geq$1 vasopressor and $\geq$1 inotrope or $\geq$1 pulmonary vasodilator (i.e., nitric oxide or epoprostenol); or

        2.   More than one CPB weaning attempt; or

        3.   Mechanical support device (i.e., RV assist device); and

    ii.   >20% relative reduction in RV fractional area change measured by two-dimensional echocardiography.

B.   Hemodynamic criteria:

    i.   CVP >18 mmHg or cardiac index <1.8 L/min/m^2, in the absence of elevated left atrial and pulmonary capillary wedge pressure >18 mmHg, tamponade, ventricular arrhythmias, or pneumothorax; and

    ii.   RV stroke work index <4 g·min^{-1}·m^2. RVSWI = 0.136 $\times$ SVI $\times$ (mPAP $-$ RAP); where SVI = stroke volume index = stroke volume/body surface area, mPAP = mean pulmonary artery pressure, and RAP = right atrial pressure.

2.3. Cases and Controls

Cases were defined as patients with postoperative RVF, c-AKI or non-congestive AKI. Controls were patients who were free of these complications during the follow up period. Controls were 1:1 matched to the cases based on age and sex. All patients received routine standard of care during the study period.

2.4. Study Procedures

All patients were followed prospectively until hospital discharge. Baseline patient characteristics, operative data and postoperative outcomes were recorded by trained research staff. The attending anesthesiologist recorded baseline RV function, and whether difficulty was encountered with CPB separation. Baseline RV function was recorded from the most recent echocardiogram within 90 days of surgery in patients with stable cardiac disease, and during the index surgical admission or intraoperatively prior to CPB in patients who presented acutely.

2.5. Biomarkers

Biomarkers were sampled at baseline immediately following anesthesia induction and postoperatively within 1 h of arrival to the ICU. In addition, serum creatinine was measured at least daily during the first 2 postoperative days. Biomarker samples were centrifuged and plasma supernatants stored at -80 °C until analysis. Plasma hs-cTnT (Roche Diagnostics, Indianapolis, IN, USA) and NT-proBNP (Roche Diagnostics) were measured using commercially available US food and Drug Administration-approved electrochemiluminescence immunoassays with a Roche Cobas e411 anaylzer. Manufacturer's normal reference value for hs-cTnT and NT-proBNP are <13.5 pg/mL (99th percentile) and <300 pg/mL, respectively [23,30]. NGAL levels were measured using a commercially available ELISA kit (Bioporto Diagnostics, Copenhagen, Denmark) and using a mean reference value in healthy volunteers of 35.4 (95% CI, 18.9–46.5) ng/mL [31].

2.6. Statistical Analysis

Statistical analyses and graphic representation were performed using SAS 9.4 (SAS Institute, Cary, NC, USA) and Graphpad Prism 6.0 (Graphpad Software, San Diego, CA, USA). Categorical characteristics were compared using X^2 or Fisher's exact test for categorical variables where appropriate. Continuous variables were compared using Student's t test or Wilcoxon rank sum test depending on normality of distribution. An analysis of variance (ANOVA) was used to compare hospital and ICU stay and ventilation duration between groups. Log transformed NGAL, NT-proBNP, and hs-cTnT were used because their distributions were not normal. A two-way, repeated measure ANOVA was used to compare the effects of time (pre-versus post surgery) and AKI/RVF status for all variables. A Bonferroni correction was used for post hoc pairwise comparison of means. We used conditional logistic regression to assess the association between individual biomarker levels and c-AKI, with and without adjustment for baseline estimated GFR (eGFR), diabetes, and surgery type. These covariates were selected *a priori* based on the strength of their known association with AKI and RVF in cardiac surgical patients [21,32]. As cases were already matched to controls based on age and sex, these covariates were not included in the model. Measure of association was odds ratio (OR) with associated 95% confidence interval (CI). In addition, linear regression was used to assess the association between biomarker levels and continuous outcomes such as length of hospital/ICU stay and duration of mechanical ventilation. The Pearson correlation coefficient was reported as measure of correlation. Area under (AUC) the receiver operator characteristic (ROC) curve was used to assess the ability of individual biomarkers to discriminate between patients who developed each of the outcomes vs. those who did not. Youden's index was used to identify the optimal ROC cutoff. We also evaluated the incremental value of these biomarkers when added to the clinical model using the method of Delong, Delong, and Clarke-Pearson [33]. $p < 0.05$ was considered statistically significant.

3. Results

3.1. Patient Characteristics

A total of 350 patients were enrolled in the study, from whom 89 cases were identified and age-sex matched to 89 controls (Supplemental Table S2). Of the cases, 36 (40.5%) developed postoperative RVF, 35 (39.3%) developed non-congestive AKI, and 18 (20.2%) developed c-AKI. Baseline characteristics of c-AKI cases and controls are shown in Table 1. Compared to matched controls, c-AKI patients were more likely to have pre-existing renal insufficiency, diabetes, and to undergo more complex surgery with longer CPB and aortic crossclamp durations. In addition, there was a trend towards higher baseline CVP and lower cardiac index in c-AKI patients. There were no differences in baseline left ventricle ejection fraction (LVEF) between c-AKI and controls.

Table 1. Characteristics of patients with congestive acute kidney injury (c-AKI) vs. controls.

	Control (n = 89)	c-AKI (n = 18)	p-Value
Baseline Characteristics			
Male	61 (68.5%)	11 (61.1%)	0.54
Age (years)	66.0 (63.8–68.2)	67.1 (61.1–73.2)	0.57
Body Mass Index (kg/m^2)	28.5 (27.4–29.7)	30.5 (27.3–33.6)	0.35
eGFR (mL/min/1.73 m^2)	89.8 (83.4–96.1)	75.2 (60.6–89.7)	0.03
Serum Creatinine (μmol/L)	84.3 (79.5–89.1)	100.7 (87.3–114.1)	0.009
Cardiac Index (L/min/m^2)	2.18 (2.03–2.33)	1.93 (1.66- 2.19)	0.08
Central Venous Pressure (mmHg)	13.9 (12.9–14.9)	16.6 (14.1–19.1)	0.06
Left Ventricle Ejection Fraction (%)	53.1 (51.4–54.9)	49.6 (44.3–54.8)	0.14
Comorbidities			
Hypertension	57 (64%)	12 (67%)	0.83
Diabetes	20 (22%)	12 (67%)	0.0002
COPD	8 (9%)	1 (6%)	1.0
Pre-existing Right Heart Dysfunction	1 (1.1%)	1 (6%)	0.31
Coronary Artery Disease	57 (64%)	11 (61%)	0.81
Medications			
ASA	54 (61%)	11 (62%)	0.97
Beta Blocker	59 (66%)	11 (62%)	0.67
ACE Inhibitor	50 (56%)	8 (44%)	0.36
Lipid Lowering agents	55 (62%)	11 (62%)	0.96

Table 1. *Cont.*

	Control (*n* = 89)	c-AKI (*n* = 18)	*p*-Value
Intraoperative Characteristics			
Surgery Type			0.0006
CABG	43 (48%)	5 (28%)	
Single Valve	33 (37%)	3 (17%)	
Combined CABG/Valve/Other	13 (15%)	10 (56%)	
Cardiopulmonary Bypass Duration (min)	89.1 (82.1–96.0)	141.1 (114.5–167.7)	0.0002
Aortic Cross Clamp Duration (min)	64.6 (58.4–70.8)	102.1 (78.8–125.4)	0.003
Postoperative characteristics			
Length of Hospital Stay (days)	11.8 (9.5–14.1)	23.3 (14.2–32.4)	0.0001
Length of Intensive Care Unit Stay (days)	2.1 (1.3–2.8)	6.1 (3.4–8.8)	<0.0001
Mechanical Ventilation Duration (hours)	9.7 (3.6–15.7)	63.0 (1.23–124.7)	<0.0001

eGFR, estimated glomerular filtration rate; CABG, coronary artery bypass graft; COPD, chronic obstructive pulmonary disease; ASA, acetylsalicylic acid; ACE, angiotensin-converting-enzyme; Data presented are expressed as n (%) or mean (95% confidence interval).

3.2. Biomarker Analysis Pre and Post Cardiac Surgery

Patients who developed c-AKI had significantly higher baseline NT-proBNP levels compared to controls (Figure 1A). In patients who developed non-congestive AKI, baseline NT-proBNP, NGAL, and hs-cTnT were significantly higher than controls (Figure 1A–C). Following surgery, NT-proBNP remained relatively unchanged while hs-cTnT and NGAL increased 2–2.5 fold in all groups (Figure 1B,C). The magnitude of postoperative increase in hs-cTnT was highest in the c-AKI group. Postoperatively, NGAL increased in those who developed RVF but remained relatively unchanged in the AKI, c-AKI, and control groups.

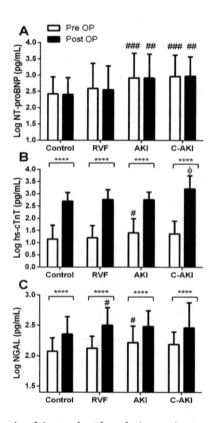

Figure 1. Baseline and postoperative biomarker levels in patients who developed congestive acute kidney injury (c-AKI) vs. controls. **** Within group differences (baseline vs. postoperative) *p* < 0.0001. # Significantly different than control *p* < 0.05, ## *p* < 0.01, ### *p* < 0.001. Φ Significantly different than control, right ventricular failure (RVF), and AKI, *p* < 0.05.

3.3. Hemodynamics Pre and Post Cardiac Surgery

Compared to controls, patients who developed c-AKI had significantly lower cardiac index at all time points (Figure 2A). Conversely, CVP decreased postoperatively from baseline in both c-AKI and control groups but remained higher in c-AKI patients throughout the postoperative period (Figure 2B). This trend was particularly evident on postoperative day 2 where CVP in c-AKI patients remained >1.5 fold higher than in the controls ($p < 0.001$).

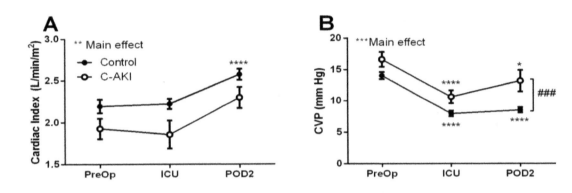

Figure 2. Cardiac index (**A**) and central venous pressure (**B**) in patients who developed congestive acute kidney injury (c-AKI) vs. controls. Hemodynamic variables were assessed preoperatively, upon admission to the intensive care unit and on postoperative day two. * Significantly different than baseline levels, $p < 0.05$; ** $p < 0.01$; *** $p < 0.001$; **** $p < 0.0001$. ### Significant difference between c-AKI and control, $p < 0.001$.

In patients with non-congestive AKI, a similar trend was observed where CVP was significantly elevated compared to controls throughout the follow up period (Supplemental Figure S1A). No significant differences in hemodynamic profiles were observed for patients who developed RVF vs. controls (Supplemental Figure S1B,D).

3.4. Biomarker and Hemodynamic Correlation

A weak positive relationship was observed between baseline log hs-cTnT and CVP ($r = 0.21$, $p = 0.006$). However, log NT-proBNP and log NGAL levels did not correlate with CVP at baseline. At baseline, cardiac index was inversely correlated with log NT-proBNP ($r = -0.2$, $p = 0.01$) and log hs-cTnT ($r = -0.19$, $p = 0.01$). In addition, there were weak-moderate inverse correlations between baseline eGFR and log hs-cTnT ($r = -0.27$, $p = 0.0002$), log NT-proBNP ($r = -0.37$, $p < 0.0001$), and log NGAL ($r = -0.28$, $p < 0.0001$). Postoperatively, a positive correlation was observed between log NT-proBNP and CVP ($r = 0.20$, $p = 0.007$), but no correlations were found between cardiac index and biomarkers.

3.5. Performance of Biomarkers vs. Traditional Parameters for c-AKI Prediction and Detection

3.5.1. Prediction of c-AKI

Higher baseline CVP was associated with c-AKI after multivariable adjustment (adjusted OR 1.20, 95% CI 1.04–1.38 for each 1 mmHg increase in CVP) (Table 2).

Table 3 and Figure 3 summarize the AUCs for individual biomarkers and traditional parameters for prediction of c-AKI. Of the baseline biomarkers, NT-proBNP had the highest AUC for predicting c-AKI (0.74, 95% CI 0.60–0.89). However, the clinical model alone (based on baseline eGFR, diabetes and surgery type) had an AUC of 0.83 (0.72–0.94), and the addition of NT-proBNP to the clinical model did not significantly improve the AUC ($p = 0.39$, Table 3). The optimal cut-off of baseline NT-proBNP for c-AKI prediction was >476 pg/mL (sensitivity 77%, specificity 72%) (Table 4).

Table 2. Association between cardiorenal biomarkers and congestive acute kidney injury.

	Unadjusted		Adjusted [a]	
	OR (95% CI)	*p* Value	OR (95% CI)	*p* Value
Baseline				
NGAL	1.37 (1.05–1.78)	0.02	1.19 (0.88–1.61)	0.25
NT-proBNP	1.17 (1.06–1.29)	0.001	1.10 (0.97–1.24)	0.12
hs-cTnT	1.06 (0.98–1.15)	0.15	0.99 (0.87–1.11)	0.81
CVP	1.12 (1.01–1.25)	0.03	1.20 (1.04–1.38)	0.01
Postoperative				
NGAL	1.11 (0.93–1.33)	0.25	1.02 (0.83–1.26)	0.86
NT-proBNP	1.21 (1.09–1.34)	0.0005	1.13 (1.00–1.29)	0.05
hs-cTnT	1.26 (1.10–1.45)	0.0009	1.22 (1.05–1.42)	0.008
CVP	1.17 (1.03–1.32)	0.01	1.15 (0.98–1.35)	0.09
Change (Postoperative–Baseline)				
ΔNGAL	1.23 (0.96–1.57)	0.09	1.26 (0.93–1.71)	0.13
ΔNT-proBNP	0.99 (0.96–1.03)	0.85	0.99 (0.94–1.05)	0.84
Δhs-cTnT	1.15 (1.07–1.24)	0.0002	1.25 (1.09–1.44)	0.001
ΔCVP	1.00 (0.91–1.10)	0.94	0.93 (0.83–1.04)	0.20

eGFR, estimated glomerular filtration rate; NGAL, neutrophil gelatinase-associated lipocalin; NT-proBNP, N-Terminal Pro-B-Type Natriuretic Peptide; hs-cTNT, high sensitivity cardiac troponin T; CVP, central venous pressure; OR, odds ratio; CI, confidence interval. [a] Biomarker models were adjusted for eGFR, diabetes and type of cardiac surgery. Baseline and postoperative biomarker levels were log transformed. Odds ratios were expressed per 0.1 unit increase in log-transformed baseline and postoperative biomarker levels and per 100 pg/mL increase for Δbiomarker levels.

Table 3. Areas under the Receiver-Operating Curve for the prediction of congestive acute kidney injury.

	Unadjusted AUC (95% CI) Biomarker Only	[a] Adjusted AUC (95%CI) Biomarker + Clinical Model
Clinical Model	-	0.83 (0.72, 0.94)
Baseline		
NGAL	0.67 (0.51–0.82)	0.84 (0.73–0.95)
NT-proBNP	0.74 (0.60–0.89)	0.84 (0.75–0.94)
hs-cTnT	0.67 (0.53–0.81)	0.82 (0.71–0.94)
CVP	0.64 (0.50–0.78)	0.88 (0.80–0.96)
Postoperative		
NGAL	0.60 (0.43–0.77)	0.83 (0.72–0.94)
NT-proBNP	0.78 (0.66–0.91)	0.86 (0.76–0.96)
hs-cTnT	0.75 (0.58–0.92)	0.88 (0.80–0.96)
CVP	0.68 (0.55–0.81)	0.87 (0.80–0.95)
Change (Postoperative-Baseline)		
ΔNGAL	0.61 (0.42–0.79)	0.82 (0.72–0.93)
ΔNT-proBNP	0.69 (0.54–0.85)	0.83 (0.71–0.94)
Δhs-cTnT	0.80 (0.64–0.96)	* 0.94 (0.89–0.99)
ΔCVP	0.49 (0.34–0.63)	0.84 (0.72–0.96)
Combined Model		
ΔHs-cTnT + Preoperative Creatinine	0.87 (0.76–0.99)	-
ΔHs-cTnT + Diabetes	0.93 (0.88–0.99)	-

eGFR, estimated glomerular filtration rate; NGAL, neutrophil gelatinase-associated lipocalin; NT-proBNP, N-Terminal Pro-B-Type Natriuretic Peptide; hs-cTNT, high sensitivity cardiac troponin T; CVP, central venous pressure; AUC, area under the receiver operative characteristic curve; CI, confidence interval. * Significantly improves AUC of the clinical model *p* < 0.05. [a] Biomarker models were adjusted for eGFR, type of cardiac surgery and diabetes.

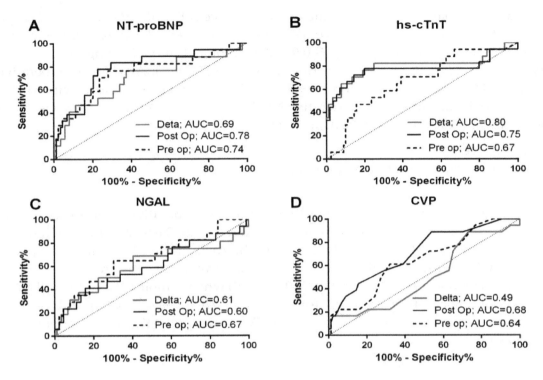

Figure 3. Receiver operating characteristic curves for N-Terminal Pro-B-Type Natriuretic Peptide (NT-proBNP) (**A**), high sensitivity cardiac troponin T (hs-cTnT) (**B**), neutrophil gelatinase-associated lipocalin (NGAL) (**C**), and central venous pressure (**D**). Dotted lines are for baseline assessments, black lines are for postoperative assessments, and red lines are for change in levels (post-preoperative). AUC, area under the curve.

Table 4. Cutoff values for predicting congestive acute kidney injury.

	Cutoff	Sensitivity	Specificity
Baseline			
NGAL (pg/mL)	140.2	64.7	69.7
NT-proBNP (pg/mL)	476.0	76.5	71.9
hs-cTnT (pg/mL)	25.0	47.1	84.3
CVP	15.5	61.1	67.8
Postoperative			
NGAL (pg/mL)	440.9	41.2	84.3
NT-proBNP (pg/mL)	599.5	72.2	79.5
hs-cTnT (pg/mL)	1089.0	66.7	84.1
CVP	10.5	44.4	84.3
Change (Postoperative-Baseline)			
ΔNGAL (pg/mL)	181.7	50.0	77.5
ΔNT-proBNP (pg/mL)	−38.8	76.5	62.5
Δhs-cTnT (pg/mL)	730.9	82.4	75.0
ΔCVP	−9.5	88.9	26.4

NGAL, neutrophil gelatinase-associated lipocalin; NT-proBNP, N-Terminal Pro-B-Type Natriuretic Peptide; hs-cTNT, high sensitivity cardiac troponin T; CVP, central venous pressure.

3.5.2. Early Detection of c-AKI

After adjusting for eGFR, diabetes, and type of surgery, postoperative NT-proBNP and hs-cTnT remained robust in detecting c-AKI (Table 2). Of note, postoperative CVP was not associated with c-AKI after risk adjustment.

ROC analysis (Table 3, Figure 3) revealed postoperative NT-proBNP and hs-cTnT as parameters with the highest AUCs for early detection of c-AKI after multivariable adjustment. Specifically, AUC for postoperative NT-proBNP was 0.78 (0.66–0.91) alone (optimal cutoff 599.5 pg/mL, sensitivity 72.2%, specificity 79.5%) and 0.86 (0.76–0.96) after risk adjustment (Table 3). AUC for postoperative hs-cTnT was 0.75 (0.58–0.92) alone (optimal cutoff 1089.0 pg/mL, sensitivity 66.7%, specificity 84.1%) and 0.88 (0.80–0.96) after risk adjustment. Postoperative NGAL alone and CVP alone only yielded moderate AUCs for detecting c-AKI (0.60 for NGAL and 0.68 for CVP).

3.5.3. Perioperative Changes in Biomarker Levels

Change in hs-cTnT levels between baseline and the postoperative period was associated with c-AKI (Tables 2 and 3). Δhs-cTnT alone yielded an AUC of 0.8 (0.64–0.96) for c-AKI detection, and was the only biomarker that significantly increased the AUC of the clinical model. Specifically, the AUC was 0.87 (0.76–0.99) when Δhs-cTnT was combined with baseline creatinine, 0.93 (0.88–0.99) when combined with diabetes status, and 0.94 (0.89–0.99) when combined with the full clinical model (Table 3). The optimal cutoff of Δhs-cTnT for detecting c-AKI was > 730.9 pg/mL (sensitivity 82%, specificity 75%; Table 4). In contrast, the ability of ΔCVP to detect c-AKI was no better than a coin toss (AUC 0.49, 95% CI 0.34–0.63).

3.6. Sample Size Calculation

A post-hoc sample size calculation was performed to validate our findings in light of the size of our cohort. An AUC of 0.70 for biomarker prediction of post cardiac surgery AKI has been deemed clinically meaningful [34]. We conservatively chose a null hypothesis AUC of 0.75. To detect an AUC of 0.93 in our Δhs-cTnT + diabetes model, our observed 18 c-AKI cases and 89 controls yielded a 86% power using a two-sided z-test at an alpha of 0.05.

3.7. Secondary Outcomes

Supplemental Table S3 summarizes the AUCs of biomarkers and CVP in predicting non-congestive AKI and postoperative RVF. At baseline, all three biomarkers had moderate accuracy for predicting non-congestive AKI (AUC 0.67 to 0.70). Postoperatively, NT-proBNP detected non-congestive AKI with moderate accuracy (AUC 0.72). ΔBiomarker levels and ΔCVP detected non-congestive AKI poorly (AUC ranging from 0.44–0.57). In contrast, none of the parameters predicted or detected RVF well (AUC 0.48–0.62).

During follow up, 3 (1.7%) patients died (2 c-AKI and 1 control) and 3 patients (1.7%) developed severe AKI requiring renal replacement therapy (2 c-AKI and 1 non-congestive AKI). Compared to controls, patients who developed c-AKI had significantly longer hospitalization, ICU length of stay and duration of mechanical ventilation (Table 1, Figure 4). Non-congestive AKI was associated longer periods of ICU stay and mechanical ventilation compared to controls. In contrast, there were no differences in observed outcomes for patients who developed postoperative RVF alone (Figure 4).

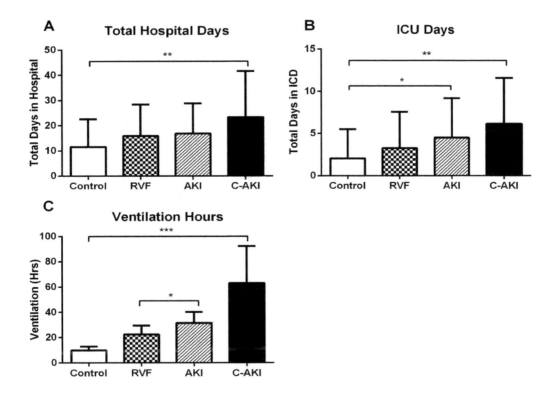

Figure 4. Lengths of stay in hospital (**A**) and ICU (**B**) and duration of mechanical ventilation (**C**) in patients who developed postoperative acute kidney injury (AKI), right ventricular failure (RVF), congestive AKI (c-AKI), and controls. Data expressed mean $\pm$ SD. * $p < 0.05$, ** $p < 0.01$, *** $p < 0.001$.

4. Discussion

This prospective nested case-control study found cardiac biomarkers hs-cTnT and NT-proBNP to be stronger predictors of c-AKI following cardiac surgery than the renal biomarker NGAL. Four major findings were derived from this study. (1) We identified the novel concept of c-AKI as a cardiorenal syndrome in the context of RVF. C-AKI was associated with prolonged mechanical ventilation and length of stay in hospital and ICU; (2) A single measurement of NT-proBNP or hs-cTnT predicted and detected c-AKI with high accuracy. In contrast, traditional measure of venous congestion such as ΔCVP had an AUC for c-AKI that was analogous to a coin flip. Specifically, baseline and postoperative NT-proBNP yielded AUCs of 0.74 and 0.78, postoperative hs-cTnT yielded an AUC of 0.75, and baseline and postoperative CVP yielded AUCs of 0.64 and 0.68, respectively; (3) Δhs-cTnT alone yielded an AUC of 0.80 for c-AKI, and the addition of diabetes increased the AUC to 0.93; (4) Neither the cardiorenal biomarkers, clinical variables, nor CVP were able to predict postoperative RVF well.

4.1. A New AKI Phenotype

Our study is novel in our definition and characterization of a congestive subtype of AKI. We found that c-AKI was associated with a higher burden of postoperative morbidity and healthcare cost than non-congestive AKI or RVF alone. The etiology of cardiac surgery-associated AKI is multifactorial involving many non-modifiable risk factors such as ischemic-reperfusion injury, inflammation and oxidative stress [14]. Unlike other AKI subtypes, c-AKI is potentially preventable and treatable, although it is often difficult to detect at an early stage. Our findings offer new insights on the role of biomarkers in the prediction and early detection of c-AKI and represent a critical first step towards characterizing postoperative c-AKI. Determining whether a biomarker-guided approach can complement current prediction, prevention and timely management strategies in the perioperative period is an important area for future investigation.

4.2. Venous Congestion and CVP

Our study is the first to prospectively characterize postoperative c-AKI with serial cardiac and renal biomarkers. Although several studies have evaluated the utility of similar biomarkers for AKI risk stratification in cardiac surgery cohorts [14,18,21,32,35], none have focused on c-AKI, which is truly a cardiorenal syndrome [15]. AKI in the context of RVF results from a complex series of cardiorenal interactions. This interaction has been believed to be primarily due to renal hypoperfusion [36], but recent evidence suggests venous congestion as a primary contributor [2,15,16,37,38]. Transrenal perfusion pressure is calculated as the mean arterial pressure minus the CVP. Clinically, in patients with acute decompensated heart failure and volume overload, the combination of low systemic pressure with elevated CVP may impair renal perfusion [15,39,40]. In a study of 145 patients admitted with acute decompensated heart failure, and using CVP as a surrogate for systemic venous congestion, Mullens et al. demonstrated that patients with low CVP (<8 mmHg) experienced significantly less decline in renal function compared to those with high CVP (>24 mmHg), independent of their cardiac index [38]. Similarly, we demonstrated that patients who developed postoperative c-AKI had elevated CVP at baseline that persisted into the postoperative period. In further support of a congestive etiology, those who developed c-AKI had LVEFs that were statistically similar to the controls and may benefit from perioperative decongestive strategies. The success of such strategies requires accurate and timely identification of venous congestion, as accumulating evidence suggests a poor correlation between CVP and circulating blood volume and an inability of CVP or ΔCVP to predict fluid responsiveness (ROC AUC value of 0.56) [16,17]. Our study corroborates these findings. Specifically, CVP detected c-AKI poorly (AUC = 0.64 for baseline CVP and AUC = 0.49 for ΔCVP). In contrast, biomarkers of cardiac function and distention (NT-proBNP) and myocardial injury (hs-cTnT) were superior to CVP for predicting and detecting c-AKI.

4.3. Congestive AKI and Cardiorenal Biomarkers

NT-proBNP and hs-cTnT are well-established prognosticators in stable and acute decompensated heart failure. NT-proBNP is a prohormone secreted by the atria and ventricles in response to volume and pressure overload. In patients with pulmonary hypertension, NT-proBNP has been shown to increase in proportion to the degree of RV distension and wall stress; whereas hs-cTnT levels increase in proportion to the severity of RV dysfunction [24,25,41]. Several studies have evaluated whether baseline and postoperative BNP could predict cardiac surgery-associated AKI with mixed results (AUC range 0.60 to 0.86) [21,34,35]. To our knowledge, only two studies have evaluated the relationship between hs-cTnT and AKI in the perioperative setting [32,34]. One study reported similar hs-cTnT and NT-proBNP changes in a pediatric cohort to those observed in our adult cohort. In addition, these authors found baseline and postoperative biomarker levels were weakly predictive of AKI (AUC for hs-cTnT: Baseline 0.57, post 0.62; AUC for NT-proBNP: Pre 0.53, post 0.57) [34]. Our study adds to this knowledge by evaluating the same biomarkers to predict RVF, c-AKI, and non-congestive AKI in adult patients. We demonstrate NT-proBNP and hs-cTnT as excellent potential biomarkers for postoperative c-AKI, but poor predictors of isolated RVF. This observation may be explained by two mechanisms. First, potential etiologies for perioperative RVF are diverse, including myocardial ischemia due to poor myocardial preservation [42], graft occlusion, or air emboli [43]. Some of these events are unanticipated complications of CPB and surgery and cannot be predicted using biomarkers or conventional means [44,45]. Second, c-AKI is the end organ manifestation of longer and more severe episodes of perioperative RVF. In our study, there was a positive correlation between hs-cTnT and CPB duration ($r = 0.44$, $p < 0.0001$). Higher postoperative hs-cTnT levels (and thus higher Δhs-cTnT) were likely secondary to complex surgery requiring prolonged CPB with prolonged myocardial ischemia that was possibly compounded by suboptimal myocardial preservation. In addition, prolonged RV ischemia and infarction leading to end organ complications are more likely with complex cardiac procedures. Future studies are needed to fully elucidate mechanisms responsible for hs-cTnT release in c-AKI and congestive states.

4.4. Secondary Outcomes

In the cardiac surgical setting, elevated pre and postoperative NT-proBNP and hs-TnT levels have been shown to be associated with prolonged ICU length of stay, mechanical ventilation, and postoperative inotropic support [35,46–49]. We showed higher preoperative hs-cTnT and postoperative NT-proBNP were associated with increased duration of mechanical ventilation and hospital and ICU stay.

4.5. Clinical Implications

Our findings have important implications for the optimization of patients who may be at high-risk for developing postoperative c-AKI. This is especially important, as unlike its non-congestive counterpart, c-AKI, may improve with diuretic, vasodilator therapies, and inotropic support [16,38]. Although both baseline and postoperative NT-proBNP levels were associated with c-AKI, baseline biomarker level may be of greater practical importance as it allows for a greater window of opportunity for preoperative optimization by postponing non-emergent surgery for decongestive therapy. We in addition demonstrated a high AUC of 0.93 (95% CI 0.88–0.99) when combining Δhs-cTnT and diabetes for the early detection of c-AKI in the immediate postoperative period, days before the confirmation of c-AKI by serum creatinine using the traditional AKIN definition. When adjusted for diabetes, each 100 pg/mL increase in Δhs-cTnT is associated with a 23% increased odds of c-AKI (adjusted OR 1.23, 95% 1.10–1.38). In addition, 37% of diabetic patients who had Δhs-cTnT values above the cutoff developed c-AKI, where as none of the non-diabetic patients with Δhs-cTnT values below cutoff developed c-AKI. This simple model helps to efficiently identify a high-risk group that is most likely to benefit from future clinical trials of intensive perioperative monitoring and targeted therapy including fluid restriction, decongestion, and inotropic support. The feasibility of these biomarker-guided trials is enhanced by the availability of NT-proBNP and hs-cTnT as accurate and affordable point of care assays that could be easily and rapidly implemented at the bedside or preoperative assessment clinics [50,51]. Significant progress has been made in the development of these point of care assays, with newer generations demonstrating comparable diagnostic accuracy as high sensitivity core-laboratory assays [50,51].

4.6. Study Limitations

This study has several limitations. Firstly, it is single center in nature. However, we recruited a representative sample of patients undergoing all major cardiac surgery, and our sample size was similar to that from other studies in the field. Secondly, c-AKI was a relatively rare event, and the small event rate limited our ability to explore the additive predictive value of biomarkers in more comprehensive clinical models. Thirdly, the number of patients experiencing dialysis or death in our study was low, limiting our ability to evaluate the association of biomarkers with these outcomes.

5. Conclusions

Our study findings support hs-cTnT and NT-proBNP as potential biomarkers for prediction of a highly morbid subtype of postoperative AKI that occurs with RVF. Baseline and postoperative NT-proBNP, postoperative hs-cTnT, and Δhs-cTnT had excellent AUCs for the prediction and early detection of c-AKI. Importantly, the addition of diabetes status to Δhs-cTnT further increased accuracy for detecting c-AKI. Our findings provide novel insights into cardiorenal physiology in the perioperative setting and may be used to monitor response to goal-directed decongestive therapy in clinical trials to mitigate c-AKI. In addition, the relatively rare incidence of postoperative c-AKI identified in our study highlights the importance of using biomarker models (i.e., Δhs-cTnT + diabetes) to identify high-risk patients for future interventional studies.

Author Contributions: L.Y.S. and L.M.M. designed the study; L.Y.S. acquired the data; J.G.E.Z. and L.Y.S. analyzed the data and drafted the manuscript; all authors participated in data interpretation, critical revision and approval of the manuscript.

References

1. Skhiri, M.; Hunt, S.A.; Denault, A.Y.; Haddad, F. Evidence-based management of right heart failure: A systematic review of an empiric field. *Rev. Esp. Cardiol.* **2010**, *63*, 451–471. [CrossRef]

2. Gambardella, I.; Gaudino, M.; Ronco, C.; Lau, C.; Ivascu, N.; Girardi, L.N. Congestive kidney failure in cardiac surgery: The relationship between central venous pressure and acute kidney injury. *Interact. Cardiovasc. Thorac. Surg.* **2016**, *23*, 800–805. [CrossRef] [PubMed]

3. Costachescu, T.; Denault, A.; Guimond, J.-G.; Couture, P.; Carignan, S.; Sheridan, P.; Hellou, G.; Blair, L.; Normandin, L.; Babin, D.; et al. The hemodynamically unstable patient in the intensive care unit: Hemodynamic vs. transesophageal echocardiographic monitoring. *Crit. Care Med.* **2002**, *30*, 1214–1223. [CrossRef] [PubMed]

4. Denault, A.Y.; Haddad, F.; Jacobsohn, E.; Deschamps, A. Perioperative right ventricular dysfunction. *Curr. Opin. Anaesthesiol.* **2013**, *26*, 71–81. [CrossRef] [PubMed]

5. Maslow, A.D.; Regan, M.M.; Panzica, P.; Heindel, S.; Mashikian, J.; Comunale, M.E. Precardiopulmonary bypass right ventricular function is associated with poor outcome after coronary artery bypass grafting in patients with severe left ventricular systolic dysfunction. *Anesth. Analg.* **2002**, *95*, 1507–1518. [CrossRef] [PubMed]

6. Haddad, F.; Denault, A.Y.; Couture, P.; Cartier, R.; Pellerin, M.; Levesque, S.; Lambert, J.; Tardif, J.-C. Right ventricular myocardial performance index predicts perioperative mortality or circulatory failure in high-risk valvular surgery. *J. Am. Soc. Echocardiogr.* **2007**, *20*, 1065–1072. [CrossRef] [PubMed]

7. Thiele, R.H.; Isbell, J.M.; Rosner, M.H. AKI associated with cardiac surgery. *Clin. J. Am. Soc. Nephrol.* **2015**, *10*, 500–514. [CrossRef] [PubMed]

8. Karkouti, K.; Wijeysundera, D.N.; Yau, T.M.; Callum, J.L.; Cheng, D.C.; Crowther, M.; Dupuis, J.-Y.; Fremes, S.E.; Kent, B.; Laflamme, C.; et al. Acute kidney injury after cardiac surgery: Focus on modifiable risk factors. *Circulation* **2009**, *119*, 495–502. [CrossRef] [PubMed]

9. Thomson, R.; Meeran, H.; Valencia, O.; Al-Subaie, N. Goal-directed therapy after cardiac surgery and the incidence of acute kidney injury. *J. Crit. Care* **2014**, *29*, 997–1000. [CrossRef]

10. Pearse, R.; Dawson, D.; Fawcett, J.; Rhodes, A.; Grounds, R.M.; Bennett, E.D. Early goal-directed therapy after major surgery reduces complications and duration of hospital stay. A randomised, controlled trial [ISRCTN38797445]. *Crit. Care* **2005**, *9*, R687–R693. [CrossRef]

11. Waikar, S.S.; Bonventre, J.V. Creatinine kinetics and the definition of acute kidney injury. *J. Am. Soc. Nephrol.* **2009**, *20*, 672–679. [CrossRef] [PubMed]

12. Shiao, C.-C.; Wu, V.-C.; Li, W.-Y.; Lin, Y.-F.; Hu, F.-C.; Young, G.-H.; Kuo, C.-C.; Kao, T.-W.; Huang, D.-M.; Chen, Y.-M.; et al. Late initiation of renal replacement therapy is associated with worse outcomes in acute kidney injury after major abdominal surgery. *Crit. Care* **2009**, *13*, R171. [CrossRef] [PubMed]

13. Karkouti, K.; Beattie, W.S.; Wijeysundera, D.N.; Rao, V.; Chan, C.; Dattilo, K.M.; Djaiani, G.; Ivanov, J.; Karski, J.; David, T.E. Hemodilution during cardiopulmonary bypass is an independent risk factor for acute renal failure in adult cardiac surgery. *J. Thorac. Cardiovasc. Surg.* **2005**, *129*, 391–400. [CrossRef] [PubMed]

14. Devarajan, P. Neutrophil gelatinase-associated lipocalin: A promising biomarker for human acute kidney injury. *Biomark. Med.* **2010**, *4*, 265–280. [CrossRef]

15. Ronco, C.; McCullough, P.; Anker, S.D.; Anand, I.; Aspromonte, N.; Bagshaw, S.M.; Bellomo, R.; Berl, T.; Bobek, I.; Cruz, D.N.; et al. Cardio-renal syndromes: Report from the consensus conference of the Acute Dialysis Quality Initiative. *Eur. Heart J.* **2010**, *31*, 703–711. [CrossRef]

16. Aronson, D.; Abassi, Z.; Allon, E.; Burger, A.J. Fluid loss, venous congestion, and worsening renal function in acute decompensated heart failure. *Eur. J. Heart Fail.* **2013**, *15*, 637–643. [CrossRef]

17. Marik, P.E.; Baram, M.; Vahid, B. Does central venous pressure predict fluid responsiveness? A systematic review of the literature and the tale of seven mares. *Chest* **2008**, *134*, 172–178. [CrossRef]

18. Bulluck, H.; Maiti, R.; Chakraborty, B.; Candilio, L.; Clayton, T.; Evans, R.; Jenkins, D.P.; Kolvekar, S.; Kunst, G.; Laing, C.; et al. Neutrophil gelatinase-associated lipocalin prior to cardiac surgery predicts acute kidney injury and mortality. *Heart* **2018**, *104*, 313–317. [CrossRef]

19. Daniels, L.B.; Barrett-Connor, E.; Clopton, P.; Laughlin, G.A.; Ix, J.H.; Maisel, A.S. Plasma neutrophil

gelatinase-associated lipocalin is independently associated with cardiovascular disease and mortality in community-dwelling older adults: The Rancho Bernardo Study. *J. Am. Coll. Cardiol.* **2012**, *59*, 1101–1109. [CrossRef]

20. Lindberg, S.; Pedersen, S.H.; Mogelvang, R.; Jensen, J.S.; Flyvbjerg, A.; Galatius, S.; Magnusson, N.E. Prognostic utility of neutrophil gelatinase-associated lipocalin in predicting mortality and cardiovascular events in patients with ST-segment elevation myocardial infarction treated with primary percutaneous coronary intervention. *J. Am. Coll. Cardiol.* **2012**, *60*, 339–345. [CrossRef]

21. Patel, U.D.; Garg, A.X.; Krumholz, H.M.; Shlipak, M.G.; Coca, S.G.; Sint, K.; Thiessen-Philbrook, H.; Koyner, J.L.; Swaminathan, M.; Passik, C.S.; et al. Preoperative serum brain natriuretic peptide and risk of acute kidney injury after cardiac surgery. *Circulation* **2012**, *125*, 1347–1355. [CrossRef] [PubMed]

22. Song, D.; de Zoysa, J.R.; Ng, A.; Chiu, W. Troponins in acute kidney injury. *Ren. Fail.* **2012**, *34*, 35–39. [CrossRef] [PubMed]

23. Januzzi, J.L.; van Kimmenade, R.; Lainchbury, J.; Bayes-Genis, A.; Ordonez-Llanos, J.; Santalo-Bel, M.; Pinto, Y.M.; Richards, M. NT-proBNP testing for diagnosis and short-term prognosis in acute destabilized heart failure: An international pooled analysis of 1256 patients: The International Collaborative of NT-proBNP Study. *Eur. Heart J.* **2006**, *27*, 330–337. [CrossRef] [PubMed]

24. Blyth, K.G.; Groenning, B.A.; Mark, P.B.; Martin, T.N.; Foster, J.E.; Steedman, T.; Morton, J.J.; Dargie, H.J.; Peacock, A.J. NT-proBNP can be used to detect right ventricular systolic dysfunction in pulmonary hypertension. *Eur. Respir. J.* **2007**, *29*, 737–744. [CrossRef] [PubMed]

25. Nagaya, N.; Nishikimi, T.; Okano, Y.; Uematsu, M.; Satoh, T.; Kyotani, S.; Kuribayashi, S.; Hamada, S.; Kakishita, M.; Nakanishi, N.; et al. Plasma brain natriuretic peptide levels increase in proportion to the extent of right ventricular dysfunction in pulmonary hypertension. *J. Am. Coll. Cardiol.* **1998**, *31*, 202–208. [CrossRef]

26. Ricci, Z.; Cruz, D.N.; Ronco, C. Classification and staging of acute kidney injury: Beyond the RIFLE and AKIN criteria. *Nat. Rev. Nephrol.* **2011**, *7*, 201–208. [CrossRef] [PubMed]

27. Holman, W.L. Interagency Registry for Mechanically Assisted Circulatory Support (INTERMACS): What have we learned and what will we learn? *Circulation* **2012**, *126*, 1401–1406. [CrossRef]

28. Denault, A.Y.; Bussières, J.S.; Arellano, R.; Finegan, B.; Gavra, P.; Haddad, F.; Nguyen, A.Q.N.; Varin, F.; Fortier, A.; Levesque, S.; et al. A multicentre randomized-controlled trial of inhaled milrinone in high-risk cardiac surgical patients. *Can. J. Anaesth. J.* **2016**, *63*, 1140–1153. [CrossRef]

29. Rudski, L.G.; Lai, W.W.; Afilalo, J.; Hua, L.; Handschumacher, M.D.; Chandrasekaran, K.; Solomon, S.D.; Louie, E.K.; Schiller, N.B. Guidelines for the echocardiographic assessment of the right heart in adults: A report from the American Society of Echocardiography endorsed by the European Association of Echocardiography, a registered branch of the European Society of Cardiology, and the Canadian Society of Echocardiography. *J. Am. Soc. Echocardiogr.* **2010**, *23*, 685–713, quiz 786–788.

30. Giannitsis, E.; Kurz, K.; Hallermayer, K.; Jarausch, J.; Jaffe, A.S.; Katus, H.A. Analytical validation of a high-sensitivity cardiac troponin T assay. *Clin. Chem.* **2010**, *56*, 254–261. [CrossRef]

31. Bolignano, D.; Lacquaniti, A.; Coppolino, G.; Donato, V.; Campo, S.; Fazio, M.R.; Nicocia, G.; Buemi, M. Neutrophil gelatinase-associated lipocalin (NGAL) and progression of chronic kidney disease. *Clin. J. Am. Soc. Nephrol.* **2009**, *4*, 337–344. [CrossRef] [PubMed]

32. Omar, A.S.; Mahmoud, K.; Hanoura, S.; Osman, H.; Sivadasan, P.; Sudarsanan, S.; Shouman, Y.; Singh, R.; AlKhulaifi, A. Acute kidney injury induces high-sensitivity troponin measurement changes after cardiac surgery. *BMC Anesthesiol.* **2017**, *17*, 15. [CrossRef] [PubMed]

33. DeLong, E.R.; DeLong, D.M.; Clarke-Pearson, D.L. Comparing the areas under two or more correlated receiver operating characteristic curves: A nonparametric approach. *Biometrics* **1988**, *44*, 837–845. [CrossRef] [PubMed]

34. Bucholz, E.M.; Whitlock, R.P.; Zappitelli, M.; Devarajan, P.; Eikelboom, J.; Garg, A.X.; Philbrook, H.T.; Devereaux, P.J.; Krawczeski, C.D.; Kavsak, P.; et al. Cardiac biomarkers and acute kidney injury after cardiac surgery. *Pediatrics* **2015**, *135*, e945–e956. [CrossRef] [PubMed]

35. Elíasdóttir, S.B.; Klemenzson, G.; Torfason, B.; Valsson, F. Brain natriuretic peptide is a good predictor for outcome in cardiac surgery. *Acta Anaesthesiol. Scand.* **2008**, *52*, 182–187. [CrossRef] [PubMed]

36. Schrier, R.W.; Bansal, S. Pulmonary hypertension, right ventricular failure, and kidney: Different from left ventricular failure? *Clin. J. Am. Soc. Nephrol.* **2008**, *3*, 1232–1237. [CrossRef] [PubMed]

37. Firth, J.D.; Raine, A.E.; Ledingham, J.G. Raised venous pressure: A direct cause of renal sodium retention in oedema? *Lancet* **1988**, *331*, 1033–1036. [CrossRef]

38. Mullens, W.; Abrahams, Z.; Francis, G.S.; Sokos, G.; Taylor, D.O.; Starling, R.C.; Young, J.B.; Tang, W.H.W. Importance of venous congestion for worsening of renal function in advanced decompensated heart failure. *J. Am. Coll. Cardiol.* **2009**, *53*, 589–596. [CrossRef]

39. Liang, K.V.; Williams, A.W.; Greene, E.L.; Redfield, M.M. Acute decompensated heart failure and the cardiorenal syndrome. *Crit. Care Med.* **2008**, *36*, S75–S88. [CrossRef]

40. Liu, P.P. Cardiorenal syndrome in heart failure: A cardiologist's perspective. *Can. J. Cardiol.* **2008**, *24*, 25B–29B. [CrossRef]

41. Daquarti, G.; March Vecchio, N.; Mitrione, C.S.; Furmento, J.; Ametrano, M.C.; Dominguez Pace, M.P.; Costabel, J.P. High-sensitivity troponin and right ventricular function in acute pulmonary embolism. *Am. J. Emerg. Med.* **2016**, *34*, 1579–1582. [CrossRef] [PubMed]

42. Allen, B.S.; Winkelmann, J.W.; Hanafy, H.; Hartz, R.S.; Bolling, K.S.; Ham, J.; Feinstein, S. Retrograde cardioplegia does not adequately perfuse the right ventricle. *J. Thorac. Cardiovasc. Surg.* **1995**, *109*, 1116–1126. [CrossRef]

43. Kevin, L.G.; Barnard, M. Right ventricular failure. *Contin. Educ. Anaesth. Crit. Care Pain* **2007**, *7*, 89–94. [CrossRef]

44. Aissaoui, N.; Salem, J.-E.; Paluszkiewicz, L.; Morshuis, M.; Guerot, E.; Gorria, G.M.; Fagon, J.-Y.; Gummert, J.; Diebold, B. Assessment of right ventricular dysfunction predictors before the implantation of a left ventricular assist device in end-stage heart failure patients using echocardiographic measures (ARVADE): Combination of left and right ventricular echocardiographic variables. *Arch. Cardiovasc. Dis.* **2015**, *108*, 300–309. [PubMed]

45. Matthews, J.C.; Koelling, T.M.; Pagani, F.D.; Aaronson, K.D. The right ventricular failure risk score a pre-operative tool for assessing the risk of right ventricular failure in left ventricular assist device candidates. *J. Am. Coll. Cardiol.* **2008**, *51*, 2163–2172. [CrossRef] [PubMed]

46. Brynildsen, J.; Petäjä, L.; Pettilä, V.; Nygård, S.; Vaara, S.T.; Linko, R.; Okkonen, M.; Hagve, T.-A.; Soininen, L.; Suojaranta-Ylinen, R.; et al. The predictive value of NT-proBNP and hs-TnT for risk of death in cardiac surgical patients. *Clin. Biochem.* **2018**, *53*, 65–71. [CrossRef] [PubMed]

47. Cuthbertson, B.H.; Croal, B.L.; Rae, D.; Gibson, P.H.; McNeilly, J.D.; Jeffrey, R.R.; Smith, W.C.; Prescott, G.J.; Buchan, K.G.; El-Shafei, H.; et al. N-terminal pro-B-type natriuretic peptide levels and early outcome after cardiac surgery: A prospective cohort study. *Br. J. Anaesth.* **2009**, *103*, 647–653. [CrossRef]

48. Domanski, M.J.; Mahaffey, K.; Hasselblad, V.; Brener, S.J.; Smith, P.K.; Hillis, G.; Engoren, M.; Alexander, J.H.; Levy, J.H.; Chaitman, B.R.; et al. Association of myocardial enzyme elevation and survival following coronary artery bypass graft surgery. *JAMA* **2011**, *305*, 585–591. [CrossRef]

49. Mohammed, A.A.; Agnihotri, A.K.; van Kimmenade, R.R.J.; Martinez-Rumayor, A.; Green, S.M.; Quiroz, R.; Januzzi, J.L. Prospective, comprehensive assessment of cardiac troponin T testing after coronary artery bypass graft surgery. *Circulation* **2009**, *120*, 843–850. [CrossRef]

50. Wilke, P.; Masuch, A.; Fahron, O.; Zylla, S.; Leipold, T.; Petersmann, A. Diagnostic performance of point-of-care and central laboratory cardiac troponin assays in an emergency department. *PLoS ONE* **2017**, *12*, e0188706. [CrossRef]

51. Fellner, S.; Hentze, S.; Kempin, U.; Richter, E.; Rocktäschel, J.; Langer, B. Analytical evaluation of a BNP assay on the new point-of-care platform respons® IQ. *Pract. Lab. Med.* **2015**, *2*, 15–21. [CrossRef] [PubMed]

Permissions

List of Contributors

Andrei Mihai Bălan, Alexandra Caziuc and Natalia Hagău
Department of Anaesthesia and Intensive Care, "Iuliu Hațieganu" University of Medicine and Pharmacy, No 3-5 Clinicilor Street, Cluj-Napoca, 400005 Cluj, Romania

Oana Antal, Elena Stefănescu and Monica Mlesnite
Department of Anaesthesia and Intensive Care, "Iuliu Hațieganu" University of Medicine and Pharmacy, No 3-5 Clinicilor Street, Cluj-Napoca, 400005 Cluj, Romania
Department of Anaesthesia and Intensive Care, Cluj Emergency Clinical County Hospital, No 3-5 Clinicilor Street, Cluj-Napoca, 400005 Cluj, Romania

Cheng-Ting Lee and Chun-Yi Wu
Division of Nephrology, Department of Internal Medicine, Taichung Veterans General Hospital, Taichung 407, Taiwan

Ming-Ju Wu
Division of Nephrology, Department of Internal Medicine, Taichung Veterans General Hospital, Taichung 407, Taiwan
School of Medicine, Chung Shan Medical University, Taichung 402, Taiwan
Rong Hsing Research Center for Translational Medicine, Institute of Biomedical Science, College of Life Science, National Chung Hsing University, Taichung 402, Taiwan
Graduate Institute of Clinical Medical Science, School of Medicine, China Medical University, Taichung 404, Taiwan

Shang-Feng Tsai
Division of Nephrology, Department of Internal Medicine, Taichung Veterans General Hospital, Taichung 407, Taiwan
Department of Life Science, Tunghai University, Taichung 407, Taiwan
School of Medicine, National Yang-Ming University, Taipei 112, Taiwan

Jia-Jin Chen and George Kou
Department of Nephrology, Kidney Research Center, Chang Gung Memorial Hospital, Taoyuan 333, Taiwan

Pei-Chun Fan, Cheng-Chia Lee and Chih-Hsiang Chang
Department of Nephrology, Kidney Research Center, Chang Gung Memorial Hospital, Taoyuan 333, Taiwan
Graduate Institute of Clinical Medical Science, College of Medicine, Chang Gung University, Taoyuan 333, Taiwan

Su-Wei Chang
Clinical Informatics and Medical Statistics Research Center, College of Medicine, Chang Gung University, Taoyuan 333, Taiwan
Division of Allergy, Asthma, and Rheumatology, Department of Pediatrics, Chang Gung Memorial Hospital, Taoyuan 333, Taiwan

Yi-Ting Chen
Department of Nephrology, Kidney Research Center, Chang Gung Memorial Hospital, Taoyuan 333, Taiwan
Department of Biomedical Sciences, College of Medicine, Chang Gung University, Taoyuan 333, Taiwan

Justyna Wajda
Department of Anatomy, Jagiellonian University Medical College, 31-034 Krakow, Poland

Paulina Dumnicka
Department of Medical Diagnostics, Faculty of Pharmacy, Jagiellonian University Medical College, 30-688 Krakow, Poland

Mateusz Sporek
Department of Anatomy, Jagiellonian University Medical College, 31-034 Krakow, Poland
Surgery Department, The District Hospital, 34-200 Sucha Beskidzka, Poland

Beata Kuśnierz-Cabala and Barbara Maziarz
Department of Diagnostics, Chair of Clinical Biochemistry, Faculty of Medicine, Jagiellonian University Medical College, 31-501 Krakow, Poland

Witold Kolber
Department of Surgery, Complex of Health Care Centers in Wadowice, 34-100 Wadowice, Poland

Anna Ząbek-Adamska
Diagnostics Department of University Hospital in Krakow, 31-501 Krakow, Poland

Piotr Ceranowicz and Marek Kuźniewski
Department of Nephrology, Jagiellonian University Medical College, 31-501 Kraków, Poland

Alexander Sarnowski, Farzad Saadat, Sam Huddart, Nial Quiney and Matthew C. Dickinson
Department of Intensive Care Medicine and Surrey Peri-Operative Anaesthesia and Critical Care Collaborative Research Group (SPACER), Royal Surrey County Hospital NHS Foundation Trust, Guildford, Surrey GU2 7XX, UK

James F. Doyle
Department of Intensive Care Medicine and Surrey Peri-Operative Anaesthesia and Critical Care Collaborative Research Group (SPACER), Royal Surrey County Hospital NHS Foundation Trust, Guildford, Surrey GU2 7XX, UK
Department of Intensive Care Medicine, Royal Brompton & Harefield NHS Foundation Trust, London SW3 6NP, UK

Theophilus L. Samuels
Department of Anaesthesia and Intensive Care Medicine, Surrey & Sussex Healthcare NHS Trust, Redhill RH1 5RH, UK

Jeremy Preece, Bruce McCormick and Robert deBrunner
Department of Anaesthesia, Royal Devon & Exeter NHS Foundation Trust, Exeter EX2 5DW, UK

Michael Swart
Department of Anaesthesia, Torbay & South Devon NHS Foundation Trust, Torquay TQ2 7AA, UK

Carol J. Peden
Department of Anaesthesia, Royal United Hospitals Bath NHS Foundation Trust, Avon BA1 3NG, UK

Sarah Richards
Department of Surgery, Royal United Hospitals Bath NHS Foundation Trust, Avon BA1 3NG, UK

Lui G. Forni
Department of Intensive Care Medicine and Surrey Peri-Operative Anaesthesia and Critical Care Collaborative Research Group (SPACER), Royal Surrey County Hospital NHS Foundation Trust, Guildford, Surrey GU2 7XX, UK
Department of Clinical & Experimental Medicine, Faculty of Health and Medical Sciences, University of Surrey, Guildford Guildford, GU2 7YS, UK

Philipp Eisenmann
Karlsruhe Institute of Technology, Institute of Organic Chemistry, Fritz-Haber-Weg 6, 76131 Karlsruhe, Germany

Claudia Muhle-Goll and Burkhard Luy
Karlsruhe Institute of Technology, Institute for Biological Interfaces 4, 76021 Karlsruhe, Germany
Karlsruhe Institute of Technology, Institute of Organic Chemistry, Fritz-Haber-Weg 6, 76131 Karlsruhe, Germany

Stefan Kölker
Division of Pediatric Neurology and Metabolic Medicine, University Children's Hospital Heidelberg, Im Neuenheimer Feld 430, 69120 Heidelberg, Germany

Burkhard Tönshoff, Alexander Fichtner and Jens H. Westhoff
Department of Pediatrics I, University Children's Hospital Heidelberg, Im Neuenheimer Feld 430, 69120 Heidelberg, Germany

Youn Kyung Kee
Department of Internal Medicine, Hangang Sacred Heart Hospital, Hallym University College of Medicine, Seoul 07247, Korea

Dahye Kim
Department of Nursing, Ewha Womans University Mokdong Hospital, Seoul 07985, Korea

Seung-Jung Kim, Duk-Hee Kang and Kyu Bok Choi
Department of Internal Medicine, School of Medicine, Ewha Womans University, Seoul 03761, Korea

Hyung Jung Oh
Research Institute for Human Health Information, Ewha Womans University Mokdong Hospital, Seoul 07985, Korea
Ewha Institute of Convergence Medicine, Ewha Womans University Mokdong Hospital, Seoul 07985, Korea

Dong-Ryeol Ryu
Department of Internal Medicine, School of Medicine, Ewha Womans University, Seoul 03761, Korea
Research Institute for Human Health Information, EwhaWomans University Mokdong Hospital, Seoul 07985, Korea
Tissue Injury Defense Research Center, College of Medicine, EwhaWomans University, Seoul 07985, Korea

Ploypin Lertjitbanjong and Kanramon Watthanasuntorn
Department of Internal Medicine, Bassett Medical Center, Cooperstown, NY 13326, USA

Charat Thongprayoon
Division of Nephrology and Hypertension, Mayo Clinic, Rochester, MN 55905, USA

Sohail Abdul Salim and Wisit Cheungpasitporn
Division of Nephrology, Department of Medicine, University of Mississippi Medical Center, Jackson, MS 39216, USA

Oisín A. O'Corragain
Department of Thoracic Medicine and Surgery, Temple University Hospital, Philadelphia, PA 19140, USA

Narat Srivali
Department of Internal Medicine, St. Agnes Hospital, Baltimore, MD 21229, USA

Tarun Bathini
Department of Internal Medicine, University of Arizona, Tucson, AZ 85721, USA

Narothama Reddy Aeddula
Department of Medicine, Deaconess Health System, Evansville, IN 47747, USA
Division of Nephrology, Department of Medicine, Deaconess Health System, Evansville, IN 47747, USA

Patompong Ungprasert
Cleveland Clinic Lerner College of Medicine of Case Western Reserve University, Cleveland Clinic, Cleveland, OH 44195, USA
Clinical Epidemiology Unit, Department of Research and Development, Faculty of Medicine, Siriraj Hospital, Mahidol University, Bangkok 10700, Thailand

Erin A. Gillaspie
Department of Thoracic Surgery, Vanderbilt University Medical Center, Nashville, TN 37212, USA

Karn Wijarnpreecha and Michael A. Mao
Department of Medicine, Mayo Clinic, Jacksonville, FL 32224, USA

Wisit Kaewput
Department of Military and Community Medicine, Phramongkutklao College of Medicine, Bangkok 10400, Thailand

Jeremy Leventhal and Paolo Cravedi
Department of Medicine, Division of Nephrology, Icahn School of Medicine at Mount Sinai, 1 Levy Place, New York, NY 10029, USA

Gianluigi Zaza
Renal Unit, Department of Medicine, University/ Hospital of Verona, 37126 Verona, Italy

Sofia Andrighetto
Department of Medicine, Division of Nephrology, Icahn School of Medicine at Mount Sinai, 1 Levy Place, New York, NY 10029, USA
Renal Unit, Department of Medicine, University/ Hospital of Verona, 37126 Verona, Italy

Tak Kyu Oh, In-Ae Song and Young-Tae Jeon
Department of Anesthesiology and Pain Medicine, Seoul National University Bundang Hospital, Seoul 13620, Korea

You Hwan Jo
Department of Emergency Medicine, Seoul National University Bundang Hospital, Seoul 13620, Korea

Ashley R. Selby
Department of Pharmacy Practice, Texas Tech University Health Sciences Center Jerry H. Hodge School of Pharmacy, Dallas, TX 75235, USA
VA North Texas Health Care System, Dallas, TX 75216, USA

Ronald G. Hall II
Department of Pharmacy Practice, Texas Tech University Health Sciences Center Jerry H. Hodge School of Pharmacy, Dallas, TX 75235, USA
VA North Texas Health Care System, Dallas, TX 75216, USA
Department of Surgery, University of Texas Southwestern Medical Center, Dallas, TX 75390, USA
Dose Optimization and Outcomes Research (DOOR) Program, Dallas, TX 75235, USA

Fabio Sallustio
Interdisciplinary Department of Medicine (DIM), University of Bari "Aldo Moro", 70124 Bari, Italy
Department of Basic Medical Sciences, Neuroscience and Sense Organs, University of Bari "Aldo Moro", 70124 Bari, Italy

Anna Gallone
Department of Basic Medical Sciences, Neuroscience and Sense Organs, University of Bari "Aldo Moro", 70124 Bari, Italy

Claudia Curci
Department of Basic Medical Sciences, Neuroscience and Sense Organs, University of Bari "Aldo Moro", 70124 Bari, Italy
Nephrology, Dialysis and Transplantation Unit, DETO, University "Aldo Moro", 70124 Bari, Italy

Francesco Pesce, Loreto Gesualdo and Vincenzo Di Leo
Nephrology, Dialysis and Transplantation Unit, DETO, University "Aldo Moro", 70124 Bari, Italy

Natanong Thamcharoen
Division of Nephrology, Beth Israel Deaconess Medical Center, Harvard Medical School, Boston, MA 02215, USA

Kanramon Watthanasuntorn, Ploypin Lertjitbanjong and Konika Sharma
Department of Internal Medicine, Bassett Medical Center, Cooperstown, NY 13326, USA

Wisit Cheungpasitporn and Sohail Abdul Salim
Division of Nephrology, Department of Medicine, University of Mississippi Medical Center, MS 39216, USA

Karn Wijarnpreecha and Paul T. Kröner
Department of Medicine, Division of Gastroenterology and Hepatology, Mayo Clinic, Jacksonville, FL 32224, USA

Michael A Mao
Department of Medicine, Division of Nephrology and Hypertension, Mayo Clinic, Jacksonville, FL 32224, USA

Na Young Kim, Hoon Jae Nam and So Yeon Kim
Department of Anesthesiology and Pain Medicine, Anesthesia and Pain Research Institute, Yonsei University College of Medicine, 50-1 Yonsei-ro, Seodaemun-gu, Seoul 03722, Korea

Jung Hwa Hong
Department of Policy Research Affairs National Health Insurance Service Ilsan Hospital, 100 Ilsan-ro, Ilsandong-gu, Goyang, Gyeonggi-do 10444, Korea

Dong Hoon Koh
Department of Urology, Konyang University College of Medicine, 158 Gwanjeodong-ro, Daejeon 35365, Korea

Jongsoo Lee
Department of Urology and Urological Science Institute, Yonsei University College of Medicine, 50-1 Yonsei-ro, Seodaemun-gu, Seoul 03722, Korea

Hyun-Kyu Yoon, Ho-Jin Lee, Seokha Yoo, Sun-Kyung Park, Yongsuk Kwon, Kwanghoon Jun and Won Ho Kim
Department of Anesthesiology and Pain Medicine, Seoul National University Hospital, Seoul National University College of Medicine, Seoul 03080, Korea

Chang Wook Jeong
Department of Urology, Seoul National University Hospital, Seoul National University College of Medicine, Seoul 03080, Korea

Jason G. E. Zelt
Department of Cellular and Molecular Medicine, Faculty of Medicine, University of Ottawa, Ottawa, ON K1H8M5, Canada

Lisa M. Mielniczuk
Department of Cellular and Molecular Medicine, Faculty of Medicine, University of Ottawa, Ottawa, ON K1H8M5, Canada
Division of Cardiology, Department of Medicine, University of Ottawa Heart Institute, 40 Ruskin Street Ottawa, ON K1Y 4W7, Canada

Sharon Chih and Peter P. Liu
Division of Cardiology, Department of Medicine, University of Ottawa Heart Institute, 40 Ruskin Street Ottawa, ON K1Y 4W7, Canada

Ayub Akbari
Division of Nephrology, Department of Medicine, The Ottawa Hospital, 1967 Riverside Dr., Ottawa, ON K1H 7W9, Canada

Jean-Yves Dupuis
Division of Cardiac Anesthesiology, Department of Anesthesiology and Pain Medicine, University of Ottawa Heart Institute, 40 Ruskin Street, Ottawa, ON K1Y 4W7, Canada

Louise Y. Sun
Division of Cardiac Anesthesiology, Department of Anesthesiology and Pain Medicine, University of Ottawa Heart Institute, 40 Ruskin Street, Ottawa, ON K1Y 4W7, Canada
School of Epidemiology and Public Health, University of Ottawa, 600 Peter Morand Crescent, Ottawa, ON K1G 5Z3, Canada

Index

Printed in the USA
CPSIA information can be obtained
at www.ICGtesting.com
JSHW051401091023
49903JS00006B/229

9 781639 277100